AF899002

UPDATES ON CANCER TREATMENT

Edited by **Leticia B. A. Rangel**
and **Ian Victor Silva**

Updates on Cancer Treatment
http://dx.doi.org/10.5772/58657
Edited by Leticia B. A. Rangel and Ian Victor Silva

Contributors

Oleg Viktorovich Bukhtoyarov, Denis Samarin, Bassam Abdul Rasool Hassan, Shouji Shimoyama, Sergio Huerta, Letícia Rangel, Wade Russu, Mario Pérez-Sayáns García, Paula Boñar Álvarez, Abel García García, Raoul Saggini, Rosa Grazia Bellomo, Zeeshan Ramzan, Karen Wonders, Peltier Alexandre, Fouad Aoun, Roland Van Velthoven, Marc Zanaty

Published by InTech

Janeza Trdine 9, 51000 Rijeka, Croatia

Publishing Process Manager Ana Pantar

Technical Editor InTech DTP team

Cover InTech Design team

First published October, 2015

Printed in Croatia

Additional hard copies can be obtained from orders@intechopen.com

Updates on Cancer Treatment, Edited by Leticia B. A. Rangel and Ian Victor Silva

p. cm.

ISBN 978-953-51-2194-7

For EU product safety concerns:
IN TECH d.o.o., Prolaz Marije Krucifikse Kozulić 3, 51000 Rijeka, Croatia,
info@intechopen.com or visit our website at intechopen.com.

Meet the editors

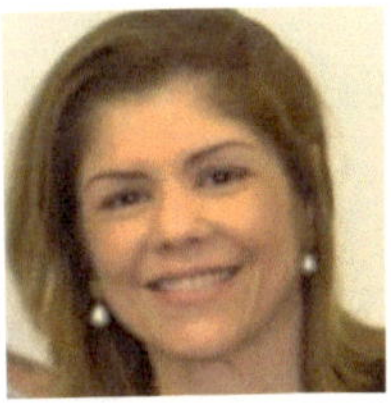

Leticia B. A. Rangel, Pharm.D., Ph.D., is an Associate Professor of the Department of Pharmaceutical Sciences, a member of the Biotechnology/RENORBIO and of the Biochemistry and Pharmacology Programs at the Federal University of Espirito Santo (UFES). As the head of the Laboratory of Cellular and Molecular Biology of Human Cancer, she coordinates projects on ovarian and breast cancers, with emphasis on the cellular and molecular basis of the diseases, and mechanisms involved in the chemoresistant phenotype of cancer cells. Her scientific network includes universities in Brazil and in the United States of America, as well as the private sector. She has been awarded by the Brazilian government in recognition to her contribution in cancer research.

Ian Victor Silva, Pharm.D., Ph.D., is an Associate Professor at the Department of Morphology, a member of the Biotechnology/RENORBIO Program at the Federal University of Espirito Santo (UFES). As the head of Aging Cell Laboratory, he coordinates projects on aging associated diseases, with emphasis on the molecular mechanisms of these illnesses. His scientific network includes universities in Brazil as well United States of America. Along with his fruitful collaboration within the academic sector, Dr. Silva also works as a consultant for the private sector, mostly as a scientific advisor for clinical trials and pharmaceutical private sector management. He has been recognized by the Brazilian government, as well as internationally, for his contribution to research on aging.

Contents

Preface

Notwithstanding the advances in the cancer research field, the related epidemiology data remain dramatic and clearly point to an urge to optimize and innovate the therapeutic approaches to fight cancer. Indeed, the elucidation of important aspects of cancer biology and human tumorigenesis has progressively enabled oncologists to provide more accurate cancer diagnosis, thus, guiding more efficiently the treatment of multiple cancer types and subtypes. Nonetheless, cancer treatment still challenges researchers and clinicians, as proven by the still impressive and increasing number of worldwide cancer-related deaths, caused either by late diagnosis of the disease, surgical limitations or radio/chemoresistance. Adding complexity to the inter-individual variables, cancer comprises multiple diseases harboring diverse genetic and epigenetic signatures, the types and subtypes of which respond differently to treatment and are associated with distinct clinical outcomes. *Updates on Cancer Treatment* is an attempt to integrate into a book volume various aspects of cancer treatment, compiling comprehensive reviews written by an international team of experts in the field.

Leticia B. A. Rangel, Pharm.D., Ph.D.
and Ian Victor Silva
Federal University of Espirito Santo
Espirito Santo, Brazil

Chapter 1

Focal High Intensity Focused Ultrasound for Prostate Cancer

Fouad Aoun, Marc Zanaty, Alexandre Peltier and Roland van Velthoven

Additional information is available at the end of the chapter

http://dx.doi.org/10.5772/60267

1. Introduction

Conventional treatment options for organ confined prostate cancer range from active surveillance to whole gland radical therapy. Active surveillance has the distinct advantage of avoiding over treatment and treatment related morbidity but carries the risk of silent progression of prostate cancer in up to 35 % of cases [1]. It may also induce no treatment related significant anxiety and uncertainty [2]. Radical therapy has the advantage of improving the overall and cancer specific survival in appropriately selected patients [3-4] but bears significant risk of treatment related functional complications that detrimentally affect quality of life [5-6]. Therefore, counseling patients for appropriate, individual treatment strategy remains challenging even for experienced physicians.

Consequently, focal therapy has emerged as an alternative option to standard therapies. The goal of this tissue preserving strategy as defined by the International Task Force on Prostate Cancer and the Focal Lesion Paradigm would be to 'selectively ablate(s) known disease and preserve(s) existing functions, with the overall objective of minimizing lifetime morbidity without compromising life expectancy [7]. A number of focal therapy energies and modalities have commonly been used [8]. Among these therapies, High Intensity Focused Ultrasound (HIFU) emerged as a valid mini invasive therapy for localised prostate cancer, using focused ultrasound to generate areas of intense heat to induce tissue necrosis. This energy delivery system originally used to treat the whole prostate is used nowadays to treat a part of the gland. Many case series have reported encouraging short term functional and oncological results of men with prostate cancer treated primarily in a focal manner [8-19]. Recently, we have published the first mid-term report (median follow up of 38 months) of focal HIFU for a clinically unilateral prostate cancer.

2. Basic physics of waves and ultrasound

To understand the basic principle of high intensity focused ultrasound as an ablative treatment modality for prostate cancer, the main properties of sound waves should be known and are summarized in figure 1 and 2.

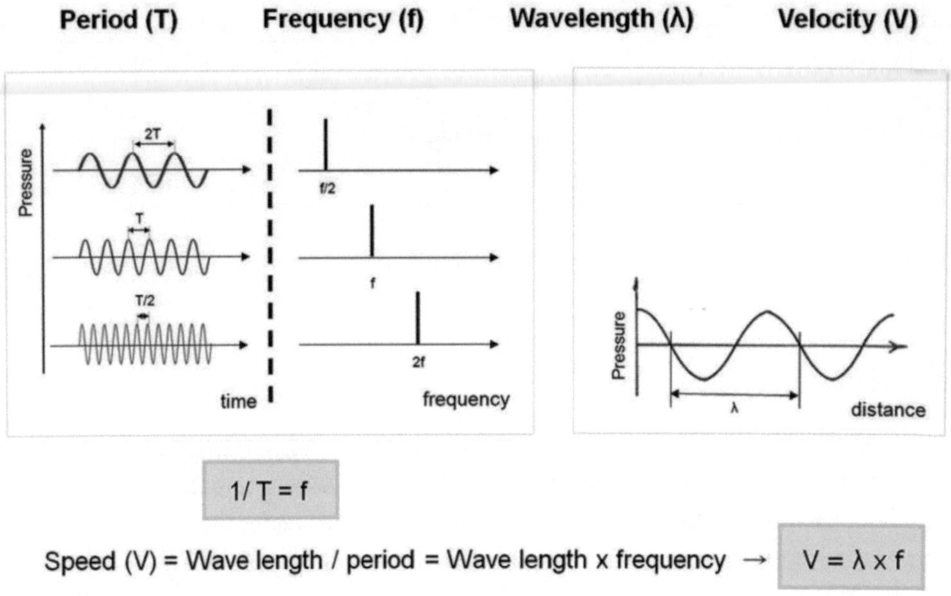

Figure 1. Physical parameters of sound physics

Sound is defined as a mechanical disturbance from a state of equilibrium that propagates through an elastic material medium in the form of vibrating waves. These vibrating waves transport energy from its source to another area as long as a medium is present. The energy transported by sound is known as acoustic energy or sonic energy. Sonic intensity (SI), defined as a time-average rate of sonic energy-flow through a unit area (SI unit: W/cm2), is proportional to sonic pressure square and has a positive correlation with the power and energy of sound. This implies that the amount of energy accumulating at a target area is larger when the sonic pressure or intensity increases. The latter parameter varies with space and time, and it is usually expressed as peak or average intensity, and both quantities can refer to either a spatial or temporal dimension (e.g. ISP = spatial peak intensity, ISATA = spatial average, temporal average intensity). The frequency of a wave is derived from the amount of cycles per unit of time. Ultrasound (US) is a form of sound that has a frequency higher than the frequency detected by human ear (> 20.000 Hz vs. 20-20.000 Hz). HIFU therapy utilizes high intensity US waves that are propagated through human tissues. In contrast to other ablative therapies, HIFU therapy operates without the need of an electrode or antenna to deliver its waves. However, the main challenge of such a technique is focusing energy-accumulation at the target area to

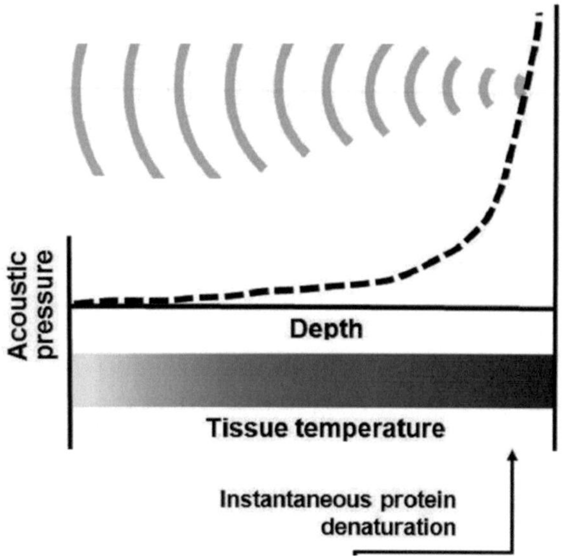

Figure 2. HIFU uses high energy US waves generated from numerous sources and focuses them to a small spot. Acoustic pressure is rapidly elevated near focus where tissue temperatures are also raised to level that is sufficient for coagulation necrosis

induce significant biological reactions without causing harm to the intervening and surrounding tissues. Recently, a phased array US transducer technique was adopted for focal HIFU treatment. It sends temporally different sets of electronic signals to each specific transducer component, thus enabling beam-steering and focusing, which can move a focal spot in virtually any direction within physically allowed ranges. This system is not only more versatile than other systems but also highly efficient without any sonic attenuation [20].

3. Biological interactions of US

Since the mid 1950, US have been extensively used for diagnostic procedures without any detrimental effect on the human body [21]. However, it must be noted that US waves used for therapeutic purposes could be potentially dangerous. In fact, it carries energy that causes biological reactions in various ways. The most important are the thermal (hyperthermia) and non thermal (acoustic cavitation) effects [22-23]. The thermal effect is tissue heating and protein denaturation can occur at a temperature of 56°C [24-25]. Protein denaturation contributes to a subsequent coagulation necrosis (thermal ablation). The effect is a function of the wave amplitude and pulse frequency. Acoustic cavitation is defined by the creation and development of bubbles or cavities. The violent oscillation and collapse in US fields of these bubbles cause a significant degree of mechanical and thermal effects. Mechanical and cavitation tissue effects are caused by high amplitudes and ultra-short pulse wave, with amplitude reaching 100 Mpa and a pulse of 1-2 ms. Moderate pressure amplitude of 10 Mpa and continuous wave of 1 s are the cause of thermal effects. Short ultrasound pulses and low amplitude up to 1 Mpa causes no significant heating, but cavitation caused by this type of waves are used in some circumstances like enhancing a drug delivery or the transient opening of the blood-brain barrier [22].

4. Mechanisms of action of high intensity focused ultrasound

The technique is based on the generation of focused ultrasound field. The focused ultrasound field is generated by a piezoelectric transducer with a center frequency of 1 to 7 MHz. The field is coupled into the body and aimed into a target region. Ultrasound waves are absorbed by tissues throughout their propagation and the acoustic energy will be converted to heat with a high energy density inside the focal zone [22]. The result is a temperature rise in the target zone within seconds to a level exceeding the threshold level of protein denaturation which is around 60 degrees. The result will be protein coagulation and coagulative necrosis [22-24]. In contrast there is a low acoustic energy density in the surrounding structures which keep them spared. This will create elliptical small volume lesions of 50-300 mm^3. Larger volume can be ablated without gaps by combining single lesions.

Between sonication a pause is necessary to prevent boiling and bubbles formations which can reflects and distort the ultrasound field and the consequence is unpredictable lesion growth and lesion formation in unwanted areas. So to ablate a large solid tumor it can take several hours. Thus HIFU is a very time consuming procedure [22]. HIFU has the advantage over other thermal ablative techniques of being a mini-invasive and non-ionizing with no long-term cumulative effects which means that it could be safely repeated. Further more it is interesting non invasive surgical tool because it can cause cell death in a tissue that is distant from the source of US [23].

5. Clinical devices in use

There are two main types of transducers used for HIFU. In general HIFU needs a high power ultrasound transducer. Such kind of transducers is made of low loss piezoceramic materials or piezocomposites working in resonant mode. The two major types are the self- focusing spherical shaped piezoceramic transducers with fixed aperture and fixed focal length which is the simplest, and the phased array transducers made up of a large number of separate transducer elements. Thereby each element is driven by a separate electric radio frequency signal with an individual phase, frequency and amplitude. The advantages of phased arrays are the possibility for an adaptive selection of elements, the fast electronic beam steering and the beam forming capability. Such transducers are much more expensive and the number of elements in such transducers can reach thousands in some special cases [22].

On the other hands we can divide the transducers into extracorporeal used for the treatment of cutaneous and abdominal tumors, transrectal as those used for the prostate, and interstitial and endoscopic ones used for the treatment of biliary or esophageal lesions [24].

http://dx.doi.org/10.5772/60267

6. Guiding/monitoring of therapy

Therapy guidance is the key for a safe and effective HIFU. Guidance is accomplished mainly with two imaging methods which are US and MRI. Imaging techniques are used with HIFU therapy not only for therapeutic guidance but it allows also therapy planning and targeting, monitoring, controlling and assessing the treatment response and follow-up [22].

6.1. Ultrasound monitoring

This is the case of most today's HIFU treatment. In general the divergent field of the diagnostic transducer and the field of therapeutic source are superposed and arranged in parallel so that the diagnostic imager provides the beam view. This eases the positioning of the therapeutic source and the identification of organ at risk [22]. Real-time visualization of the targeted volume is feasible with decoupling of US image and focused US.

US are able to detect cloud of gas bubbles that are formed as results of cavitation and tissue heating. The detection of bubble could be an indication for the position of the thermal focus, but this cannot be used to assess and control lesion formation.

US are not able to perform temperature mapping. Some try to use some parameters such as speed of sound, or attenuation or reflection coefficient as indicators for temperature variations, but with modest success.

The major advantages of US are, first they share same physical mechanism so a good assessment of the beam pass is possible. Then it allows the use of conventional materials for the therapy unit so that the diagnostic US transducer can be easily integrated in the therapeutic source that allows for a small and flexible devices with lower prices [22].

6.2. MR-monitoring

The advantages of MRI over US are the capacity of giving a morphological image for planning, targeting and thermal monitoring. It can also assess the shape and size of the induced tissue lesion at the end of therapy. Contrast enhanced T1 imaging are employed. The induced lesions prove hypointense reflecting the loss of perfusion. Major disadvantage is the need for an MR compatible HIFU therapy unit and the cost of the MR scanner. Limitations are the confined space for patient access and the need of a complex and expensive technology [22].

6.3. MR thermometry

A different method exists to measure the temperature related changes with the MR. Mainly four methods have been described: T1, diffusion, proton density, and proton resonance frequency shift. The most frequently used method is the proton resonance frequency shift (PRFS). The proton resonance frequency shift can be measured directly or by phase mapping which consists of observing the phase shift induced by temperature change. Phase mapping is easier to do than direct assessment. Therefore phase mapping is the most common approach used for temperature mapping [22].

7. HIFU Therapy for prostate cancer: Its role in focal therapy

HIFU for the treatment of localized prostate cancer was developed in 1990. Nowadays there are two available devices for the treatment of prostate cancer: the Ablatherm™ (EDAP TMS S.A., Vaulx-en-Velin, France) and the Sonablate™ (Focus Surgery, Inc, Indianapolis, Indiana, USA) [26].

Both of them have a simultaneous imaging technique coupled to the treatment device. They differ by patient positioning and the degree of manual control of power. Currently, the technique is used among many cancer centers despite the fact that available guidelines do not recommend it for the treatment of localized prostate cancer. In 2010, the Cancer Care Ontario group excluded HIFU from its recommendations due to lack of randomized controlled clinical trials and short follow up [27]. The NICE guidelines in 2012 considered HIFU as an experimental technique with further studies needed in order to conclude [28]. In 2014, the FDA bans the use of HIFU for whole-gland primary treatment of clinically localized prostate cancer. At present, high quality evidence on efficacy and safety of HIFU is based on uncontrolled case series with a significant overlap of patients among series. There are no direct comparisons with active surveillance or whole gland radical therapies. Furthermore, the technique is not standardized and patient selection is not unanimous. The ideal candidate is defined as a patient aged > 70 years of age, with clinical stage T1-T2 N0M0, a Gleason score<7, a PSA level <15 ng/ml and a prostate volume of <40 ml, in particular if the patient is unsuitable for or refuse radical therapy [26]. A prostate volume of >40 ml and the presence of large calcifications are a contraindications for HIFU. In such cases where the volume exceed 40 ml a TURP or a cytoreductive androgen deprivation therapy or a 5 alpha reductase inhibitor before HIFU is recommended to reduce the volume of the prostate. The number of HIFU treatment per patient varies between one and five. The median follow up time is short with the longest series reporting data after a median follow up of 94 months [29].

HIFU could be used as a primary treatment or as a salvage therapy in recurrent prostate cancer after radiotherapy failure. The field could involve a whole gland ablation or a more focal therapy. For technical considerations, Hemiablation HIFU of an entire lobe delivered with intention to treat is currently used for focal therapy. The technique was demonstrated to be feasible and functional and disease control outcomes were encouraging at 3 years of follow up.

8. The principle rationale of tissue preservation is harm reduction and functional preservation

Adverse events affecting the urinary tract are reported in 2-58% of whole gland HIFU therapy in the literature. Rectal toxicities ranged from 0 to 15%. Erectile dysfunction is reported in 0 to 39% of cases [30]. Toxicity rates are believed to be lower after focal therapy. In our case series, 31 consecutive patients with unilateral organ confined prostate cancer were primarily treated by hemiablation HIFU. Early self-resolving LUTS were the most common complications and no rectal toxicities were reported. The strategy was well tolerated in the genitourinary functional domains: all patients were pad free continent despite a high number of apical lesions (n=12) and only 25% of men in our cohort of relatively elderly patients (average age 71 years) who were potent preoperatively reported having ED post hemiablation. The procedure could possibly be delivered in an ambulatory care setting [19].

9. Monitoring of patients after focal HIFU

In the literature, there is no consensus on whether cancer control in focal therapy should be considered the absence of any cancer or the absence of clinically significant cancer and whether this should be limited to the treated or untreated area. In addition there is no standard follow up protocol for the assessment of clinical failure. In our opinion, histologic confirmation of complete ablation within the treated area appears to be essential in focal therapy. That's why any positive biopsy in the treated lobe independently of the percentage of core involvement should be considered a clinical failure. In contrast, controlateral positive biopsy should not be considered as a clinical failure but as a technical limitation. As a surrogate, although PSA testing is accepted as a valid outcome in standard therapy, there are no validated biochemical measures in tissue preservation. Furthermore, PSA values are difficult to interpret in the follow up because many factors influence post treatment values (the proportion of initial PSA that was due to tumor, amount of residual prostate tissue, progression of BPH, TURP...). Definitions that are currently used and validated for biochemical failure in whole gland radiation therapy (ASTRO, Phoenix, Stuttgart...) are used, without any evidence or validation, in whole gland HIFU and focal therapy [31]. Phoenix criteria should not be considered as response criteria to define failure but as a threshold to offer biopsy. We believe that a specific PSA based definition is unlikely to be derived and multiparametric MRI will play a major role in the future in the definition of failure if it is validated against histology outcomes.

10. Oncologic outcomes

Following whole gland ablation therapy, negative biopsy rates at 3 month of 51-96% and 64-87% with Ablatherm and Sonablate respectively were reported [32-36]. Overall survival rates and prostate cancer specific survival rates were 90% and 100% at 5 years and 83% and 98% at 8 years, respectively. The actuarial biochemical failure–free survival rates at 5 and 7 years were 77% and 69%, respectively. The actuarial disease–free survival rate at 5 and 7 years were 66% and 59%, respectively [32-36]. Biochemical success or failure rate was stratified against risk category according to the D'Amico classification in the majority of reports and was uniformly more favourable for the low and intermediate risk category compared to the high risk category. Some authors have argued that HIFU is a coagulative technology that unlike radiation therapy results in complete cell destruction independently of Gleason score. However, high grade tumours in prostate cancer are associated with increased neoangiogenesis responsible of a heat sink phenomenon that is tissue cooling by blood flow that causes thermal loss. The tissue under ablation in high grade tumour may be inadequately ablated and is a high risk site for persistent residual progressive disease and metastatic spread. Following focal therapy, we demonstrated a biochemical recurrence free survival of 100%, 89%, 82.7% at 1, 2 and 3 years respectively, with an overall and cancer specific survival of 100% [19].

11. Limitations and Future perspectives

As any other interventional technique, there are some limitations for HIFU that must be mentioned. First, there are factors to take into account such as collateral damage to the tissues and the fact that the technique is operator dependent [37]. Second, the lack of comparative trials precludes any conclusion regarding the added value of HIFU treatment compared to active surveillance or radical therapies. Urological societies recommend using focal HIFU in controlled trials in order to provide the needed answers. In the future, the use of focal HIFU will not be limited to prostate cancer but will widespread to other applications. The two most interested research topics are focused ultrasound mediated targeted drug delivery and the transient and reversal opening of the blood-brain barrier

Author details

Fouad Aoun*, Marc Zanaty, Alexandre Peltier and Roland van Velthoven

*Address all correspondence to: fouad.aoun@bordet.be

Department of Urology, Free University of Brussels (ULB), Brussels, Belgium

References

[1] Marberger M, Barentsz J, Emberton M, Hugosson J, Loeb S, Klotz L, Koch M, Shariat SF, Vickers A. Novel approaches to improve prostate cancer diagnosis and management in early-stage disease. BJUI 2012;109(2):1-7.

[2] Kazer MW, Psutka SP, Latini DM, Bailey DE. Psychosocial aspects of active surveillance. Curr Opin Urol. 2013 May;23(3):273-7.

[3] Wilt TJ, Brawer MK, Jones KM, et al. Radical prostatectomy versus observation for localized prostate cancer. N Engl J Med. 2012 Jul 19;367(3):203-13.

[4] Boorjian SA, Eastham JA, Graefen M, et al. A critical analysis of the long-term impact of radical prostatectomy on cancer control and function outcomes. Eur Urol 2012;61(4):664-675.

[5] Resnick MJ, Koyama T, Fan KH, et al. Long-term functional outcomes after treatment for localized prostate cancer. N Engl J Med 2013;368(5):436-445.

[6] Turpen R, Rosser CJ. Focal therapy for prostate cancer: revolution or evolution? BMC Urology 2009;9:2.

[7] Valerio M, Ahmed HU, Emberton M et al. The Role of Focal Therapy in the Management of Localised Prostate Cancer: A Systematic Review. Eur Urol. 2013 Jun 6. pii: S0302-2838(13)00557-5.

[8] Onik G, Vaughan D, Lotenfoe R. The "male lumpectomy": focal therapy for prostate cancer using cryoablation results in 48 patients with at least 2-year follow-up. Urol Oncol. 2008;26:500–505.

[9] Lambert EH, Bolte K, Masson P. Focal cryosurgery: encouraging health outcomes for unifocal prostate cancer. Urology. 2007;69:1117–1120.

[10] Muto S, Yoshii T, Saito K. Focal therapy with high-intensity-focused ultrasound in the treatment of localized prostate cancer. Jpn J Clin Oncol. 2008;38:192–199.

[11] Ward JF, Jones JS. Focal cryotherapy for localized prostate cancer: a report from the national Cryo On-Line Database (COLD) Registry. BJU Int. 2011 published online Oct 28.

[12] El Fegoun AB, Barret E, Prapotnich D. Focal therapy with high-intensity focused ultrasound for prostate cancer in the elderly. A feasibility study with 10 years follow-up. Int Braz J Urol. 2011;37:213–219.

[13] Ahmed HU, Hindley RG, Dickinson L et al. Focal therapy for localised unifocal and multifocal prostate cancer: a prospective development study Lancet Oncol 2012; 13(6): 622–632.

[14] Barret E, Ahallal Y, Sanchez-Salas R et al. Morbidity of focal therapy in the treatment of localized prostate cancer Eur Urol, 2013;63(4):618–622.

[15] Ahmed HU, Freeman A, Kirkham A et al. Focal therapy for localized prostate cancer: a phase I/II trial. J Urol, 2011;185(4):1246–1254.

[16] Bahn DK, Silverman P, Lee F, Badalament R, Bahn ED, Rewcastle JC. Focal prostate cryoablation: initial results show cancer control and potency preservation. J Endourol, 2006;20(9):688–692.

[17] Ellis DS, Manny TB, Rewcastle JC. Cryoablation as primary treatment for localized prostate cancer followed by penile rehabilitation. Urology 2007, 69(2): 306–310

[18] Bahn D, de Castro Abreu AL, Gill IS et al. Focal cryotherapy for clinically unilateral, low-intermediate risk prostate cancer in 73 men with a median follow-up of 3.7 years. Eur Urol, 62 (1) (2012), pp. 55–63.

[19] van Velthoven R, Aoun F, Limani K, Narahari K, Lemort M and Peltier A Primary Zonal High Intensity Focused Ultrasound for Prostate Cancer: Results of a Prospective Phase IIa Feasibility Study Prostate Cancer Volume 2014, Article ID 756189, 6 pages http://dx.doi.org/10.1155/2014/756189

[20] Hynynen K, McDannold N. MRI-guided focused ultrasound for local tissue ablation and other image-guided interventions. In:Wu J, Nyborg WL, eds. Emerging therapeutic ultrasound, 1st ed. Singapore: World Scientific Publishing, 2006:167-218

[21] Dalecki D. Mechanical bioeffects of ultrasound. Annu Rev Biomed Eng 2004;6:229-248

[22] Jenne, J.W., T. Preusser, and M. Gunther, High-intensity focused ultrasound: principles, therapy guidance, simulations and applications. Z Med Phys, 2012. 22(4): p. 311-22.

[23] Cordeiro, E.R., et al., High-intensity focused ultrasound (HIFU) for definitive treatment of prostate cancer. BJU Int, 2012. 110(9): p. 1228-42.

[24] ter Haar GR. Therapeutic application of ultrasound. Prog Biophys Mol Biol 2007;93:111-129.

[25] ter Haar GR. Therapeutic and surgical applications. In: Hill CR, Bamber JC, ter Haar GR, eds. Physical principles of medical ultrasound, 2nd ed. West Sussex: John Wiley & Sons, 2004:407-456.

[26] Rebillard, X., et al., High-intensity focused ultrasound in prostate cancer; a systematic literature review of the French Association of Urology. BJU Int, 2008. 101(10): p. 1205-13.

[27] Lukka H, Waldron T, Chin J, Mayhew L, Warde P, Winquist E, Rodrigues G, Shayegan BHigh-intensity focused ultrasound for prostate cancer: a practice guideline. Can Urol Assoc J. 2010 Aug;4(4):232-6.

[28] NICE guidelines 2012: Focal therapy using high-intensity focused ultrasound for localised prostate cancer. Issued in guidance.nice.org.uk/ipg424

[29] Limani K, Aoun F, Holz S, Paesmans M, Peltier A, van Velthoven R. Single High Intensity Focused Ultrasound Session as a Whole Gland Primary Treatment for Clinically Localized Prostate Cancer: 10-Year Outcomes. Prostate Cancer 2014,http://dx.doi.org/10.1155/2014/186782

[30] Warmuth M, Johansson T, Mad P. Systematic review of the efficacy and safety of high-intensity focussed ultrasound for the primary and salvage treatment of prostate cancer. Eur Urol. 2010 Dec;58(6):803-15.

[31] Roach M 3rd, Hanks G, Thames H Jr, et al. Defining biochemical failure following radiotherapy with or without hormonal therapy in men with clinically localized prostate cancer: recommendations of the RTOG-ASTRO Phoenix Consensus Conference. Int J Radiat Oncol Biol Phys. 2006; 65:965–974.

[32] Blana A, Robertson CN, Brown SC, Chaussy C, Crouzet S, Gelet A, Conti GN, Ganzer R, Pasticier G, Thuroff S, Ward JF. Complete high-intensity focused ultrasound in

prostate cancer: outcome from the @-Registry. Prostate Cancer Prostatic Dis. 2012 Sep;15(3):256-9.

[33] Pfeiffer D, Berger J, Gross AJ. Single application of high-intensity focused ultrasound as a first-line therapy for clinically localized prostate cancer: 5-year outcomes. BJU Int. 2012 Dec;110(11):1702-7

[34] Thüroff S, Chaussy C. Evolution and outcomes of 3 MHz high intensity focused ultrasound therapy for localized prostate cancer during 15 years. J Urol. 2013 Aug; 190(2):702-10.

[35] Pinthus JH, Farrokhyar F, Hassouna MM, Woods E, Whelan K, Shayegan B, Orovan WL. Single-session primary high-intensity focused ultrasonography treatment for localized prostate cancer: biochemical outcomes using third generation-based technology. BJU Int. 2012 Oct;110(8):1142-8.

[36] Crouzet S, Rebillard X, Chevallier D, Rischmann P, Pasticier G, Garcia G, Rouviere O, Chapelon JY, Gelet A.Multicentric oncologic outcomes of high-intensity focused ultrasound for localized prostate cancer in 803 patients. Eur Urol. 2010 Oct;58(4):559-66.

[37] Baumunk D, Andersen C, Heile U, et al, High-intensity focussed ultrasound in low-risk prostate cancer - oncological outcome and post interventional quality of life of an inexperienced therapy centre in comparison with an experienced therapy centre. Aktuelle Urol. 2013 Jul;44(4):285-92.

Chapter 2

Kinase Inhibitors — Targeted Personalized Cancer Therapy

Wade A. Russu

Additional information is available at the end of the chapter

http://dx.doi.org/10.5772/60417

1. Introduction

Cancer arises when a group of cells of a specific tissue type acquires genetic alterations which allow them to grow in an uncontrolled manner eventually invading surrounding tissue and/or traveling to other sites in the body disrupting the normal bodily functions and can result in death. Often the type of acquired genetic alteration in the cancer cell is one which causes the over or under production of a protein important to the regulation of cell growth, or the production of a mutant form of such a protein that is overactive or less active (or not active) or that has a different function than the normal form of the protein. This alteration in expression pattern or altered function contributes to the cancerous state.

The science and art of molecular biology applied to tumor cell lines has provided much information about how mutations contribute to the development of cancers. One group of proteins that are often mutated in cancers are receptor tyrosine kinases. These proteins sit on the cell surface and bind to molecules such as growth factors and result in the growth, maintenance and multiplication of cells. When an activating mutation occurs in a receptor tyrosine kinase the growth factor signal is no longer needed and the cell grows and multiplies uncontrollably, contributing to a cancerous state. While mutations in receptor tyrosine kinases has garnered much attention, and many drugs have been developed targeting them, these kinases are by no means the only relevant kinase family to cancer.

In the past decade there has been rapid growth in the number of FDA approved cancer drugs within the class known as kinase inhibitors. Some kinase inhibitors have become first line targeted therapy for certain tumor types. For example, imatinib (Gleevec) is used effectively to treat Philadelphia chromosome positive (Ph+) chronic myeloid leukemia (CML). The Philadelphia chromosome encodes the mutant BCR-Abl kinase, an oncogenic driver for CML.

Unfortunately, resistance to kinase inhibitors can develop through up-regulation of the target kinase, or mutation of the target kinase resulting in decreased drug binding.

In the most ideal sense of targeted therapy for cancer, kinase inhibitors have the potential to fulfill the goal of personalized cancer therapy. Studies have shown kinase inhibitors targeting specific kinases that drive a proportion of patients' tumors can provide better outcomes for those patients. Combine this outcome with the possibility of mutant selective kinase inhibitors which may leave tissue that expresses wild-type kinase largely unaffected and provide a potentially better safety profile.

2. Kinase structure and function

Protein kinase function was first observed in 1954 by Burnett and Kennedy who discovered an enzyme that phosphorylates casein [1]. Protein kinases are a group of protein enzymes that phosphorylate protein and other targets in the cell in order to modulate these target proteins' function. Protein kinases are often target proteins themselves. Protein kinases catalyze the transfer of a phosphate group from adenosine triphosphate (ATP) to amino acid sidechains that bear a hydroxyl group on target proteins, namely serine, threonine, and tyrosine. The phosphorylation of one of these amino acid sidechains can drastically change the local physicochemical environment as the relatively small polar unionized hydroxyl group is transformed into the relatively large polar ionized phosphate group. This change in the local environment can initiate a conformational change in the newly phosphorylated target protein, in an attempt to find a new low energy conformation, which may modulate the function of the target protein. The phosphorylation event may serve to activate or inhibit target protein enzyme function, or simply modify the target proteins' surface to modulate protein/protein interactions. For example, Src homology 2 (SH2) domain containing proteins recognize certain phospho-tyrosine sequences within protein targets which enable them to perform their adaptor or scaffolding function [2].

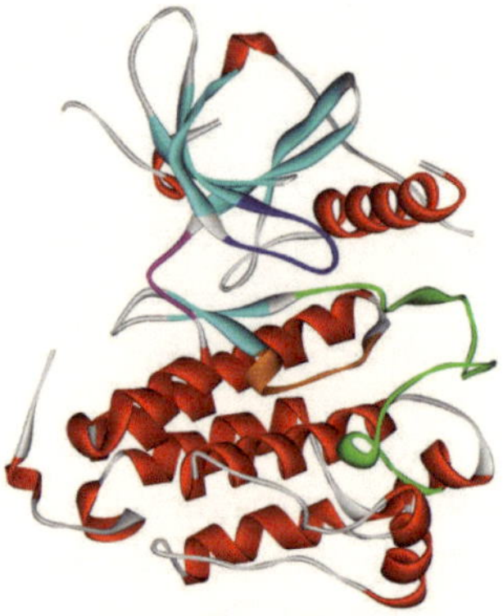

Figure 1. The EGFR kinase domain with color coded structural elements. Cyan; N-terminal lobe. Red; C-terminal lobe. Blue; P-loop. Magenta; hinge. Green; activation loop. Orange; catalytic loop.

http://dx.doi.org/10.5772/60417

Protein kinases are classified into groups based on sequence similarity [3]. The AGC group is named for protein kinases A, G and C. The CaM group is named for calcium/calmodulin-dependent kinases. The CK1 group is named for casein kinase 1. The CMGC group is named for cyclin dependent, mitogen-activated, glycogen synthase, and CDK-like kinases. The STE group is named for sterile phenotype kinase. The TK group is named for tyrosine kinases, and the TKL group is named for tyrosine kinase-like kinases. The groups are further broken down to individual protein kinase families and these families may be further broken down to sub-families. For example, within the TK group is the family called epidermal growth factor receptor (EGFR) tyrosine kinase. The EGFR family includes members EGFR (Her1/ErbB1), Her2/ErbB2, Her3/ErbB3 and Her4/ErbB4. These family members have a high degree of sequence similarity and function.

All protein kinases have a somewhat homologous kinase domain that adopts a common tertiary structure [4]. Figure 1 represents the epidermal growth factor receptor (EGFR) kinase domain and will serve to identify the various secondary structural elements of kinase domain structure and function. Starting from the N-terminus, the basic structural elements of a kinase domain include an N-terminal lobe, composed mostly of beta-sheet structure, and a C-terminal lobe, composed mostly of alpha-helix structure. The two lobes are connected by a hinge region. Of particular interest are the conserved mobile elements of the kinase domain which contribute to kinase function.

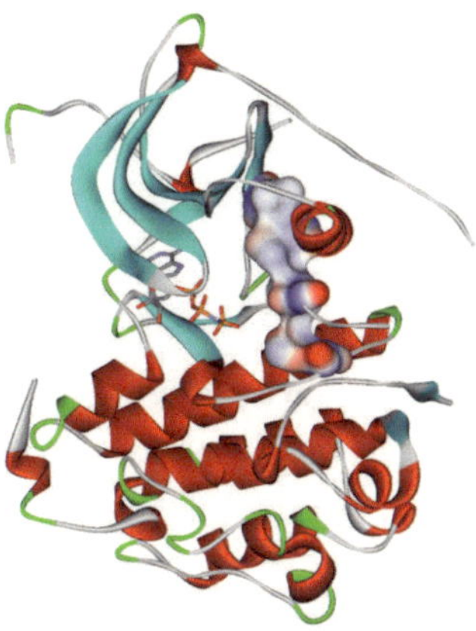

Figure 2. EGFR kinase domain (ribbon) in the active conformation bound to an ATP analog (stick). The active conformation is characterized by alignment of key amino acid sidechains that form a hydrophobic spine (surface representation).

Conformational mobility is essential for kinase function. A number of flexible loop regions are important for the ability to interconvert between active and inactive conformations. These loop regions include the activation loop (A-loop), catalytic loop, nucleotide binding loop (P-loop), and the hinge region. The P-loop is a long loop that joins two anti-parallel beta-strands that are a part of the N-terminal lobe beta-sheet structure of the kinase domain. This loop typically contains a number of glycine residues that are able to access a large range of phi and psi angles and enable considerable conformational flexibility. In the inactive conformation the P-loop may be largely disordered. In the active kinase conformation the P-loop may resemble more of a classic beta-turn and is able to interact with the triphosphate group of bound ATP. The A-loop includes one or more tyrosine residues that when phosphorylated induce the conversion from the inactive to the active kinase conformation. The A-loop is long, containing around 27 amino acid residues that may fold into a number of isolated single turn helices. The A-loop has a conserved DFG sequence, where in the non-phosphorylated inactive kinase conformation the phenylalanine sidechain is oriented toward the triphosphate binding area of the ATP binding site, the so called DFG-out conformation. In the phosphorylated active kinase conformation, the DFG phenylalanine sidechain is oriented toward the interior of the protein, the so-called DFG-in conformation [5-7]. While the DFG orientation related to active and inactive kinase conformations is clear in some cases it is not clear in others, and is not as general in differentiating active and inactive conformations as first thought. It has subsequently been found through surface comparison of x-ray derived crystal structures of both active and inactive forms of specific kinases, that the assembly of a hydrophobic spine through sidechain interaction of discontiguous amino acids within the N-lobe, C-lobe and activation loop regions offers a better structural definition of kinase activation for all kinase families [8]. Figure 2 demonstrates the hydrophobic spine assembly of a representative kinase. Both active and inactive kinase conformations are able to bind ATP. However, only the active kinase conformation can perform the kinase function on substrates.

Protein kinases are important to many biological processes, as is evidenced by the more than 500 kinases encoded in the human genome. Kinases are involved in processes ranging from modulation of intracellular trafficking of proteins, to assembly of complicated multiprotein complexes, to gene expression. Kinase modulation of gene expression through signal transduction is of particular interest for cancer therapy.

The underlying cause of cancer is genomic instability. The emergence of a tumor cell typically requires multiple mutations in the genome that both activate oncogenes and inactivate tumor suppressor genes. These mutations synergize to transform a cell to a state of uncontrolled growth, proliferation, and enhanced survival. Mutations and/or epigenetic alterations that increase expression of, or produce constitutive active forms of some kinase proteins are known to drive the proliferation and/or survival of some tumors [9]. The types of kinases that are often mutated in tumor cells, although not exclusively, are found in signal transduction pathways. These pathways are kinase cascades that transmit extracellular signals to the nucleus and ultimately affect gene expression patterns. When a kinase in such a pathway is mutated where it is constitutively active, the extracellular signal is no longer needed and the pathway is always active and not regulated. Alternatively, epigenetic alterations or an increase in copy number of a protein kinase gene may cause overexpression of the kinase to increase activation of a signaling pathway. For example, a significant portion of non-small cell lung cancers (NSCLC) over express or have EGFR mutations. This causes over active signaling through one or more of the Ras/Raf/ERK, PI3K/AKT/mTOR, and STAT pathways that lead to increased growth, proliferation, motility and survival of the tumor cells.

The KIT receptor tyrosine kinase, or stem cell factor receptor, is a good example for representing the different types of mutations that occur in kinases that contribute to the development of cancer. KIT possesses an extracellular domain, a juxtamembrane domain, and a kinase domain. Point mutations have been observed to occur in all domains of KIT [10]. The most common mutations occur in the juxtamembrane domain followed by the extracellular domain, and finally the kinase domain. Within the kinase domain mutations occur within the ATP binding site and the activation loop. Multiple muatations may occur within a tumor cell. All of these mutations produce constitutive active KIT. For example, juxtamembrane mutations result in the disruption of the autoinhibited form of the kinase, which results in a similar conformation to the phosphorylated activated kinase [11] Additionally, a KIT isoform with a GNNK insert in the extracellular domain has been identified that, once phosphorylated remains so for longer than the isoform that does not contain this insert, increases survival of myeloma cells [12, 13]. Overexpression of wildtype KIT may also drive tumor development. Overexpression may be due to an increase in gene copy number and/or hypomethylation of the gene promoter region.

The link between the development of some tumors, and aberrant modulation of certain protein kinases-either wildtype of mutant- has been established. Some of these aberrations, such as the BCR-Abl protein, represent driver mutations that have lead to the successful translation of experimental protein kinase inhibitors into the clinic for therapeutic treatment of cancer patients.

3. Kinase inhibitors

The natural product staurosporin was one the first small molecules discovered that inhibits the function of protein kinases [14]. Staurosporin is a non-selective inhibitor and is not amenable to development as a drug. However, one staurosporin-like molecule, midostaurine is in clinical development for oncology indications such as indolent systemic mastocytosis [15].

Imatinib, the first marketed kinase inhibitor for treatment of cancer, was discovered by scientist at Ciba-Geigy in the 1990s. It was determined that imatinib inhibited the function of the BCR-Abl fusion kinase that drives chronic myeloid leukemia [16]. Since this time (and perhaps before) the primary rational approach to design of kinase inhibitors has been to target the ATP binding site. The first experimentally determined structure of a small molecule bound to the ATP binding site of a kinase appeared in the year 2000 [17]. This structure was groundbreaking, in that it showed imatinib to be buried deeply in the ATP binding site of the kinase thus locking it in an inactive conformation. This structure provided data that could be used for a structure based design approach of future kinase inhibitors. The structure revealed a pose of imatinib in the ATP binding site that is today designated the type II binding mode.

Clinically used ATP site binding direct kinase inhibitors fall within two categories that describe their binding modes. Type I inhibitors may bind both active and inactive conformations of a particular kinase target. Type II kinase inhibitors bind only inactive conformations of a kinase. Both type I and II inhibitors bind in the ATP binding site and make use of hydrogen bonds to the amide backbone of hinge region amino acid residues. The difference between type I and II inhibitors is that type II inhibitors typically penetrate deeper into the pocket accessing what is termed an allosteric binding site, the effect of which is to displace the C-helix and locking the kinase in an inactive conformation. Knowledge of binding geometries has been applied to kinase inhibitor design projects.

The majority of kinase inhibitor design projects have focused on ATP competitive inhibitors targeting the ATP binding site. The popularity of such programs have spurred the growth of contract research screening services that screen potential inhibitors in a high throughput format for binding to the ATP binding site and/or inhibition of target kinase function [18]. Design programs may be conducted in a variety of manners from high throughput screening of compound libraries to fragment based and/or structure guided design. One approach is to start from known privileged fragments or templates - chemical moieties that appear in numerous kinase inhibitors - such as the quinazoline ring system [19]. The quinazoline ring system appears in many experimental kinase inhibitors, clinical candidates (tandutinib), and kinase inhibitor drugs such as afatinib, vandetinib, lapatinib, erlotinib and gefitinib (see Table 1).

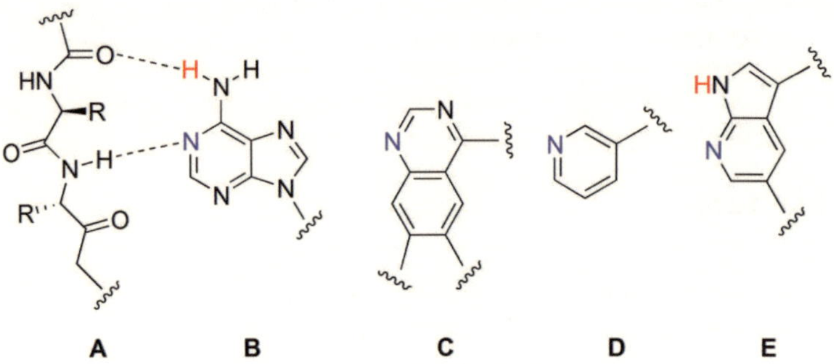

Figure 3. Kinase hinge peptide backbone (A) hydrogen bonding pattern to ATP heterocycle (B) and other heterocycles found in drug molecules. (C) quinazoline, e.g. erlotinib. (D) pyridine, e.g. imatinib. (E) pyrrolopyridine, e.g. vemurafenib. Dashed lines represent hydrogen bonds.

It appears that a unifying characteristic of kinase inhibitors that bind to the ATP binding site is a heterocyclic moiety that serves as a mimic of the adenine ring system and forms Van der Waals contacts with hydrophobic groups of the floor and ceiling of the ATP binding site as well as one or more hydrogen bonds with the amide backbone of hinge region amino acid residues. Figure 3 describes how ATP and some heterocycles found in kinase inhibitors form their hydrogen bonding patterns to the hinge region. Because the ATP binding site is conserved among kinases, kinase inhibitors tend to be promiscuous and inhibit numerous kinases other than their primary target. How the final kinase inhibitor is adorned about its hinge binding moiety contributes to its overall shape and possible intermolecular interactions, ultimately determines its degree of selectivity for its intended target.

Another unifying theme of kinase inhibitors is that their binding to their kinase targets displaces the alignment of the hydrophobic spine that is formed by kinase activation [8].

Besides the occupation of the ATP binding site by the kinase inhibitor, disallowing binding and use of ATP, the kinase inhibitor disrupts the formation of the hydrophobic spine necessary for attainment of the active conformation (Figure 4). This observation leads to the inevitable question of whether inhibitors, that disrupt the hydrophobic spine, but do not bind to the ATP binding site, may be developed.

Considering the mountain of published research and plethora of X-ray diffraction and NMR derived structures of kinase inhibitors bound to their target kinases, the design of kinase inhibitors is fairly well understood. The remaining challenges for drug designers, in the area of kinase inhibitors, are concerned with selectivity. Selectivity is a potential problem for kinase inhibitors, thus far, because most target the highly conserved ATP binding site. Targeting a single family of kinases, let alone a single member of a family, is difficult because of the inherent promiscuity of this drug class. An even more difficult challenge is targeting a cancer relevant mutant kinase selectively with respect to the wild type kinase. The selective targeting of a mutant kinase that drives the proliferation and survival of a patients' tumor has great promise not only in potential survival benefit but also reduction in drug side effects.

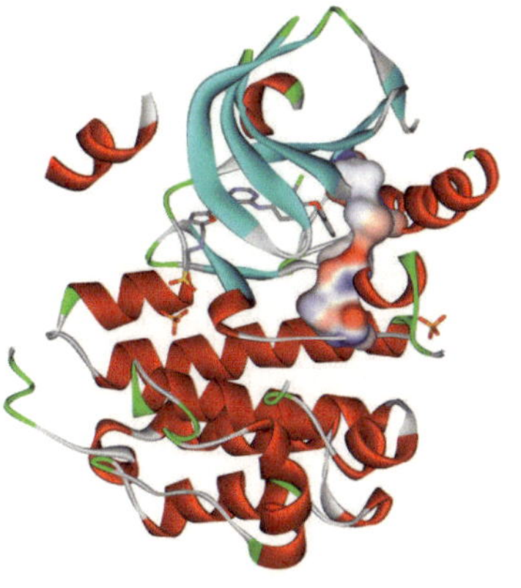

Figure 4. EGFR kinase domain (ribbon) bound to kinase inhibitor lapatinib (stick). Note that the amino acid sidechains that form the hydrophobic spine (surface) are bowed out of alignment.

Common side effects caused by kinase inhibitors include rash, fatigue, and gastrointestinal disturbances such as nausea, vomiting, diarrhea, or constipation. For example, patients receiving therapy with EGFR inhibitors may experience severe acneiform eruption and diarrhea which may be dose limiting [20]. Additionally, the EGFR inhibitor gefitinib has been associated with interstitial lung disease, especially in patients with underlying pulmonary diseases [21]. The more promiscuous kinase inhibitors such as sunitinib and sorafenib exhibit some cardiotoxicites such as hypertension, LVEF and QT prolongation [22]. Additional less severe side-effects may be experienced by patients receiving kinase inhibitors such as hair depigmentation which accompanies KIT inhibitors [23]. Even though kinase inhibitors are considered targeted therapy the patient will experience side effects that can be associated with the mechanism of action, off target effects and intrinsic chemical effects. Almost as common as side effects are associated with anticancer drugs so is tumor resistance. And just as other anticancer drugs may encounter tumor resistance, a kinase inhibitor may also encounter resistance either acquired or intrinsic.

Tumor resistance to anticancer drugs can be a challenging battle even though a lot has been learned about the mechanisms that allow tumor cells to escape the chemical assault. One major mechanism of tumor resistance to kinase inhibitors is mutant forms of the target kinase, either preexisting or acquired during or after treatment, that reduce the kinase inhibitors binding affinity. Early clinical experience with imatinib identified patients that developed resistance after an initial response to the drug due to mutation of the ACR-Abl kinase that prevented imatinib binding [24, 25]. Experience with KIT inhibitors has revealed drug resistant mutations in this kinase [10]. Pharmacokinetic mediated tumor resistance to kinase inhibitors include, polymorphisms in drug metabolizing enzymes and transporters. For example, CML patients with low human organic cation transporter-1 (hOCT1) activity have suboptimal response to imatinib but not to nilotinib [26, 27]. Other mechanisms of tumor resistance to kinase inhibitors may include unique features of the tumors microenvironment and activation of alternative signaling pathways. For a more comprehensive discussion of tumor resistance to kinase inhibitors the reader is directed to the references [28, 29].

Since the year 2001 there have been no less than 24 small molecule, ATP site binding kinase inhibitors approved by the USFDA for oncology indications (Table 1). As the concept of oncogene addiction is explored more and a better understanding of the role of kinases in oncology is realized, the class of kinase drugs may be ideally situated to have a profound effect on personalized cancer medicine.

Structure	Generic Name	Target(s)	Indication(s)
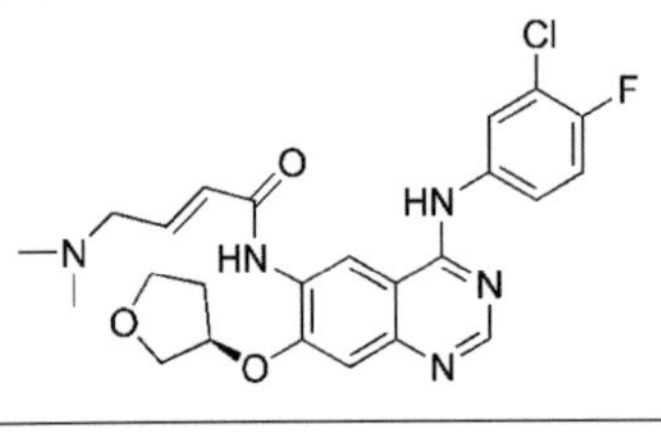	afatinib	EGFR	NSCLC
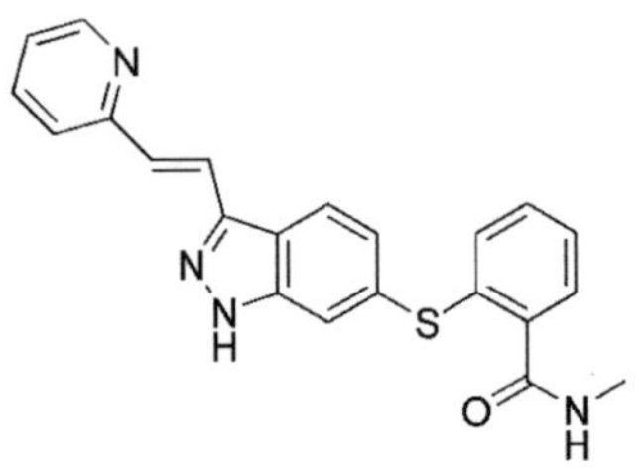	axitinib	VEGFR 1/2/3	RCC
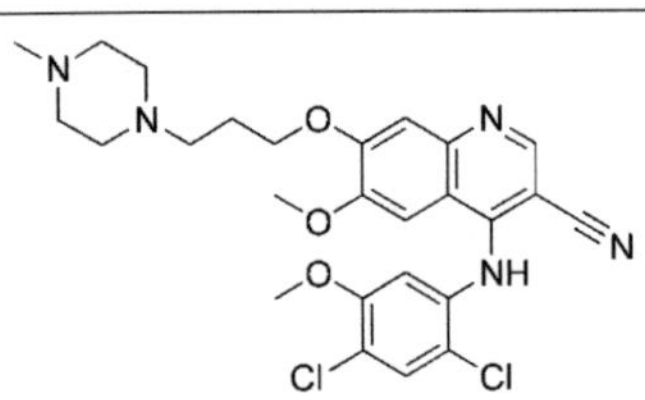	bosutinib	BCR-Abl, Hck, Lyn, Src	CML

http://dx.doi.org/10.5772/60417

Structure	Generic Name	Target(s)	Indication(s)
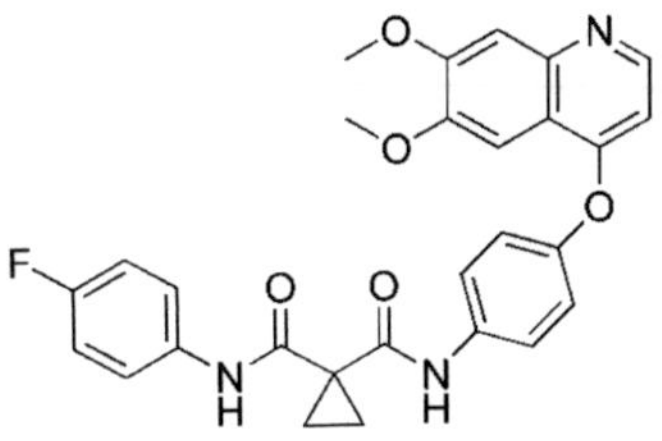	cabozantinib	RET, MET, VEGFR 1/2/3, KIT, TRKB, Flt-3, AXL, TIE-2	MTC
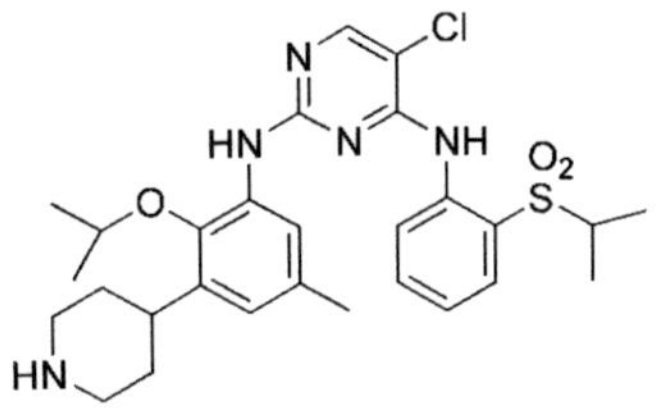	ceritinib	ALK, IGF-1R, InsR, ROS1	ALK-positive NSCLC
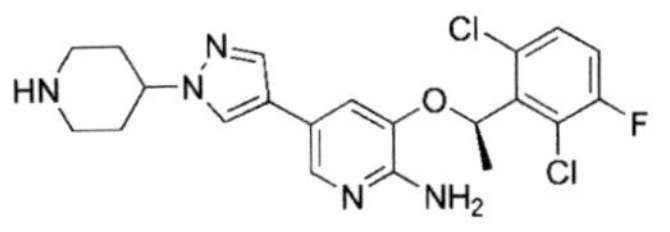	crizotinib	ALK, c-Met, ROS	ALK-positive NSCLC
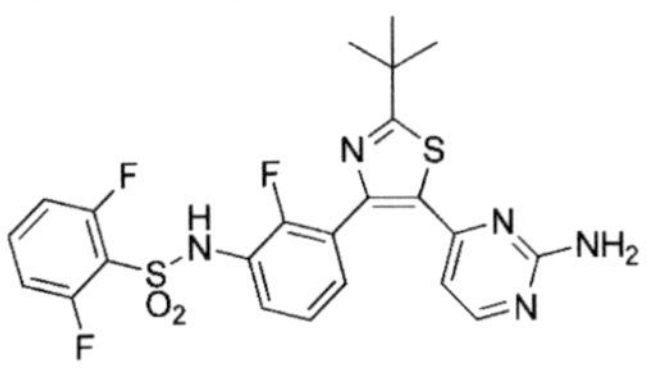	dabrafenib	B-RAF	melanoma
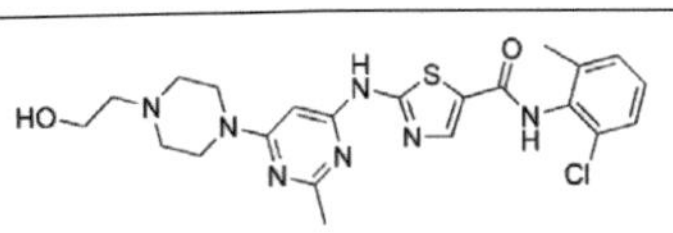	dasitinib	BCR-Abl, SRC, LYN, YES, FYN, KIT, EPHA2, PDGFRb	CML
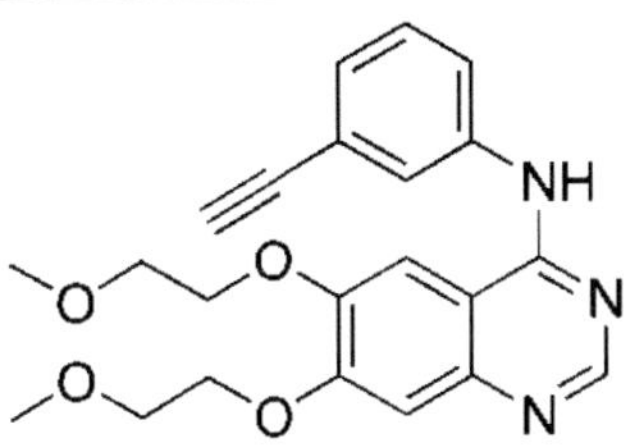	erlotinib	EGFR	NSCLC, pancreatic cancer
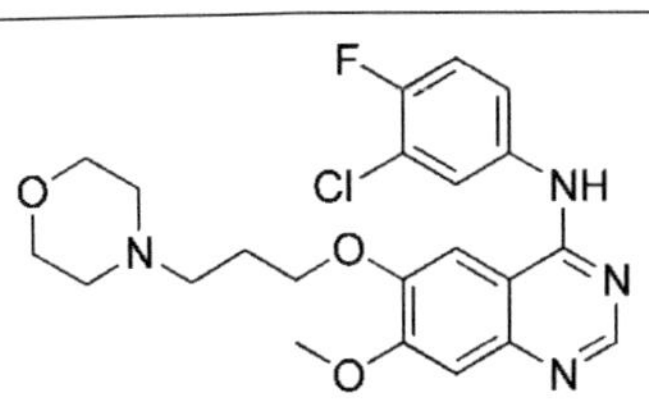	gefitinib	EGFR	NSCLC

Structure	Generic Name	Target(s)	Indication(s)
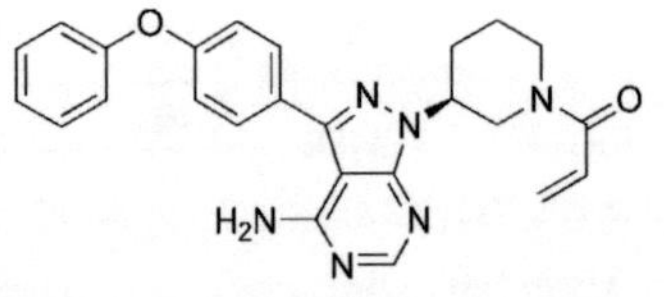	ibrutinib	BTK	CLL, mantle cell lymphoma
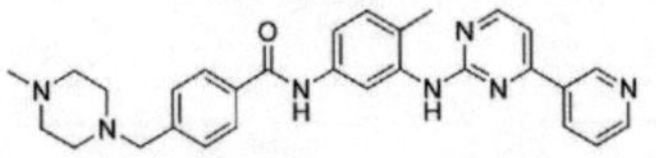	imatinib	BCR-Abl, PDGFR, KIT	CML, ALL, GIST, ASM
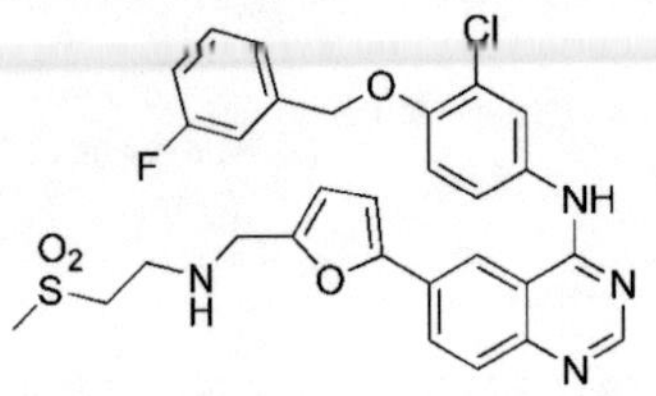	lapatinib	EGFR, ERBB2	Breast cancer
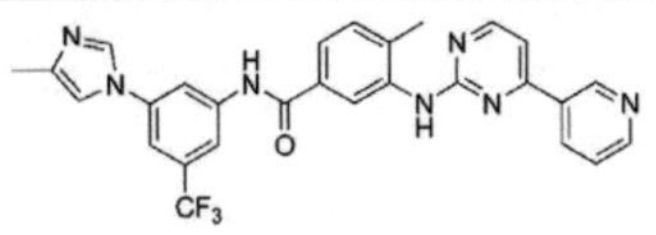	nilotinib	BCR-Abl, PDGFR	CML
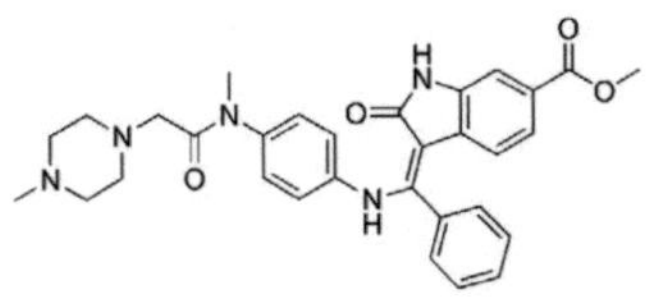	nintedanib	VEGFR, FGFR, PDGFR	IPF
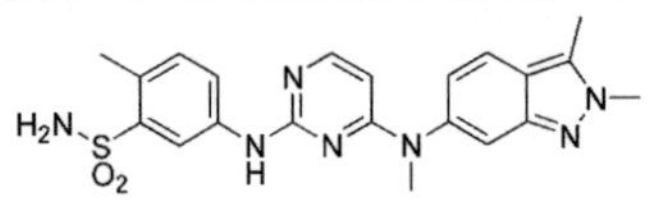	pazopanib	VEGFR, PDGFR, FGFR, KIT, Lck, FMS, ITK	RCC, soft tissue sarcomas
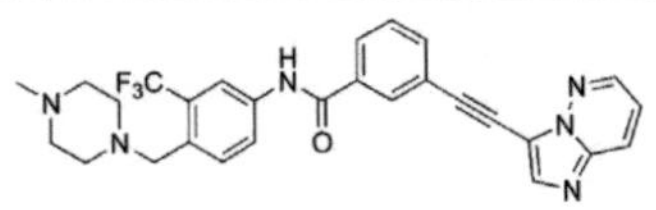	ponatinib	BCR-Abl, VEGFR, PDGFR, Src, KIT, Flt3, RET, Tie2	CML, Ph+ All
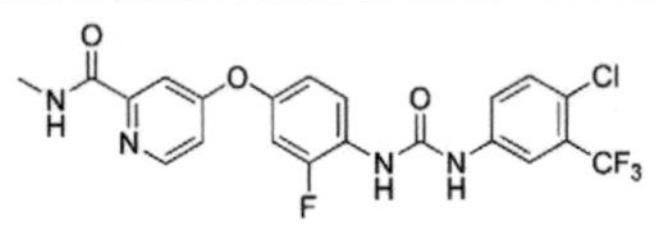	regorafenib	VEGFR, BCR-Abl, B-Raf, PDGFR, FGFR, Tie2	CRC
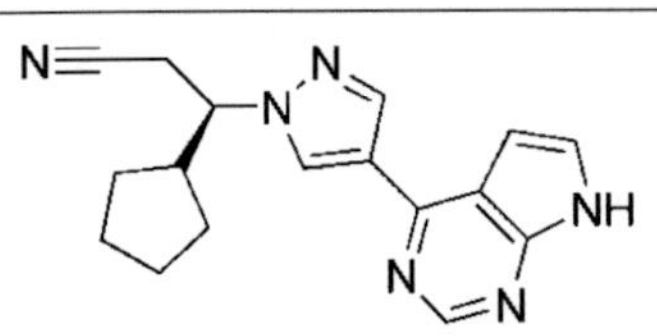	ruxolitinib	JAK	myelofibrosis
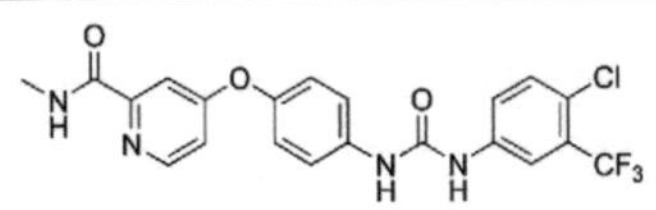	sorafenib	Multi-kinase inhibitor	RCC, DTC

Structure	Generic Name	Target(s)	Indication(s)
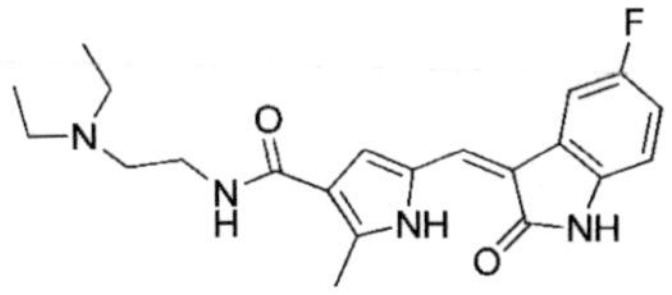	sunitinib	Multi-kinase inhibitor	RCC, GIST, pancrease cancer, neuro-endocrine tumors
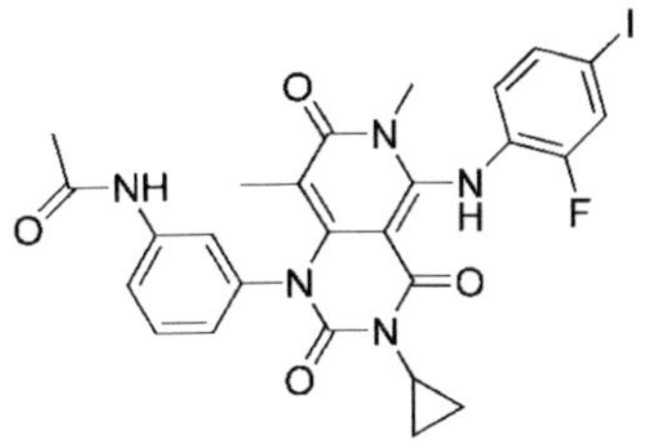	trametinib	MEK	melanoma
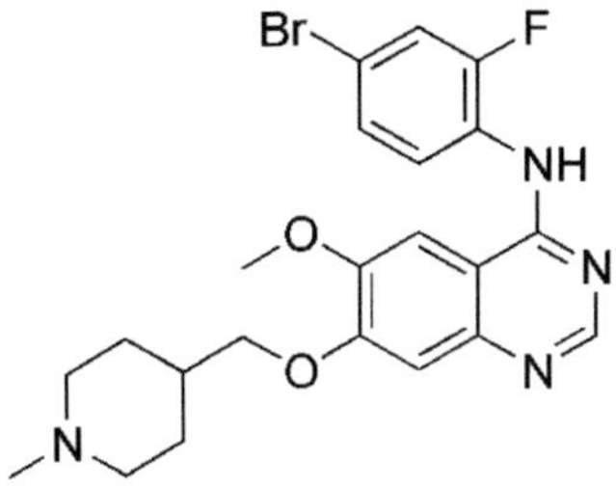	vandetanib	EGFR, VEGFR, RET, Brk, Src, Tie2	MTC
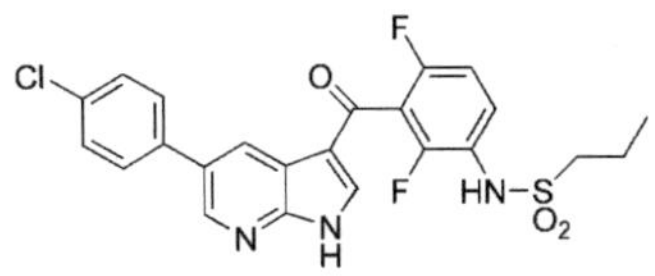	vemurafenib	Raf kinases	melanoma

Table 1. USDA approved kinase inhibitors for oncology indication.

4. Personalized medicine and kinase inhibitors

The basic concept of personalized cancer medicine is to match the patient with an appropriate therapeutic regimen that will provide the best outcome [30]. This can be accomplished on a variety of different levels. With regard to a pharmacological approach, the traditional way patients are assigned to therapy is based on tumor type, that is, what anatomical site at which the tumor resides and/or what type of histopathology the tumor cells derive from. Once these pieces of information were obtained the patient would be assigned a pharmacotherapy regimen that provided the best statistical outcome based on collective experience. This approach has worked as well as can be expected, and exceedingly well in some tumor types considering the diseases' high mortality. However with modern scientific advances and strive toward better outcomes, an even more personalized approach has emerged.

A modern approach to personalized cancer pharmacotherapy can be considered on three basic levels which can be applied individually or combined. These three levels are the patient's pharmacogenetics, the tumor's genomics and/or proteomics, and the tumor's response to drug exposure. Patient pharmacogenetics refers to the patients genetics that are relevant to effects on pharmacokinetics of drugs, for example, polymorphisms in drug metabolizing enzymes. Tumor genomics and/or proteomics refers to specific genetic abnormalities that effect specific gene expression and is thought to contribute to tumor development or maintenance. The application of any or all of these pieces of information may improve the outcome of pharmacotherapy for the patient.

The application of pharmacogenomics to personalized therapy can be exemplified by application to tamoxifen therapy for the breast cancer patient. Tamoxifen acts as an anti-estrogen on breast tissue and is used for treatment of estrogen receptor positive (ER+) breast cancer. It has been determined that tamoxifen is converted in vivo to 4-hydroxytamoxifen, which is a much more active anti-estrogen agent. It was subsequently found that this transformation is accomplished by the drug metabolizing enzymes cytochrome P-450 (CYP) isofroms 2D6 and 2C19 [31]. Patients that were receiving tamoxifen therapy and concurrently receiving selective serotonin reuptake inhibitor (SSRI) drugs, known to inhibit CYP 2D6, experienced poor outcomes because of the failure to convert tamoxifen to 4-hydroxtamoxifen. A significant percentage of the population carry a genetic polymorphism in the CYP 2D6 gene which results in poor metabolism with respect for the CYP 2D6 isoform and will not receive the full benefit of tamoxifen therapy [32]. Consequently a readily available genomic test is available for patients that can identify those who are not good candidates for tamoxifen therapy, because they have a specific 2D6 polymorphism, so that they can be directed to alternatives.

Advances in genomics and proteomics have enabled selection of patients that may benefit from targeted therapies for certain tumor types. Analysis of tumor cells on the protein level using immunohistochemistry (IHC) can identify cells that express relevant protein targets. An example of the application of this approach is the detection of c-erbB2 (Her2/Neu) receptor in breast cancer patients which can direct them toward trastuzumab therapy. Specific gene mutations in tumor cells may be detected using techniques of RT-PCR, DNA microarray, and fluorescence in situ hybridization (FISH) that can be used to direct patients to therapy that may be beneficial. For example, a study demonstrated the utility of screening non-small cell lung cancer patients for amplification of the epidermal growth factor receptor (EGFR). Patients with amplified EGFR receiving an EGFR kinase inhibitor (gefitinib) had longer median progression free survival (PFS) and overall survival (OS), compared to those who did not have amplified EGFR [33, 34]. Furthermore, of those patients who responded to gefitinib therapy 77% had EGFR gene amplification, whereas only 33% of non-responders had EGFR gene amplification. This study demonstrates the utility of identifying patients with mutations that drive tumor growth and survival and matching them with appropriate targeted therapy. The study also highlights the shortcoming of single gene determination directed therapy in that 33% of non-responders also had EGFR amplification.

A potentially more invasive and perhaps technically challenging approach is to directly test samples of the patient's tumor against available drugs. This approach of using personalized xenografts to direct patient therapy was demonstrated in a patient with advanced pancreatic patient [35]. After initial surgery metastases were discovered and adjuvant gemcitabine therapy failed to halt progression. A personalized mouse xenograft model was developed from the patient's tumor tissue and was found to respond to the DNA alkylating agents, mitomycin C and cisplatin. The patient was assigned to mitomycin C treatment and subsequently cisplatin and achieved a partial response with duration of 50+ months. Genomic analysis of the patient's tumor tissue revealed inactivation of the PALB2 gene, which is involved with repair of double strand DNA breaks. It seems logical that the patient's tumor responded to the DNA alkylating agents that would cause double stranded DNA breaks.

The genomic approach has been applied to kinase inhibitors from the beginning of their introduction to the arsenal of pharmacotherapy options. Imatinib, the first kinase inhibitor to be marketed is targeted at a specific genomic alteration, a chromosomal translocation producing the Philidelphia chromosome (Ph) that expresses a mutant gene product, the BCR-Abl kinase. This kinase is constitutively active, and is the driver of nearly all chronic myeloid leukemias (CML). Therefore, patients with CML and are Ph+ can be matched to imatinib therapy. Imatinib therapy has been fairly successful for CML patients. It has been shown that patients who achieve complete cytogenic response at 2 years on imatinib therapy tend to maintain the durable response and do not have mortality significantly different than the general population [36].

Because the effectiveness of kinase inhibitors require that the target kinase to be a driver of, expressed in, or aberrantly expressed in, or be mutated in the tumor cells, it is important to know the status of the target within the specific patient's tumor in order to best assign the patient to kinase inhibitor therapy. To this end specific diagnostic tests have been developed to help guide selection of kinase inhibitor therapy. Indeed, twelve of the approved kinase inhibitors' prescribing information assume diagnostic testing be performed, and of those, four require a diagnostic test for prescription. Table 2 lists six such diagnostics recognized by the USFDA [37].

5. Emerging kinase targets

Because kinase enzymes are involved in numerous biological processes it is not surprising that many of them have become therapeutic targets for various disease sates including cancers. As noted above, drug development of kinase inhibitors for oncology indications has accelerated in the last decade with no sign of slowing. This acceleration has been spurred by emergent technologies and advances in molecular and systems biology, proteomics, and genomics. The continued advancement of understanding of the molecular changes that occur in the development of a cancer has helped identify likely therapeutic targets. Some of the more recently identified targets include the BTK, CDK8, and DNA-PK.

Although a Bruton's tyrosine kinase (BTK) inhibitor (ibrutinib) was recently approved for clinical use, BTK is a relatively new kinase target. BTK plays a role in B-cell receptor signaling, proliferation, differentiation, and survival. Ibrutinib works by irreversible inhibition of BTK through covalent modification of the enzyme. In a clinical trial in mantle cell lymphoma (MCL) patients, who had three prior therapies, an overall response rate of 69% and a progression free survival of 13.9 months were observed. Ibrutinib is approved for second line treatment of MCL and chronic lymphocytic leukemia (CLL) [38].

Drug (generic name)	Diagnostic Product	Diagnostic Product Use
afatinib	Therascreen EGFR RGQ PCR Kit	Detects EGFR exon 19 deletions and exon 21 substitution mutations. Intended for selection of NSCLC patients who may benefit from afatinib therapy.
crizotinib	VTSIS ALK Break Apart FISH Probe Kit	Detection of ALK gene rearrangements. Prescription use only, intended for selection of NSCLC patients eligible for crizotinib treatment.
dabrafenib and tramatenib	THxID BRAF Kit	Detection of BRAF(V600E) and (V600K) mutations in melanoma tissue. Intended to aid selection of melanoma patients who may benefit from treatment with dabrafenib and/or trametinib.
erlotinib	Cobas EGFR Mutation Test	Detects EGFR exon 19 deletions and exon 21 substitution mutations. Intended for selection of patients with metastatic NSCLC who may benefit from afatinib therapy.
imatinib mesylate	DAKO C-KIT PharmDx	Quantitative c-Kit detection in GIST and normal tissues. Intended to aid selection of GIST patients who may be eligible for imatinib mesylate treatment.
vemurafenib	COBAS 4800 BRAF V600 Mutation Test	Detection of BRAF (V600E) mutation in melanoma. Intended to aid selection of melanoma patients who may benefit from vemurafenib therapy.

Table 2. US FDA Cleared or Approved In Vitro Companion Diagnostic Tools for Kinase Inhibitors.

Cyclin dependent kinase 8 (CDK8) was recently identified as a colorectal cancer oncogene [39]. It was discovered that 47% of colorectal cancer samples demonstrated copy number gain of the chromosomal region carrying the CDK8 gene. It has also been shown that 76% of colorectal cancers showed positive expression of nuclear CDK8, and that increased positive expression

http://dx.doi.org/10.5772/60417

rate correlated with increased clinical stage [40]. Additionally, expression of CDK8 transformed NIH 3T3 cells, however a kinase inactive version did not. Experimental knockdown of CDK8, in colorectal cancer cell lines with high CDK8 expression levels, induced a decrease in cell proliferation. While most CDKs regulate cell cycle progression CDK8 and some others play a role in transcription regulation. Assembly of CDK8 with other key protein partners forms a mediator complex which can activate β-catenin dependent transcription. Furthermore it was shown that CDK8 function represses E2F1 activity, a known negative regulator of β-catenin [41]. Of note is the fact that knockdown of CDK8 in some colorectal cancer cell lines does not completely diminish β-catenin levels, which suggests that other genetic determinants of resistance must be identified to exclude patients that would not benefit from a future CDK8 targeted therapeutic.

DNA-dependent protein kinase (DNA-PK) is another emerging oncology kinase target. Being that the development of cancer is due to genomic instability that results in the acquiring of genetic mutations that drive tumor formation, it should be no surprise that tumor cells may have defective DNA repair pathways that result in a mutator phenotype. It is no wonder that the first class of anti-cancer drugs were DNA alkylating agents that cause irreparable damage to DNA of tumor cells, although with severe side effects and risk of secondary tumors arising from DNA damaged normal cells. A less devastating targeted approach to induce irreparable DNA damage in tumor cells, while sparing normal cells, is to target still operating DNA repair pathways that are critical to the tumor cells survival. In other words disable a DNA repair pathway that will synergize with an already disabled pathway. For example, DNA-PK is critical for repairing double strand DNA breaks through the non-homologous end joining (NHEJ) pathway. A second pathway for repairing double strand breaks is the homologous recombination pathway, which is impaired in tumor cells with mutations in genes such as BRCA1 and BRCA2 as well as others. Targeting tumors with impaired homologous recombination by inhibiting the NHEJ pathway with DNA-PK inhibitors should, in theory, cause activation of cell death pathways as double strand DNA-breaks build-up in the cells [42, 43]. Normal cells should be able to withstand the assault due to both pathways being operable.

6. Summary

Kinase inhibitors have enormous potential to facilitate improved outcomes for some cancer patients especially in the context of personalized medicine. The personalized approach that implements genomic analysis to identify potential driver kinases in patient tumor samples will enable matching the patient with the best kinase inhibitor for the best outcome. The identification of drug resistant mutations in the targeted kinase will be critical in order to avoid treatment that is not likely to be beneficial to the patient. Also critical, is the identification of relevant polymorphisms in drug metabolizing enzymes and transporters that may affect pharmacokinetics of the kinase inhibitor, in order to assure adjustments are made to achieve optimum drug exposure. These considerations along with proper management of side effects can maximize patient benefit from targeted personalized cancer therapy with kinase inhibitors.

Nomenclature

ALL-acute lymphoblastic leukemia; ASM-aggressive systemic mastocytosis; CLL-chronic lymphocytic leukemia; CML-chronic myeloid leukemia; CRC-colorectal cancer; DTC-differentiated thyroid carcinoma; GIST-gastrointestinal stromal tumor; IPF-idiopathic pulmonary fibrosis; MTC-medullary carcinoma of the thyroid; NSCLC-non-small-cell lung cancer; RCC-renal cell carcinoma.

Author details

Wade A. Russu

Address all correspondence to: wrussu@pacific.edu

Thomas J. Long School of Pharmacy and Health Sciences, University of the Pacific, Stockton, CA, USA

References

[1] Burnett G, Kennedey E. P. The Enzymatic Phosphorylation of Proteins. Journal of Biological Chemistry 1954; 211: 969-980.

[2] Songyang Z, Shoelson S. E, Chaudhuri M, Gish G, Pawson T, Haser W. G, King F, Roberts T, Ratnofsky S, Lechleider R. J, Neel B. G, Birge R. B, Fajaro J. E, Chou M. M, Hanafusa H, Schaffhausen B, Cantley L.C. SH2 Domains Recognize Specific Phosphopeptide Sequences. Cell 1993; 72: 767-778.

[3] Kostich M, English J, Madison V, Gheyas F, Wang L, Qiu P, Greene J, Laz T. M. Human members of the eukaryotic protein kinase family. Genome Biology 2002; 3(9): research0043.1-0043.12.

[4] Scheeff E. D, Bourne P. E. Structural Evolution of the Protein Kinase-Like Superfamily. PLoS Computational Biology 2005; 1(5): e49.

[5] Hubbard S. R, Mohammadi M, Schlessinger J. Autoregulatory mechanisms in protein-tyrosine kinases. Journal of Biological Chemistry 1998; 273: 11987-11990.

[6] Huse M, Kuriyan J. The conformational plasticity of protein kinases. Cell 2002; 109: 275-282.

[7] Foster R, Griffith R, Ferrao P, Ashman L. Molecular basis of the constitutive activity and STI571 resistance of Asp816Val mutant KIT receptor tyrosine kinase. Journal of Molecular Graphics and Modeling 2004; 23: 139-152.

[8] Kornev A. P, Haste N. M, Taylor S. S, Eyck L.F. Surface comparison of active and inactive protein kinases identifies a conserved activation mechanism. Proceedings of the National Academy of Sciences of the USA 2006; 103(47): 17783-17788.

[9] Blume-Jensen P, Hunter T. Oncogenic kinase signalling. Nature 2001; 411: 355-365.

[10] Gramza A. W, Corless C. L, Heinrich M. C. Resistance to Tyrosine Kinase Inhibitors in Gastrointestinal Stromal Tumors. Clinical Cancer Research 2009; 15(24); 7510-7518.

[11] Mol C. D, Dougan D. R, Schneider T. R, Skene R. J, Kraus M. L, Sheibe D. N, Snell G. P, Zou H, Sang B.-C, Wilson K. P. Structural basis for the autoinhibition and STI-571 inhibition of c-Kit tyrosine kinase. Journal of Biological Chemistry 2004; 279: 31655-31663.

[12] Theou N, Tabone S, Saffroy R, Le Cesne A, Julie C, Cortez A, Lavergne-Slove A, Debuire B, Lemoine A, Emile J-F. High expression of both mutant and wild-type allels of c-kit in gastrointestinal stromal tumors. Biochemica et Biophysica Acta 2004; 1688: 250-256.

[13] Montero J. C, Lopez-Perez R, San Miguel J. F, Pandiella A. Expression of c-Kit isoforms in multiple myeloma: differences in signaling and drug sensitivity. Haematologica 2008; 93(6): 851-859.

[14] Tamaoki T, Nomoto H. Takahashi I, Kato Y, Morimoto M, Tomita F. Staurosporin, a potnt phospholipid/Ca++ dependent protein kinase. Biochemical Biophysical Research Communications 1986; 135: 397-402.

[15] ClinicalTrials.gov. Midostaurin in Indolent Systemic Mastocytosis. ClinicalTrials.gov Identifier: NCT01920204. https://clinicaltrials.gov/ct2/show/NCT01920204 (accessed January 23, 2015).

[16] Druker B. J, Tamura, S, Buchdunger E, Ohno S, Segal G. M, Fanning S, Zimmermann J, Lydon N. B. Effects of a selective inhibitor of the Abl tyrosine kinase on the growth of Bcr-Abl positive cells. Nature Medicine 1996; 2: 561-566.

[17] Schindler T, Bornmann W, Pellicena P, Miller W.T, Clarckson B, Kuriyan J. Structural Mechanism for STI-571 inhibition of Abelson tyrosine kinase. Science 2000; 289: 1938-1942.

[18] Karaman M. W, Herrgard S, Treiber D. K, Gallant P, Atteridge C. E, Campbell B. T, Chan K. W, Ciceri P, Davis M. I, Edeen P. T. A quantitative analysis of kinase inhibitor selectivity. Nature Biotechnology 2008; 26: 127-132.

[19] Shallal H. M, Russu W. A. Discovery, synthesis, and investigation of the antitumor activity of novel piperazinylpyrimidine derivatives. European Journal of Medicinal Chemistry 2011; 26: 2043-2057.

[20] Cappuzzo F, Bartolini S, Ceresoli G. L, Tamberi S, Spreafico A, Lombardo L, Gregorc V, Toschi L, Calandri C, Villa E, Crino L. Efficacy and tolerability of gefitinib in pre-

treated elderly patients ith advanced non-small cell lung cancer (NSCLC). British Journal of Cancer 2004; 90: 82-86.

[21] Inoue A, Saijo Y, Maemondo M, Gomi K, Tokue Y, Ebina M, Kikuchi T, Moriya T, Nukiwa T. Severe acute interstitial pneumonia and gefitinib. Lancet 2003; 361: 137-139.

[22] Mellor H. R, Bell A. K, Valentin J.-P, Roberts R. R. A. Cardiotoxocity Associated with Targeting Kinase Pathways in Cancer. Toxicological Sciences 2011; 120(1): 14-32.

[23] Botchkareva, N. V, Khlgatian M, Longley B. J, Botchkareva V. A, Gilchrest B. A. SCF/c kit signaling is required for cyclic regeneration of the hair pigmentation unit. FASEB Journal 2001; 15: 645-658.

[24] Gorre M. E, Mohammed M, Ellwood K, Hsu N, Paquette R, Rao P. N, Sawyers C. L. Clinical Resistance to STI-571 Cancer Therapy Caused by BCR-ABL Gene Mutation or Amplification. Science 2001; 293: 876-880.

[25] Shah, N. P, Nicoll J. M, Nagar B, Gorre M. E, Paquette R. L, Kuriyan J, Sawyers C. L. Multiple BCR-ABL kinase domain mutations confer polyclonal resistance to the tyrosine kinase inhibitor imatinib (STI571) in chronic phase and blast crisis chronic myeloid leukemia. Cancer Cell 2002; 2: 117-125.

[26] White D. L, Saunders V. A, Dang P, Engler J, Zannettino A. C, Cambareri, A. C, Quinn S. R, Manley P. W, Hughes T. P. OCT-1-mediated influx is a key determinant of the intracellular uptake of imatinib but not nilotinib (AMW107): reduced OCT-1 activity is the cause of low in vitro sensitivity to imatinib. Blood 2006; 108: 697-704.

[27] White D. L, Saunders V. A, Dang P, Engler J, Venables A, Zrim S, Zannettino A, Lynch K, Manley P. W. Hughes T. Most CML patients who have suboptimal response to imatinib have low OCT- activity: higher doses of imatinib may overcome the negative impact of low OCT-1 activity. Blood 2007; 110: 4064-4072.

[28] Chen Y.-f, Fu L.-w. Mechanisms of acquired resistance to tyrosine kinase inhibitors. Acta Pharmaceutica Sinica B 2011; 1(4): 197-207.

[29] Barouch-Bentov R. Mechanisms of Drug-Resistance in Kinases. Expert Opinion on Investigational Drugs 2011; 20(2): 153-208.

[30] Diamandis M, White N. M. A, Yousef G. M. Personalized Medicine: Marking a New Epoch in Cancer Patient Management. Molecular Cancer Research 2010; 8(9): 1175-1187.

[31] Johnson M. D, Zuo K. H, Lee K. H, Trebley J. P, Rae J. M, Weatherman R. V, Desta Z, Flockhart D. A, Skaar T. C. Pharmacological characterization of 4-hydroxy-N-desmethyl tamoxifen, a novel active metabolite of tamoxifen. Breast Cancer Research and Treatment 2004; 85: 151-159.

[32] Newman W. G, Hadfield K. D, Latif A, Roberts S. A, Shenton A, McHague C, Lalloo F, Howell S, Evans D. G. Impaired tamoxifen metabolism reduces survival in familial breast cancer patients. Clinical Cancer Research 2008; 14: 5913-5918.

[33] Bell D. W, Lynch T. J, Haserlat S. M, Harris P. L, Okimoto R. A, Brannigan B. W, Sgroi D. C, Muir B, Riemenschneider M. J, Iacona R. B, Krebs A. D, Johnson D. H, Giaccone G, Herbst R. S, Manegold C, Fukuoka M, Kris M. G, Baselga J, Ochs J. S, Haber D. A. Epidermal growth factor receptor mutations and gene amplification in non-small lung cancer: molecular analysis of the IDEAL/INTACT gefitinib trials. Journal of Clinical Oncology 2005; 23: 8081-8092.

[34] Kimura H, Kasahara K, Kawaishi M, Kunitoh H, Tamura T, Holloway B, Nishio K. Detection of Epidermal Growth Factor Receptor Mutations in Serum as a Predictor of the Response to Gefitinib in Patients with Non-Small-Cell Lung Cancer. Clinical Cancer Research 2006; 12: 3915-3921.

[35] Villarroel M. C, Rajeshkumar, N. V, Garrido-Laguna I, Jesus-Acosta A. D, Jones S, Maitra A, Hruban R. H, Eshleman J. R, Klein A, Laheru D, Donehower R, Hidalgo M. Personalizing Cancer Treatment in the Age of Global Genomic Analysis: PALB2 Gene Mutations and Response to DNA Damaging Agents in Pancreatic Cancer. Molecular Cancer Therapeutics 2011; 10(1): 3-8.

[36] Gambocorti-Passerini C, Antolini L, Mahon F.-X, Guilhot F, Deininger M, Fava C, Nagler A, Casa C. M. D, Morra E, Abruzzese E, D'Emilio A, Stagno F, Coutre P. l, Hurtado-Monroy R, Santini V, Martino B, Pane F, Piccin A, Giraldo P, Assouline S, Durosinmi M. A, Leeksma O, Pogliani E. M, Puttini M, Jang E, Reiffers J, Valsecchi M. G, Kim D.-W. Multicenter Independent Assessment of Outcomes in Chronic Myeloid Leukemia Patients Treated With Imatinib. Journal of the National Cancer Institute 2011; 103(7): 553-561.

[37] Compiled from: http://www.fda.gov/MedicalDevices/ProductsandMedicalProcedures/InVitroDiagnostics/ucm301431.htm (accessed January 23, 2015).

[38] Wang M. L, Rule S, Martin P, Goy A, Auer R, Kahl B. S, Jurczak W, Advani R. H, Romaguera. E, Williams M. E, Barrientos J. C, Chmielowska E, Radford J, Stilgenbauer S, Dreyling M, Jedrzejczak W. W, Johnson P, Spurgeon S. E, Li L, Zhang L, Newberry K, Ou Z, Cheng N, Fang B, McGrivy J, Clow F, Buggy J. J, Chang B. Y, Beaupre D. M, Kunkel L. A, Blum K. A. Targeting BTK with Ibrutinib in Relapsed or Refractory Mantle-Cell Lymphoma. New England Journal of Medicine 2013; 369: 507-516.

[39] Firestein R, Bass A. J, Kim S. Y, Dunn I. F, Silver S. J, Guney I, Freed E, Ligon A. H, Vena N, Ogino S, Chheda M. G, Tamayo P, Finn S, Shrestha Y, Boehm J. S, Jain S, Bojarsky E, Mermel C, Barretina J, Chan J. A, Baselga J, Tabernero J, Root D. E, Fuchs C. S, Loda M, Shivdasani R. A, Meyerson M, Hahn W. C. CDK8 is a colorectal cancer oncogene that regulates β–catenin activity. Nature 2008; 455: 547-551.

[40] Seo J.-O, Han S. I, Lim S.-C. Role of CDK8 and β–catenin in colorectal adenocarcinoma. Oncology Reports 2010; 24: 285-291.

[41] Morris E. J, Ji J. Y, Yang F, Di Stefano L, Herr A, Moon N. S, Kwon E. J, Haigis K. M, Naar A. M, Dyson N. J. E2F1 represses beta-catenin transcription and is antagonized by both pRB and CDK8. Nature 2008; 455, 552-556.

[42] Gurley K. E, Kemp C. J. Synthetic lethality between mutation in Atm and DNA-PK(cs) during murine embryogenesis. Current Biology 2001; 11: 191-194.

[43] Curtin N. J, DNA repair dysregulation from cancer driver to therapeutic target. Nature Reviews Cancer 2012; 12: 801-817.

Chapter 3

Advanced Cancer Treatment – An Original Approach

Oleg Bukhtoyarov and Denis Samarin

Additional information is available at the end of the chapter

http://dx.doi.org/10.5772/60213

1. Introduction

Advanced cancer is a malignant disease that has spread to other places in the body and usually cannot be cured or controlled with treatment. The treatment and care of advanced cancer patients is focused on the management and relief of symptoms, improving the patient's comfort and quality of life. Such patients are given symptomatic treatment. At the same time the status of anti-tumour immunity is a key link in the carcinogenesis chain of advanced cancer. This means that anti-tumour immunity could be considered as a target for pathogenically justified immunotherapy. It is also known that the activity of anti-tumour immunity determines the survival of patients with cancer. It should be mentioned that an active development of immunotherapy had promised drastic changes in the management of cancer, as well as an increase in survival of patients living with cancer. However, that expectation has not yet been fulfilled. Clinical studies show that an initially compromised anti-tumour immunity of patients living with cancer cannot be surely recovered by means of immunotherapy. At the same time the use of immunotherapy in some cancer patients could be dangerous as well as useless due to the possibility of the stimulation of cancer development, for example through the induction of Treg cells [1]. At first sight an idea to administer pathogenically justified immunotherapy to patients with advanced cancer seems in appropriate. However, it could be accepted if applied with immunotherapy for advanced cancer patients based on deterministic positions of cellular/molecular and/or genetic levels.

The systemic view in the whole body approach to treatment suggests mandatory consideration of the state of higher nervous activity (mental state), which provides a serious influence on the development and outcome of cancer disease. For instance, 'depression is worsening the potentially short lives of patients living with cancer' [2]. In this regard we assumed that some patients with advanced cancer suffer from psychogenically determined immunosuppression as an outcome of untreated psychoemotional disorders that have occurred before a diagnosis of cancer. In fact, those patients went through massive psychotraumatic events that accumulated through the massive stress connected with a first diagnosis of cancer. We also assumed that the immunotherapy of advanced cancer patients with a psychogenic medical history should be preceded with an effective correction of psychoemotional disorders in order to avoid a psychogenic immunosuppressive influence. The objective of this work is the development and implementation of a psychoimmunological approach to the treatment of advanced cancer patients with a psychogenic medical history.

1.1. Theoretical justification for a psychoimmunological approach to the treatment of advanced cancer patients with a psychogenic medical history

Today there is no doubt that immune dysfunctions are the backbone of tumour pathogenesis. This immune dysfunction, along with destruction of the cellular genetic apparatus in the malignant cells, occurs in the form of the cell component of the immune system dysfunction along with the malfunction of cell control and cell differentiation mechanisms, immune tolerance, and inability to provide an effective immune response to a developing tumour [3, 4]. In this connection it was logical to use the wide range of immunotherapy methods in modern oncology. Despite being a new step in malignant tumour treatment it has not solved the problem of its effective treatment [5, 6].

At the same time, laboratory and clinical trials have shown linked and multi-functional interconnections between the two most important integrative systems of the human organism, which are the immune and the nervous systems [7-9], which formed the basis of the development of modern scientific trends of the psychoneuroimmunology and psychoimmunology of cancer [10]. The conclusions of the scientific research on the influence of chronic psychoemotional stress (CPES) to an organism of healthy and unhealthy individuals, including those with cancer, are most interesting from the practical point of view. Nowadays the somatic outcomes of CPES are well known: the CPES is able to damage the cell's DNA and inhibit DNA repair through the activation of endogenous mutagens, which are the reactive species of oxygen, nitrogen, etc. This leads to genome instability [11, 12]. CPES is always followed by immunosuppression, a decrease in the quantity and cytotoxic activity of CD8+ and NK-cells, and dysfunction of their supervising functions, processes of apoptosis, activation of proinflammatory cytokines and sustentation of the non-cropped areas of chronic inflammation [13-15]. All of these lead to a concentration of malignant cells in the body with an increase in their invasive potentiality [16]. CPES is linked with a high risk of development, progress and recurrence of malignant tumours, and the high mortality rate of cancer patients [17, 18]. The CPES also leads to hippocampal neuronal degeneration as well as amygdala atrophy [19], prolonged hyperactivity of the hypothalamo-pituitary-adrenocortical axis [20], and accelerated aging of the human body [21]. Therefore, the extensive and deep somatic damaging effect of CPES suggests a significant role of psychogenic factors in the development, recurrence and progression of cancer disease in some cancer patients with a psychogenic medical history. On the basis of the above, it is logical to assume that it is difficult to eliminate the factors compromising the immune system due to psychogenic influence and the suppression of anti-tumour immunity without effective elimination of persistent tonic descending influences of the central nervous system and the higher nervous activity to the body of cancer patients with a psychogenic medical history. The confirmation of the dependency of anti-tumour immune activity to higher nervous activity is presented by therecently discovered phenomenon of the spontaneous increase in anti-tumour activity of the immune system after the effective relief of psychoemotional disorders in cancer patients with a psychogenic medical history [22].

Thereby, advanced cancer patients with a psychogenic medical history require a special pathogenesis-based psychoimmunological cancer treatment in order to restore their mental condition, increase their quality of life, activate an anti-tumour immunity and to block the progression of cancer. The main content of psychoimmunological cancer treatment consists of compliance with a strict sequence of two stages of cancer treatment: psycho-correction and immunoactivation. The main objective of the first stage of cancer treatment (psycho-correction) is an effective and sustainable elimination of CPES effects that appear in different psychoemotional disorders such as anxiety, depression, etc. The main objective of the second stage of cancer treatment (stage of immunoactivation) is the activation of specific anti-tumour immunity.

2. Material and methods

This study had local ethical committee approval (the Ethical committee of the Institute of Clinical Immunology, Siberian Branch, Russian Academy of Medical Sciences, Novosibirsk, Russian Federation, protocol № 29, August 18, 2004). All patients gave written informed consent.

2.1. Characteristics of advanced cancer patients

The special psychoimmunological cancer treatment was offered to 17 patients with advanced cancer (13 women and four men). These patients, over seven years (2005-2012),were selected by us from the cancer patients using the following criteria: 1) the progression of the disease, despite the ongoing standard combination therapy of cancer provided, 2) the presence of distant metastases (stage IV of cancer), 3) the obvious massive psychotrauma that occurred in the lives of patients before being diagnosed with cancer (psychogenic medical history), and 4) informed consent of cancer patients for carrying out cancer treatment. A special clinical case was associated with patient № 9 (Table 1), who strictly refused to take a standard combination therapy for cancer, but expressed the strong desire to receive psychological and psychotherapeutic aid. Individual characteristics of cancer patients are presented in Table 1.

Patient №	Age	Sex	Cancer types	Primary tumour localization	Metastasis localization	Stage	Comorbidities	Treatment
1	42	F	Melanoma	Right shoulder	Brain	IV	-	SUR, CHT
2	29	F	Melanoma	Anterior chest wall	Liver	IV	-	SUR, CHT HYP
3	47	F	Melanoma	Anterior abdominal wall	Brain	IV	Urinary stone disease	SUR, CHT

Patient №	Age	Sex	Cancer types	Primary tumour localization	Metastasis localization	Stage	Comorbidities	Treatment
4	43	M	Melanoma	Uveal	Liver	IV	-	SUR, CHT
5	46	F	Melanoma	Back skin	Porta hepatis	IV	Hypertensive heart disease	SUR, CHT
6	51	M	Melanoma	Anterior abdominal wall	Subcutaneous hands & feet	IV	Chronic cholecystitis	SUR, CHT
7	38	F	Melanoma	Skin of temporal region	Retroperito-neum	IV	-	SUR, CHT
8	53	M	Melanoma	Back skin	Subcutaneous hands & feet	IV	Stomach ulcer	SUR, CHT
9	55	F	Melanoma	Neck skin	Supraclavicular & axillary lymph nodes	IV	-	Refuse standard treatment
10	76	F	Kidney cancer	Right kidney	Both lungs, mediastinal & neck lymph nodes, ribs	IV	Hypertensive heart disease, coronary artery disease	SUR, CHT
11	58	F	Kidney cancer	Right kidney	Left kidney	IV	Hypertensive heart disease	SUR, CHT
12	53	F	Stomach cancer	Stomach	Porta hepatis	IV	-	SUR, CHT
13	28	M	Stomach& pancreas cancer	Stomach& pancreas	Paraaortic lymph nodes	IV	-	SUR, CHT
14	50	F	Breast cancer	Left breast	Skull, ribs, sternum, clavicles, spine, pelvis	IV	-	SUR, CHT, RT
15	54	F	Breast cancer	Right breast	Ribs, shoulder joint	IV	Hypertensive heart disease	SUR, CHT
16	45	F	Ovarian cancer	Right ovarian	Mediastinal lymph nodes	IV	-	SUR, CHT
17	48	F	Lung cancer	Right lung	Left lung	IV	-	SUR, CHT

SUR – surgery; CHT – chemotherapy; RT – radiotherapy; HYP – hyperthermia

Table 1. Characteristics of advanced cancer patients (n=17)

2.2. Psychogenic medical history investigation

Psychogenic medical histories were taken for each patient in the clinical trial (anamnesis morbi) during the first visit, and these histories included the presence of massive psychotraumatic events (death of close person, divorce, etc.) with the development of helplessness and despair.

2.3. The mental status examination of advanced cancer patients

The mental status examination of cancer patients was conducted by the psychiatrist with supplemental usage of the following psychometric test systems (e.g., Symptom Checklist 90 (SCL-90) and rates: Somatization, Obsessive-Compulsive, Interpersonal Sensitivity, Depression, Anxiety, Hostility, Phobic Anxiety, Paranoid Ideation, Psychoticism, Global Severity Index. The psychiatrist detected the presence or absence of mental disorders in cancer patients in accordance with International Classification of Diseases (ICD-10). Normal values of SCL-90 parameters for healthy people are presented in Table 2 [23]. The mental status examination was administered in the following stages of research: 'before' – before psycho-correction; 'after' – after hypnotherapy session; and 'one month later' –hypnotherapy sessions one month later.

2.4. The pharmacotherapy of psychoemotional disorders

The pharmacotherapy of mental disorders in advanced cancer patients was conducted immediately after diagnosis. Antidepressants (tianeptine, venlafaxin), anxiolytics (afobazolum, microdoses of diazepam) and their combination were used. The psychotropic drugs were prescribed for a period of three to six months to enhance and prolong the therapeutic effect of hypnosuggestive psychotherapy (HSP).

2.5. Method of hypnosuggestive psychotherapy

The method of hypnosuggestive psychotherapy is based on strict successive, interconnected, figurative, pathogenically substantiated suggestive influences in hypnotic states. This method has previously been described in detail [24]. It includes: 1) Establishment of hypno-rapport between patient and physician; 2) Hypnotic de-actualization of psychotraumatic emotions and experience including the fact of cancer diagnosis; 3) Hypnotic lockout of dreams connected with known stress situations which are regularly reproduced in sleep with the corresponding psycho-vegetative reactions – this is needed for the subject's exhaustion of psychogenic disorders and to prevent their lingering course; 4) Hypnotic reproduction of a personal 'health standard' or 'health syndrome' – a key session of the whole course of HSP. This 'syndrome' is based on using the known phenomenon of hypnotic hypermnesia (increased memory under hypnosis), generally used for the restoration of psychogenic abnormalities of memory. However, it is possible to restore the memory of the heartbeat, respiratory rate, glycaemic rate, enzyme reaction activity, stereotype of digestive system functions, etc. from a specific time in the past. The patient recollects the concrete day (date, month, year) from the past – the 'model standard' of his health when there was no tumour and he felt well, mentally and physically. In a hypnotic state suggestions were conducted using the images required to retrieve the 'records' that are well known to the body as 'health standard' from the memory of cancer patients. It should be noted that in this key session HSP hypnotic suggestions related to the activation of a great desire and the need for further self-realization in their lives were conducted. In fact, these suggestions were aimed at restoring of life purpose dominant loss [25]; 5-6). The last HSP sessions focused on patients' education in self-hypnosis (autohypnosis) under suggestive influence. The patients were then given detailed instructions to use self-hypnosis for the prolongation of the medicinal effect, as well as keeping the psychic and vital tone of cancer patients. The duration of the individual course of the HSP was 14-16 days.

2.6. Anti-cancer diagnostic skin test for evaluation of specific anti-tumour activity of the immune system (non-stimulated native activity) in advanced cancer patients

The anti-tumour activity of the immune system was assessed by a skin test of the delayed type hypersensitivity (DTH) reaction on tumour-associated antigens (TAA), which were used as a lysed human melanoma cell line BRO [26] of 25,000 cells in a test (see Figure 1). Human melanoma cell line BRO was obtained at the Institute of Cytology of the Russian Academy of the Sciences (St. Petersburg, Russia). We investigated the DTH skin reaction after the intradermal administration on the forearm at 9, 12 and 24 hours, to identify the peak responses. The peak response in most cases (the diameter of redness in mm) was observed after 12 hours. Selection of the human melanoma cell line BRO was determined by the need to use in one test the maximum range of TAA, in order to assess the anti-tumour activity of the immune systems of patients with different cancers. As shown above, there exist all kinds of TAA characteristics of solid tumours on the melanoma cells [27].

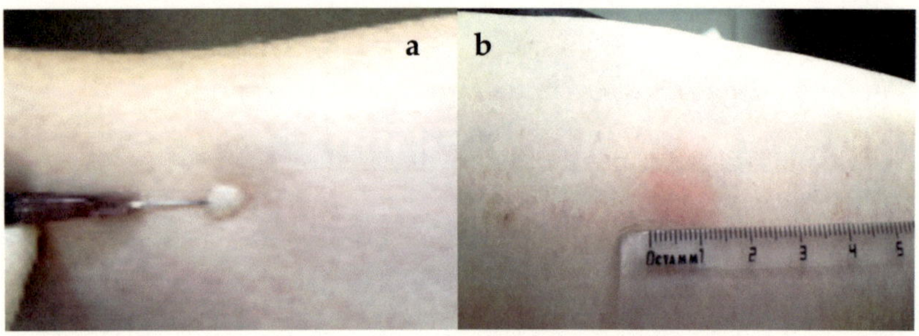

Figure 1. Anti-cancer diagnostic skin test: evaluation of specific anti-tumour activity of the immune system in advanced cancer patients (Patient № 11 after psycho-correction). (a) Intradermal introduction of tumour-associated antigens: lysed cells of human melanoma line BRO 25×10^3 per doze (50 μL); (b) Evaluation of DTH skin reaction on TAA (12 hours later): 0-5 mm – low activity, 5-10 mm – average activity, >10 mm – high activity.

The selection of the minimal quantity of TAA for the anti-cancer diagnostic DTH skin test (according to our preliminary studies) was used in order to obtain a physiological specific anti-tumour immunological response (non-stimulated native DTH skin reaction on TAA) as well as to exclude the possibility of the vaccine's effect on the diagnostic test itself. In comparison with our colleagues, who used the DTH skin reaction on the TAA of human melanoma cell lines in a study of the clinical efficacy of the anti-tumour polyvalent vaccine 'CancerVax' (USA) (developed from three allogeneic human melanoma cell lines) [28], we used a diagnostic dose that was nearly 100 times smaller (2.5×10^4 cells vs. 2.4×10^6 cells). In addition, our patients did not receive any immunotropic therapy during the study. The selected dose does not cause allergic and other pathological reactions. It is known that the delayed-type hypersensitivity reaction is a specific immune response and begins to manifest in eight to 12 hours after ingestion of antigen, and in most cases the reaction reaches a peak after 48-72 hours [29].

In our case the peak responses, due to the absence of prior immunization of cancer patients and the largest contribution of cellular reactions in the DTH skin test, were achieved early (within 12 hours) [30]. An evaluation of a specific anti-tumour activity of the immune system in advanced cancer patients was conducted through the research phases: 'before' – before psycho-correction, 'after' – after completing a course of hypnotherapy and 'one month later' – after one month following the completion of the course of hypnotherapy.

2.7. Preparation of tumour-associated antigens for diagnostic test - DTH skin reaction

The lysed cells of the human melanoma cell line BRO were used as the TAA for diagnostic test. The human melanoma cell line BRO were maintained in RPMI 1640 supplemented with 10% heat-inactivated foetal calf serum, L-glutamine (2 mmol/ml), 25 mmol HEPES buffer, and 25 μg/ml gentamicin at 37°C in 5% CO_2 humidified air. Cells were detached from the dish by treating with trypsin-EDTA followed by washing three times with Dulbecco's phosphate-buffered saline, precipitated by centrifuging, counted, and diluted with 0.9% saline solution with 0.1% EDTA. Cells were lysed by repeated (eight times) freezing and stored at -80ºC until use. As a diagnostic test 2.5×10^4 lysed cells line BRO in 50 microliters were used.

2.8. Preparation of tumour-associated antigens for epicutaneous activation of specific anti-tumour immunity

The lysed cells of the human melanoma cell line BRO were used as the TAA for epicutaneous activation of specific anti-tumour immunity. The human melanoma cell line BRO was maintained in RPMI 1640 supplemented with 10% heat-inactivated foetal calf serum, L-glutamine (2 mmol/ml), 25 mmol HEPES buffer, and 25 μg/ml gentamicin at 37°C in 5% CO_2 humidified air. Cells were detached from the dish by treating with trypsin-EDTA followed by washing three times with Dulbecco's phosphate-buffered saline, precipitated by centrifuging, counted and diluted with 0.9% saline solution with 0.1% EDTA. Cells were lysed by repeated freezing (eight times) and stored at -80ºC until use. The one epicutaneous activation of specific anti-tumour immunity was performed with the use of a 2.5×10^6 lysed cells line BRO in 0.5 ml.

2.9. Preparation of tumour-associated antigens for extracorporeal activation of specific anti-tumour immunity

Lysed placental domestic pig cells were used as the TAA for extracorporeal activation of specific anti-tumour immunity. They were obtained by careful mechanical homogenization of placenta without trypsin. Cells were diluted in saline solution supplemented with 0.1% EDTA and 25 μg/ml gentamicin up to a concentration of 50×10^6 placental cells in 1.0 ml. Cells were lysed by repeated freezing (eight times) and stored at -80ºC until use.

2.10. Extracorporeal activation of specific anti-tumour immunity

A peripheral blood mononuclear cell(PBMC), separated from 25 ml of heparinized cancer patient blood was diluted in RPMI 1640 and supplemented with 20% autological plasma, L-glutamine (2 mmol/ml), 25 mmol HEPES buffer, and 25 μg/ml gentamicin. PBMC in concentration 4 × 10^6 cells/ml was placed in a cell culture dish in the proportion 1-2 × 10^6 cells/sm^2. The lysed domestic pig placental cells were used as the antigen at a proportion of 1/6 (lysed cells of pig placenta/PBMC). This proportion was found to be optimal in previous research. Further PBMC with added antigen was placed into a CO_2 incubator and incubated at 37°C in 5% CO_2 humidified air. The incubation time was six to eight hours for antigen processing by monocytes of PBMC. The PBMC was collected after completion of incubation by rubber policeman and was triplewashed in the phosphate buffer solution with the addition of 5% autological plasma of the cancer patient. The washed incubated PBMC was diluted in 2 ml of autological plasma from the cancer patient and shared between two 1 ml syringes. Incubated PBMC was administered subcutaneously in the subscapular fossa area and in the area of the lower abdomen laterally from the umbilicus (palm width sinistral or dextral). A total of three procedures were provided, the second after two weeks and the third after one month from the first procedure.

2.11. Epicutaneous (scarification) activation of specific anti-tumour immunity

The superficial line scarifications were applied after skin disinfection on the area of 4 cm^2 with a gap in between lines of 2-3 mm wide by blood lancet (scarificator) (see Figure 2). The damaged area was covered by sterile patch underneath which a solution with TAA (2.5 × 10^6 lysed cells line BRO in 0.5 ml) was administered by syringe. The subclavicular and subscapular areas were used for the epicutaneous application of TAA. The exposition of patch was left for three days. Four sessions of epicutaneous activation of specific anti-tumour immunity were administered with a 14-day break and three sessions were provided with a 30-day break.

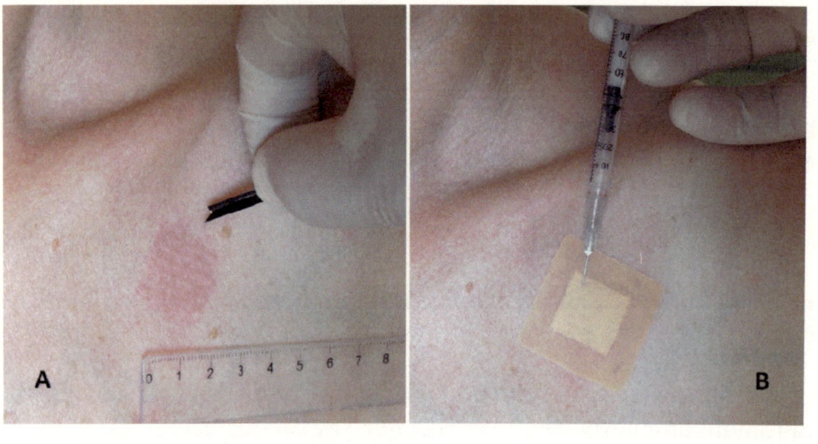

Figure 2. Epicutaneous (scarification) activation of specific anti-tumour immunity. (A) The superficial line scarifications plotted after skin disinfection by blood lancet (scarificator); (B) Patch (with viscose bandage) is superimposed on the network of surface scarification and impregnation of bandage patch by solution of tumour-associated antigens.

2.12. Statistical analysis

The statistical data processing was performed using 'BioStat 2009 Professional 5.8.4', which is publicly available. The level of statistical significance (so-called alpha level for a p-value) was accepted as 0.05. All parameters of investigation were normally distributed (by Kolmogorov-Smirnov test), so in general the parametric tests were used. In order to compare two independent statistical samples, the non-parametric Mann-Whitney test was used. The relationship study between psychometric (SCL-90) and immunological (DTH skin reaction on TAA) parameters was carried out using Pearson's correlation test.

3. Results

3.1. Mental disorders in advanced cancer patients with psychogenic medical history

Clinical studies of 17 advanced cancer patients with a psychogenic medical history showed that 100% had a variety of psychoemotional comorbidity disorders, predominantly anxiety and depression spectrum disorders. The disorders distribution was based on the International Classification of Diseases (ICD-10): generalized anxiety disorder (F41.1) – 3 (patients № 1, 13, 17), mixed anxiety and depressive disorder (F41.2) – 2 (patients № 4, 6), post-traumatic stress disorder (F43.1) – 1 (patient № 7), prolonged depressive reaction (F43.21) – 4 (patients № 3, 8, 12, 16), mixed anxiety and depressive reaction (F43.22) – 6 (patients № 2, 5, 9, 10, 11,14) and organic anxiety disorder (F06.4) – 1 (patient № 15), which in our opinion was a complication chemotherapy. The results of clinical studies of the mental state of advanced cancer patients in general have been confirmed by the data of psychometry (Table 2, the indicators 'before').

3.2. Psycho-correction stage is the first stage of psychoimmunological advanced cancer treatment

The clinical benefits after completion of HSP have been noted in all advanced cancer patients. This was confirmed by the results of psychometry and comparative analysis, which showed significant improvement in almost all of the parameters studied (Table 2). Along with a significant improvement in the mental state of cancer patients a spontaneous increase in the specific anti-tumour activity of the immune system was observed, as determined by DTH skin reaction on TAA ($p<0.0008$). The sustainability of mental and immunological changes was the main criterion in the decision to move to the next stage of psychoimmunological cancer treatment which is the stage of immunoactivation. In this regard, the studied parameters at the 'one month later' stage after completion of the HSP indicated the stability or instability of earlier positive changes. However, in a comparative analysis of indices in the overall group of cancer patients at stages 'after' and 'one month later' this deterioration was not evident (Table 2).

However, a careful study of the indicators at the stage 'one month later' detected a clear split of cancer patients into two groups by the intensity of DTH skin reaction on TAA (Table 3). The

Indicators	Normative values†	Comparative analysis 'before-after' and 'after-one month later'				
		Before (B) Mean ± s.e.m.	After (A) Mean ± s.e.m.	1 month later Mean ± s.e.m.	P B-A	P A-1 mon.
Somatization	0.44 ± 0.03	1.31 ± 0.16	0.67 ± 0.12	0.79 ± 0.15	0.0001	*
Obsessive-compulsive	0.75 ± 0.04	1.14 ± 0.12	0.62 ± 0.10	0.76 ± 0.11	0.002	*
Interpersonal sensitivity	0.66 ± 0.03	1.12 ± 0.20	0.53 ± 0.10	0.63 ± 0.11	0.006	*
Depression	0.62 ± 0.04	1.45 ± 0.16	0.54 ± 0.09	0.84 ± 0.12	0.0002	0.004
Anxiety	0.47 ± 0.03	1.10 ± 0.15	0.35 ± 0.09	0.49 ± 0.09	0.0002	*
Hostility	0.60 ± 0.04	0.74 ± 0.12	0.32 ± 0.07	0.43 ± 0.08	0.007	*
Phobic anxiety	0.18 ± 0.02	0.55 ± 0.14	0.23 ± 0.08	0.23 ± 0.07	0.045	*
Paranoid ideation	0.54 ± 0.04	0.73 ± 0.16	0.43 ± 0.12	0.50 ± 0.14	*	*
Psychoticism	0.30 ± 0.03	0.67 ± 0.11	0.31 ± 0.07	0.41 ± 0.08	0.0006	*
Global Severity Index	0.51 ± 0.02	1.06 ± 0.12	0.48 ± 0.07	0.61 ± 0.10	0.0002	*
DTH skin reaction on TAA, mm	not defined	4.59 ±1.52	11.4 ±2.45	7.35 ±2.06	0.0008	0.003

Mean ± s.e.m. – means and standard errors means; *P>0.05; † - Normative values for healthy people (Tarabrina N.V., 2001)

Table 2. Psychometric indicators (SCL-90) and DTH skin reaction on TAA in advanced cancer patients before, after, and one month later after completion of HSP sessions (n=17)

DTH skin reaction was less than 5 mm in one group of patients, and was greater than 5 mm in the other group. It was found that cancer patients in these groups differed substantially in almost all psychometric parameters. The group of patients with a DTH skin reaction of less than 5 mm (11 of 17 patients) was characterized by the deterioration of psychometric indicators, which allowed us to identify this group of patients as a group with an unstable effect of correction of psychoemotional disorders (patient № 1, 3, 4, 5, 6, 7, 8, 12, 13, 15, 17).

Clinically, these patients had worsening of general and mental health, in spite of the use of antidepressants, anxiolytics, and the conduction of self-hypnosis sessions. Another group of patients whose DTH skin reaction was more than 5 mm (six patients) differed by maintenance of the previously achieved positive effects of psycho-correction with appropriate psychometric characteristics. The last group was identified by us as a group of patients with a stable effect of psycho-correction (patients number 2, 9, 10, 11, 14, 16). The close relationship of specific anti-tumour activity of the immune system with the higher nervous activity of cancer patients was confirmed by the correlation analysis between the DTH skin reaction on TAA and psychometric parameters of SCL-90 at all stages of observation (Table 4).

Indicators	Normative values†	Unstable effect (n=11) Mean ± s.e.m.	Stable effect (n=6) Mean ± s.e.m.	P
Somatization	0.44 ± 0.03	1.05 ± 0.18	0.32 ± 0.13	0.014
Obsessive-compulsive	0.75 ± 0.04	0.95 ± 0.13	0.42 ± 0.15	0.024
Interpersonal sensitivity	0.66 ± 0.03	0.86 ± 0.11	0.20 ± 0.08	0.005
Depression	0.62 ± 0.04	1.10 ± 0.12	0.35 ± 0.11	0.003
Anxiety	0.47 ± 0.03	0.68 ± 0.10	0.13 ± 0.07	0.003
Hostility	0.60 ± 0.04	0.50 ± 0.09	0.31 ± 0.15	*
Phobic anxiety	0.18 ± 0.02	0.33 ± 0.10	0.05 ± 0.03	*
Paranoid ideation	0.54 ± 0.04	0.71 ± 0.18	0.11 ± 0.04	0.009
Psychoticism	0.30 ± 0.03	0.57 ± 0.10	0.12 ± 0.07	0.007
Global Severity Index	0.51 ± 0.02	0.82 ± 0.11	0.23 ± 0.07	0.004
DTH skin reaction on TAA, mm	not defined	1.91 ±0.53	17.3 ±2.55	0.0009

Mean ± s.e.m. – means and standard errors means; *P>0.05; † - Normative values for healthy people (Tarabrina N.V., 2001)

Table 3. A comparative analysis of the studied parameters in cancer patients with unstable and stable effects of correction of psychoemotional disorders

Indicators	DTH skin reaction on TAA, mm					
	Before		After		One month later	
	r	P	r	P	r	P
Somatization	0.13	*	-0.40	*	-0.64	0.006
Obsessive-compulsive	-0.27	*	-0.35	*	-0.73	0.0008
Interpersonal sensitivity	-0.09	*	-0.58	0.014	-0.82	0.0001
Depression	-0.09	*	-0.44	*	-0.78	0.0002
Anxiety	-0.10	*	-0.51	0.037	-0.74	0.0006
Hostility	-0.06	*	-0.29	*	-0.51	0.039
Phobic anxiety	-0.16	*	-0.28	*	-0.57	0.017
Paranoid ideation	-0.31	*	-0.37	*	-0.59	0.013
Psychoticism	-0.22	*	-0.53	0.030	-0.66	0.004
Global Severity Index	-0.14	*	-0.60	0.012	-0.76	0.0003

* P>0.05

Table 4. The correlation analysis between the DTH skin reaction and psychometric indicators of SCL-90 in advanced cancer patients with a psychogenic medical history on stages of observation (n=17)

The dynamics of the relationship showed that the medical and psychotherapeutic effect on the higher nervous activity of the cancer patients was accompanied by a cumulative increase in the significant negative correlations between the specific anti-tumour activity of the immune system and the mental wellbeing of cancer patients. The greatest number of correlations was observed month after the completion of HSP. Cancer patients with a sustained effect of psycho-correction (patient № 2, 10, 11, 14, 16) were proposed for a second stage of psychoimmunological cancer treatment (stage of immunoactivation), except for patient № 9.

3.3. Stage of immunoactivation: the second stage of psychoimmunological advanced cancer treatment

The stage of immunoactivation lasted for five months and, along with the procedures of activation of specific anti-tumour immunity, advanced cancer patients took psychotropic medications and performed self-hypnosis sessions. Each procedure of epicutaneous activation of specific anti-tumour immunity was accompanied by local reactions such as redness, pain, and local itching at the injection site. All cancer patients observed pain in the area of metastatic tumour formation (including previously undiagnosed) as well as pain in the regional lymph nodes on the third day, sometimes an increased body temperature up to 37ºC, and deterioration of health in the form of weakness, lethargy, and sleepiness. In order to relieve these reactions, patients received Nise (nimesulide) tablets 100 mg, twice per day for five to seven days. Procedures of extracorporeal activation of specific anti-tumour immunity were also accompanied by systemic reactions, but were clinically less severe than with procedures of epicutaneous activation. In addition, local reactions were observed such as redness, pain and itching at the site of local administration.

3.4. Catamnesis

The advanced cancer patients experiencing unstable clinical effects of the correction of the psychoemotional disorders (patient № 1, 3, 4, 5, 6, 7, 8, 12, 13, 15, 17) died within two to five months of the psycho-correction stage being over, except patient № 5 who died after one year. These advanced cancer patients are likely to have had more pronounced somatopsychic disorders that were not consistently removed with psycho-correction techniques and failed to influence anti-tumour immunity. Among the advanced cancer patients that were subjected to psychoimmunological cancer treatment (patient № 2, 10, 11, 14, 16) the following results were observed.

Patient № 2 is alive (five years catamnesis). The signs of haemangioma were revealed in the place of former liver metastasis (Ultrasound data) in one year following the psychoimmunological cancer treatment.

Patient № 10 is alive, and catamnesis was two years without substantial negative dynamics. Multiple foci of fibrosis and calcification were discovered by computed tomography.

Patient № 11 is alive, and catamnesis was 6.8 years after psychoimmunological cancer treatment had finished. A very interesting fact was revealed during the research. After massive stress (she found out about her daughter's drug addiction), a quick development of the cancer

http://dx.doi.org/10.5772/60213

disease was observed and within seven days the size of the metastasis in the only kidney increased from 38 × 23 mm to 41 × 32 mm. After the effective relief of psychoemotional disorders, metastasis regression to 12 × 11 mm was observed.

Patient № 14 is alive, and catamnesis was 1.1 years. Multiple foci of osteosclerosis without negative dynamics were observed (on computed tomography).

Patient № 16 is alive, catamnesis was four years. Negative dynamics were not observed, pneumosclerosis foci and extensive fibrotic process were observed in the mediastinum (on computed tomography).

3.4.1. Clinical case (patient № 9)

We have observed the unique clinical case of the cancer patient with malignant melanoma, who refused to receive mutilating surgery and chemotherapy but approached us for psychological help.

Patient № 9, 55 years old, an accountant. In autumn 2004, melanoma localized on the neck on the left side was histologically verified. The patient turned to us on 20 January 2005. It was examined that the patient had a primary focus (40 x 35 mm) and multiple metastases in the neck (20 mm), supraclavicular (35 mm) and axillary (20 mm) lymph nodes on the left (see Figure 3).

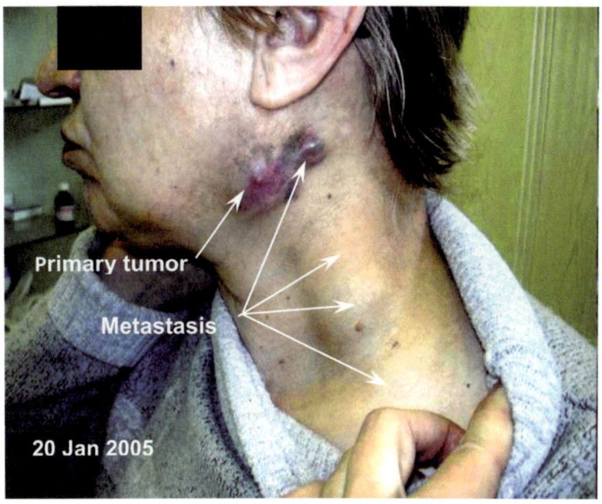

Figure 3. Localization of malignant neck melanoma, patient № 9.

Ultrasound examination of the primary tumour revealed the depth of tumour invasion in the tissues of the neck to be 25 mm.

After examination the patient was diagnosed with a psychogenic medical history (she lives with a disabled husband, who is an alcoholic), mixed anxiety and depressive reaction (F43.22) and the lack of inhibition of specific anti-tumour activity of the immune system, defined by the absence of DTH skin reaction on TAA. We observed that patients with a similar localization of melanoma die within four to six months due to profuse bleeding from the tumour foci and frequent metastasis to the brain. From 21 January to 4 February 2005 the patient underwent a course of hypnotherapy consisting of four treatment sessions and two sessions of self-hypnosis training. After treating the patient with HSP (5 February 2005), along with an improvement in general state of health and relief of anxiety and depressive disorders, positive changes were seen in a number of objective indicators.

Thus, DTH skin reaction on TAA increased from 15 mm (before HSP) to 40 mm (after HSP) and maintained for two days, the absolute number of peripheral blood lymphocytes increased three times: from 709 to 1 mm^3 (before HSP) to 2244 in 1 mm^3 (after HSP).In addition there was a change of the vegetative (autonomic) nervous system, which was assessed by heart rate variability (HRV) [31]. HRV is the assessment of individual differences in emotional reactions, particularly in relation to social processes and mental health [32]. The total energy spectrum analysis (TP of HRV) increased 20-fold: from 213 ms^2 (before HSP) to 4260 ms^2 (after HSP). In addition there was a reduction in the ratio of LF/HF (normalized units) five-fold: from 2.76 (before HSP) to 0.53 (after HSP), indicating a change of state of sympathicotonia to the state of parasympathicotonia and this is a confirmation of the clinical fact of depression relief [33]. After the completion of HSP the patient conducted daily self-hypnosis sessions in accordance with our proposed programme, the content of which was aimed at forming a dense impermeable capsule around the tumour foci, which like a 'plaster cocoon walls up, squeezes and strangles tumour foci'. After several self-hypnosis daily sessions lasting one hour each of the pronounced swellings of the left side of the neck and supraclavicular area with transition to the chest were observed (see Figure 4); body temperature rose up to 38ºC; and itching of the tumour foci appeared.

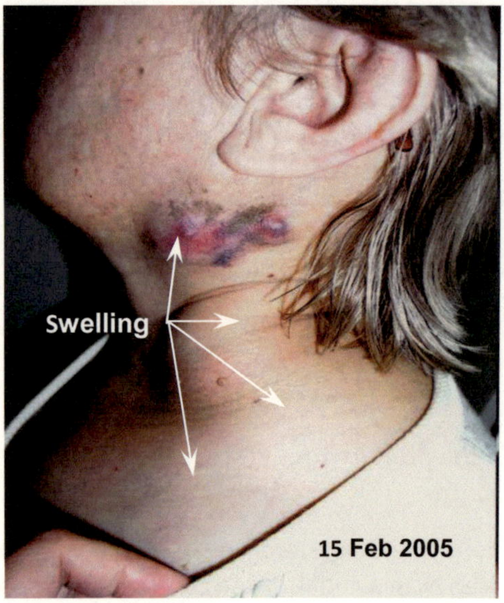

Figure 4. Pronounced swelling of the neck tissues after organic-oriented self-hypnosis sessions

The patient reported that 'stifling of the tumour' started. Within eight days the swelling completely disappeared, along with a decrease in the size of metastatic lymph nodes in the neck, supraclavicular and axillary regions. The patient continued, nearly on a daily basis, to use self-hypnosis according to an organic-oriented suggestive programme 'stifling of tumour foci'. Nine months after the beginning of organic-oriented therapeutic autosuggestion (03 November 2005), the patient underwent ultrasound examination of the tumour foci.

The results showed regression of metastatic lymph nodes in the neck, in the supraclavicular and axillary regions. A fibrous capsule (see Figure 5) formed deep in the tissues of the neck throughout the borders of the tumour invasion of the primary tumour focus, which actually corresponds to the content of curative autosuggestion.

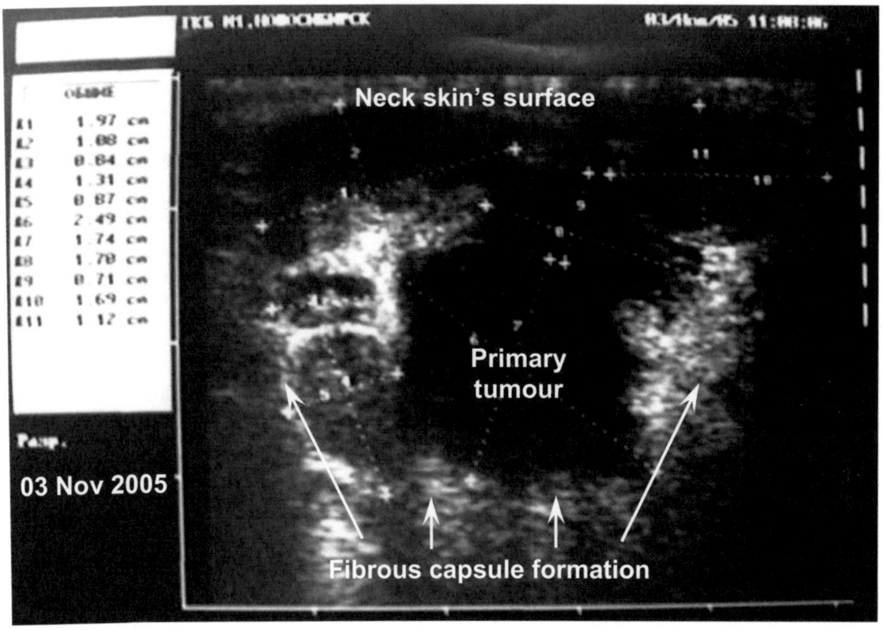

Figure 5. Fibrous capsule around the primary tumour in the depth of the neck tissues after self-hypnosis sessions (ultrasound data).

Further observation showed that endophytic growth of the primary tumour focus changed to exophytic growth (tumour acquired an exophytic form on the leg with a base of 23 mm) with the regression of metastatic lymph nodes in the neck, in supraclavicular and axillary regions (see Figure 6).

Hereinafter, a slow progression of the cancer process with a gradual increase of phenomena cachexia was observed. The patient died on 14 April 2008. Despite the expected death, it can be stated that the cancer patient had been able to live an active life for three years without surgeryon the neck melanoma.

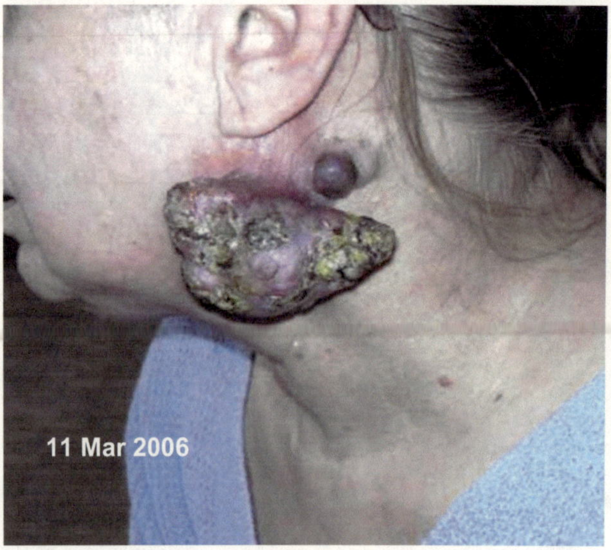

Figure 6. Exophytic growth of melanoma with metastasis regression in the lymph nodes of the neck and supraclavicular area against self-hypnosis treatment sessions

4. Features of our approach

4.1. The peculiar properties of mental disorders in advanced cancer patients with a psychogenic medical history

The study of psychogenic medical history showed that all patients were in a state of obvious emotional stress before cancer diagnosis (on average for one and a half years), which was caused by psychotraumatic events such as death of a close person, divorce, frequent family conflicts, change of residence, work and the presence of a disabled person in family. This long-term emotional tension was accompanied by the formation of the feeling of helplessness, hopelessness, and despair. We can assert that these future cancer patients, long before the diagnosis of cancer, already had psychogenically caused psychoemotional and psychosomatic disorders. The diagnosis of cancer itself is an additional massive and inexhaustible psychotrauma, causing emotionally paralyzing fear, or so-called 'Damocles syndrome' [34].

Cancer patients with a psychogenic medical history are those with a double massive psychotrauma. Advanced cancer patients with a psychogenic medical history undoubtedly form somatopsychic disorders along with cancer progression, so these patients were observed with a combination of psychosomatic and somatopsychic disorders that were clinically difficult to differentiate. The main feature of psychiatric disorders that we have found in cancer patients with a psychogenic medical history is that, despite the urgency of the massive psychotrauma and other conditions for the development of neuroses (known as neurotic 'Jaspers' triad'), cancer patients show a condition that is opposite to neurosis and can be defined as a state of 'deneurotization'. This phenomenon is clinically manifested by blurry, non-deployed with denial to accept, so cancer patients themselves do not consider their mental condition to be sick but quite natural and situationally understandable, though very painful subjectively. This deneurotization syndrome is hard to define according to DSM-IV or ICD-10. In addition, some advanced cancer patients are observed with conditions of dissociative disorders that manifest themselves through an inconsistency of psychometric assessments to clinical studies. In other words, psychoemotional disorders in a clinical study are obvious, but psychometric parameters are within the normal limits, and vice versa. Deneurotization and dissociative disorders can insidiously hide the true extent of the level of psychopathology in advanced cancer patients and may be the cause of undiagnosed mental disorders. Thus, the study of psychiatric morbidity through a self-reported screening instrument without clinical examination does not provide a fair view of psychopathology in cancer patients.

4.2. HSP as a method of choice for the quick correction of mental disorders in advanced cancer patients

For the fastest and most effective correction of psychoemotional disorders in advanced cancer patients, a combination approach was selected that involves the simultaneous use of psychotropic drugs and hypnotherapy. This approach was driven by the severity of the psychopathology of advanced cancer patients and the possibility of rapid progression of the cancer disease. It should be noted that hypnotherapy differs from other methods of psychotherapy by its high efficiency and velocity of clinical benefit achievement, including in oncology [35]. Thus, comparative analysis has shown that after 600 sessions of psychoanalysis 38% of patients reported feeling better, after 22 sessions of behavioural therapy 72% of patients reported a positive result, and after six sessions of hypnotherapy 93% of patients referred to the desired effect [36].

Our 26 years of clinical experience confirm the major clinical capabilities of hypnosuggestive psychotherapy in the correction of mental and psychosomatic disorders. In particular, we first discovered the phenomenon of psychogenic mobilization of CD34+CD38- stem cells [37] and an increase in telomere length in peripheral blood mononuclear cells in cancer patients during hypnotherapy [38]. Later, this phenomenon was to some extent confirmed by other researchers using psychosocial telephone counselling intervention [39]. It should be noted that because of the state of hyper-suggestiveness of advanced cancer patients there is a risk of the formation of hypnotic dependence (hypnomania), so the number of HSP sessions was limited to six sessions of hypnotherapy.

4.3. DTH skin reaction on TAA as a biomarker of removing mental disorders in cancer patients

It can be assumed that the spontaneous increase in the specific anti-tumour activity of the immune system, as determined by DTH skin reaction on TAA, reflects a relief of the psychogenic immunosuppressive effects of higher nervous activity on the anti-tumour activity of the immune systems of advanced cancer patients. In fact, the DTH skin reaction appeared to be a kind of biological marker of the presence or absence of psychoemotional disorders in advanced cancer patients with a psychogenic medical history. It can be assumed that the initial absence of correlation between the DTH skin reaction and psychometric parameters was likely caused by the disintegration processes in the organism of advanced cancer patients inter alia by the violation of the interaction of the two main integrative systems of the body, which are the nervous and immune systems. The systemic impact (medication and psychotherapy) on higher nervous activity in cancer patients is accompanied by the gradual recovery of damaged linkages between the nervous and immune systems of the body. These data indicate a significant effect of higher nervous action on the anti-tumour activity of the immune system of advanced cancer patients with a psychogenic medical history.

4.4. Features of immunoactivation

The main task of the immunoactivation stage was to stimulate the specific anti-tumour immunity of advanced cancer patients by immunological methods after a spontaneous increase of their immune system's anti-tumour activity resulting from the sustained relief from psychoemotional disorders. Presumably, the effective activation of the specific anti-tumour immunity had to have a positive impact on the course of the cancer disease. We have therefore developed a method of epicutaneous (scarification) activation of specific anti-tumour immunity and an extracorporeal activation method using a small amount of peripheral blood. Both methods in preliminary studies have shown high effectiveness and safety in clinical practice (unpublished data). It should be noted in particular that the very low dose of TAA administered per epicutaneous led to systemic reactions in the whole body. It can be assumed that such a clinical effect was due to the specific systemic immune responses associated with the capture of TAA by antigen-presenting epidermal Langerhans cells and the migration of these cells to regional lymph nodes and antigen-presenting TAA. The latest data indicate a greater potential of CD8+ cell activation by Langerhans cells [40]. The antigen-presenting TAA in the lymph nodes leads to activation and clonal expansion of antigen-specific T cells and the subsequent development of specific inflammation in metastatic tumour foci. We observed the systemic clinical manifestations of these processes on the third day.

4.5. Mind and tumour encapsulation

Scientific and clinical evidence shows that cancer has always been primarily a local tissue process. Ideally the focus of the tumour should be immunogenic, and is supposed to be recognized by the immune system as allogeneic, and thus localized (delimitated) and destroyed by the cell-effectors of specific anti-tumour immunity. In this case, the encapsulation process is a universal natural mechanism of localization of anything allogeneic in the body. This fully applies to the localization of malignant tumour formation. A fibrous capsule of a different density around the tumour foci has always been observed in experimental animals. It is interesting that the structure of the extracellular macromolecule matrix in capsules around the malignant and benign tumours does not differ [41]. In clinical practice, we often see a favourable course of cancer regardless of the tissue localization when a dense fibrous capsule is formed around the tumour foci. In fact, the formation of a fibrous capsule is associated with low levels of cancer recurrence, and a capsule can serve as a mechanical and chemical barrier to metastasis [42]. Other authors in clinical practice found that the encapsulation of the tumour was an

http://dx.doi.org/10.5772/60213

important favourable prognostic factor for survival without signs of cancer disease [43]. In this regard, we have developed an organic-oriented treatment programme for self-hypnosis, which could presumably have a decreased trophic effect on tumour tissue and contribute to the induction of tumour encapsulation. The examined clinical case confirms what is known about the significant impact of the brain and higher nervous activity on cancer [44]. Furthermore, this case presents new data on the possible nutritional (trophic) effects on tumour tissue and on suppressing the cancer process by deliberate action on higher nervous activity in cancer patients.

4.6. 'Cancer reparative trap': the pathophysiology of cancer in cancer patients with a psychogenic medical history

Analysis of the literature led to the conclusion of the existence of the physiological inhibition of specific anti-tumour immunity in the reparative process (see Figure 7).

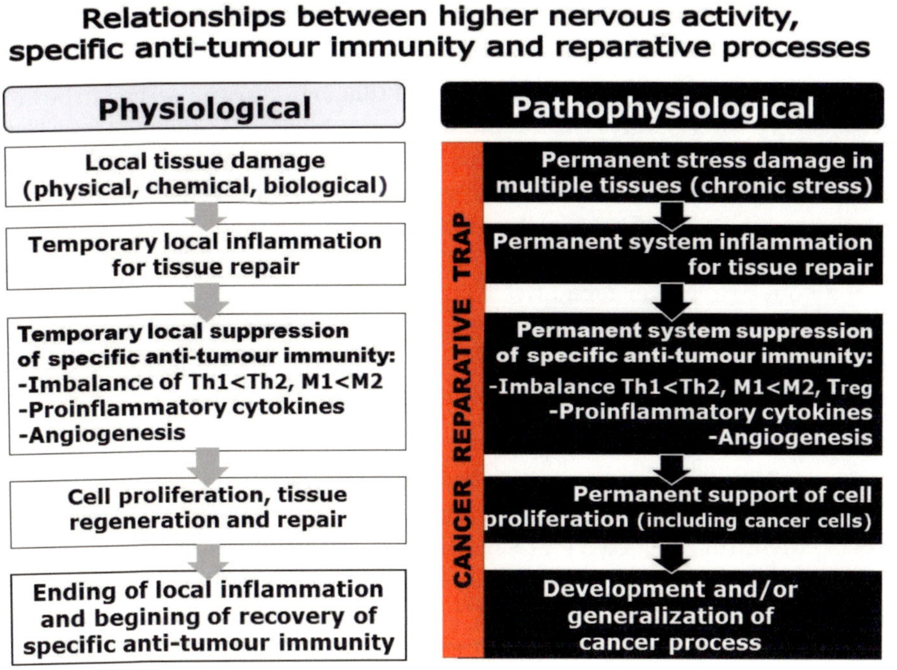

Figure 7. The pathophysiology of cancer in cancer patients with psychogenic medical history.

This local inhibition is observed in local tissue damage as a result of chemical, physical or biological exposure. For the successful healing of tissue damage, local inflammation with known cell, cytokine and vascular reactions develops in the focus. The key factor for successful tissue repair is temporary local suppression of specific anti-tumour immunity in order to avoid the elimination of proliferating cells in the damaged tissue. After completing the repair process, the local inflammation is reduced and the activity of anti-tumour immunity is restored. This natural physiological mechanism of tissue repair may become pathophysiological, i.e., as a result of chronic psychoemotional stress in the body, many foci of the stress microdamages of different tissues, which cause the formation of numerous foci of inflammation, are constantly formed. Because of the large number of inflammatory lesions in the body, there is a constant imbalance of immune reactions in the direction of maintaining reparative processes. This imbalance is accompanied by the constant systemic oppression of specific anti-tumour immunity. Under these conditions cancer tumour cells are able to grow, while the existing tumour in the body creates the possibility of the spreading of cancer. It can be stated that, in cancer patients with a psychogenic medical history, psyche is the leading factor in the development and metastasizing of cancer.

The leading role of the central nervous system in the generalization of cancer has also been shown in an animal model: in the paper of Erica Sloan and colleagues from Monash University, Melbourne, Australia, a 30-fold increase in metastasis to distant tissues from primary tumours was demonstrated in stressed mice [45]. In general, the presented cancer pathophysiological process in cancer patients with a psychogenic medical history can be called a *'cancer reparative trap'* when permanent tissue damage requires constant repair with the appropriate suppression of anti-tumour immunity.

It should be noted in particular that permanent tissue damage is also observed to be influenced by the organism's chemical, physical and biological carcinogens. Thereby, cancer is a disease of an organism that is located in the reparative trap. Any additional damage in the body of an advanced cancer patient with a psychogenic medical history, including surgery, chemotherapy, or radiation therapy, enhances the phenomenon of a 'cancer reparative trap'. The elimination of mental disorders in cancer patients with psychogenic carcinogenesis leads the patient's body out of a 'cancer reparative trap' by creating the conditions for managing the cancer process and increasing the efficiency of standard cancer therapy.

4.7. The role of the mind in the generalization of the cancer process

The cellular and molecular factors and mechanisms of cancer's generalization have been presented in detail; the determinants of invasiveness and the invasion-metastasis cascade have been studied [46]; and the tumour-induced immunosuppressive network has been shown [47]. There is also evidence that biobehavioural risk factors such as social adversity, depression, and stress are involved in cancer progression [48, 49]. As mentioned above, researchers found a 30-fold increase in cancer spread throughout the bodies of stressed mice, compared with those that were not stressed. Chronic stress acts as a kind of fertilizer that feeds breast cancer progression, significantly accelerating the spread of the disease in animal models [45, 50].It can be argued with a certain degree of confidence that chronic stress is also a kind of fuel for the growth and generalization of human cancer. The results of this study suggest that the decisive role in the generalization of the cancer process for the category of advanced cancer patients with a psychogenic medical history is the psychogenic factor. This factor is shown in the form of psychogenically determined mental disorders (depressive and/or anxiety disorders), which activate and maintain the cellular and molecular mechanisms of carcinogenesis, and open the way to the generalization of the cancer process (see Figure 8).

As can be seen in Figure 8, psychoemotional disorders (depressive and/or anxiety disorders) in cancer patients during CPES are accompanied by the disintegration of the major systems in the brain [51], in particular the persistent presence of the sympathetic-adrenal-medullary and hypothalamic-pituitary-adrenal systems prevalence (fight or flight response). In the CPES state the central nervous system exerts downward tonic effect on the 'target organs', accompanied by permanent disturbances of micro-circulation to form in the tissue where the cell's damage occurred (including DNA damage) by the products of oxidative-nitrosative stress (endogenous mutagens). Permanent tissue damage in the body simultaneously accompanied sanogenetic processes in order to repair damaged tissue with mandatory reciprocal inhibition of anti-tumour immunity for tissue healing. This is due to the fact that, with the restoration of normal tissue, proliferating cells always express a number of tumour-associated antigens; in case of the high activity of anti-tumour immunity repair processes would be difficult, since normal proliferating cells would be recognized as tumour-transformed.

The reparative focus of the immune systems of cancer patients with a psychogenic medical history is shown in a shift of balance T-helper-1/T-helper-2 lymphocyte subpopulations in the predominance of T-helper-2 lymphocyte subpopulations and a significant increase in the tissues of alternatively activated macrophages (M2 macrophages). These M2 macrophages secrete IL-10, CCL17, CCL22, CCL18, IL-1RA, and IL-1R decoy. M2 macrophages are active workers of the host, promoting the scavenging of debris, angiogenesis, remodelling, and repair of wounded/damaged tissues [52].

It is known that alternatively activated macrophages in tumour foci orient the immune response towards the activation of repair processes in cancer centres, supporting them in inflammation and angiogenesis, i.e., determining tumour growth and metastasis [53]. In tumour foci M2 macrophages take up to 50% of the tumour mass [54]. It should be particularly noted that the induction of M2 macrophages is influenced by stress hormones – corticosteroids [52]. Thus, there is every reason to believe that the growth of the tumour and the generalization of cancer in the body of patients with a psychogenic medical history are determined by the phenomenon of the reparative focus (direction) of their immune system.

Our clinical observations suggest that cancer patients in general (and with a psychogenic medical history in particular) suffer colds, bacterial and fungal diseases no more and for no longer than healthy people. This points to the selective suppression of anti-tumour immunity but not completely compromising the immune system of cancer patients. Moreover, almost all cancer patients note a common or even accelerated healing of wounds, cuts, and scratches. These clinical data also reflect the reparative orientation of the immune system of cancer patients. In our view, the need to prove empirically the categorical prohibition of any cancer patient physiotherapy, enhancing tissue repair processes in the body, is connected with this phenomenon. The abovementioned fully applies to some psychotherapy. In particular, for cancer patients with psychoemotional disorders that have not been eliminated, the use of various relaxation techniques as well as self-hypnosis a hypnotic inductions of warmth, improvement of blood supply and other trophically-oriented hypnotic inductions, result in the rapid progression of the cancer process. Moreover, cancer patients with psychoemotional disorders that have not been eliminated who relax at the spa, make tourist trips and so on to relieve stress, relax, escape, and recover, often experience progression of the cancer process shortly after returning home.

Thus, the generalization of cancer in cancer patients with a psychogenic medical history depends on the availability of psychoemotional disorders that have not been eliminated

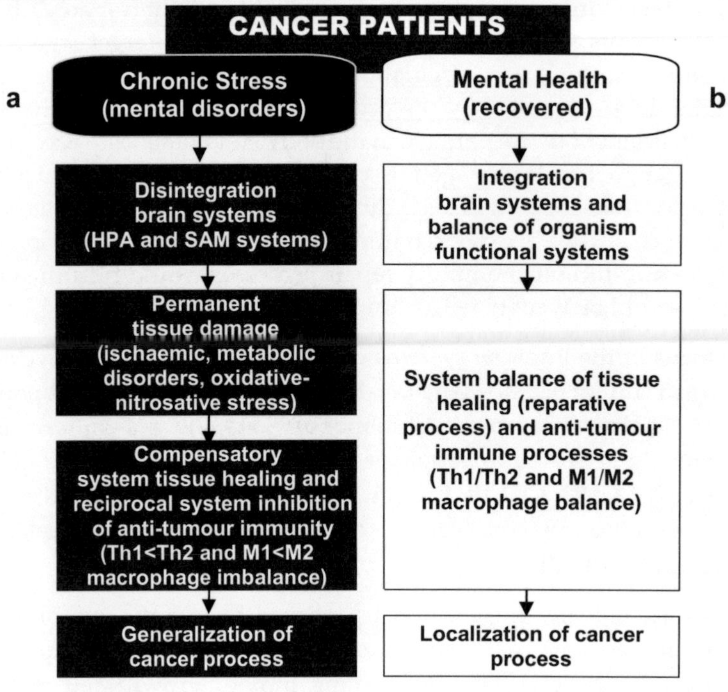

Figure 8. The role of chronic stress (mental disorders) in the generalization of the cancer process in patients with psychogenic medical history. (a) Psychoemotional disorders (anxiety, depression) as a result of chronic stress in cancer patients with psychogenic medical history are accompanied by permanent damage to body tissues and compensatory systemic activation of sanogenetic processes to repair damaged tissue. These system recovery processes are inevitably accompanied by systemic suppression of anti-tumour immunity, paving the way for the generalization of the cancer process; (b) Sustainable relief of psychoemotional disorders in cancer patients restores the natural system activity of anti-tumour immunity and promotes the localization of the cancer process.

associated with compromising their anti-tumour immunity. In this regard, early detection and relief of psychoemotional disorders in cancer patients with a psychogenic medical history could prevent the transition of these patients to the category of advanced cancer patients. At the same time, advanced cancer patients with a psychogenic medical history may have a more favourable prognosis after they receive pathogenetically substantiated psychoimmunological treatment.

5. Further research

Clinical practice shows that there are always those with frequent inexplicable recurrences of cancer, resistance to cancer therapy, rapid generalization of the cancer process and common side effects of cancer treatment. Many of these cancer patients are likely to be those with a psychogenic medical history. In order to conduct the successful treatment of such difficult cancer patients, the efficient impact on higher nervous activity of extensive drug and non-drug resources is required. The psychogenic factor is a major pathogenic

http://dx.doi.org/10.5772/60213

factor in cancer patients with a psychogenic medical history (psychogenic carcinogenesis), which operates continuously at all stages of cancer, unlike chemical, physical and biological carcinogenesis. This is particularly important for clinical practice, since it makes it possible to develop a new approach to pathogenesis-based therapeutic-diagnostic and rehabilitation cancer therapies (see Figure 9).

At the diagnostic stage, the group of cancer patients for which the psychogenic factor is pathogenetically significant can be distinguished. For this patient group we earlier proposed the clinical criteria of psychogenic carcinogenesis and developed a diagnostic test for the evaluation of the specific anti-tumour activity of the immune system [25]. At this stage, as in the subsequent stages of cancer, the integrative-oncology approach is required, involving psychiatric or clinical psychological assistance.

At the therapeutic stage, the purposeful detection of mental disorders in cancer patients and their efficient elimination in combination with the standard therapy of cancer is required. It is necessary to develop new drugs in order to conduct standard cancer therapy with a simultaneous impact on higher nervous activity in cancer patients. The development of new drugs and approaches to block the reparative orientation of the immune system in cancer patients is also required. Perhaps this will be the application of low doses of cytotoxic drugs in combination with nonsteroidal anti-inflammatory drugs and other drug combinations.

New approaches to advanced cancer management

Diagnostic stage

Detection of cancer patients group for which the psychogenic factor is pathogenetically significant (criteria of psychogenic carcinogenesis: evaluation of specific anti-tumour activity of the immune system + psychogenic medical history + mental state assessment in cancer patients).

Stage of treatment (classical treatment)

I. Identification and elimination of mental disorders in cancer patients during the cancer treatment.

II. Development and application of new anti-cancer drugs combinations:
1. Chemotherapy drug + psychotropic drug
2. Chemotherapy drug + neuroprotective drug
3. Chemotherapy drug + psychotropic drug + neuroprotective drug
4. Immunotropic drug + psychotropic drug

III. Development and application drugs for blocking of «cancer reparative trap» including conditions after surgery, chemo- and radiotherapy:
For example: Cytostatic drug (low doses) + NSAIDs and other combinations.

Additional cancer treatment and stage of cancer rehabilitation

Anti-relapse psycho-immunological treatment for cancer patients with psychogenic medical history (psychogenic carcinogenesis).

Figure 9. Future promising clinical approaches to advanced cancer treatment.

At the additional cancer treatment stage and stage of cancer rehabilitation it is necessary to preserve mental health and the specific anti-tumour activity of the immune system. In this regard, we have developed and tested an anti-relapse psychoimmunological approach to the treatment of advanced cancer patients with a psychogenic medical history using a special method of hypnotherapy and original techniques of epicutaneous and extracorporeal activation of specific anti-tumour immunity.

Thus, the early diagnosis of cancer patients with psychogenic medical history and the use of pathogenesis-based cancer treatment will allow reducing financial costs and improving the results of cancer treatment.

6. Conclusion

The present study revealed there to be a special group of advanced cancer patients by the presence of their psychogenic medical history, comorbid psychoemotional disorders, and suppressed specific anti-tumour activity of the immune system. The above mentioned characteristics, we believe, are the clinical criteria of psychogenic (stressful) carcinogenesis [25]. Therefore, the comorbid psychoemotional disorders of this group of advanced cancer patients have a major influence on the course and outcome of the cancer disease. These patients need to receive a special psychoimmunological treatment, consisting of two strictly sequential steps: elimination of psychoemotional disorders, and activation of specific anti-tumour immunity. At the same time, the impossibility of the sustained relief of psychoemotional disorders in advanced cancer patients at the first stage of cancer treatment excludes a further transition to the immunoactivation stage, and can be considered to be an adverse prognostic factor with regard to the lives of these patients. The results of this study are preliminary and require further clinical evidence on a larger contingent of patients with cancer, and may be interesting to various professionals involved in treating advanced cancer patients.

Acknowledgements

The authors gratefully acknowledge Alexey Palchevsky (Kaliningrad, Russian Federation) for financial support and Andrei Kovalevskii MD (Kazakhstan), RMT (Canada) for the Russian/English translation and proofreading of this article.

Author details

Oleg Bukhtoyarov[1,2*] and Denis Samarin[2]

*Address all correspondence to: bukhtoyarov@mail.ru

1 Department of Psychological Studies, Scientific-Research Institute of the Russia's Federal Penitentiary Service, Moscow, Russian Federation

2 Laboratory of Psychoimmunology, Immanuel Kant Baltic Federal University, Kaliningrad, Russian Federation

References

[1] Curiel TJ. Tregs and rethinking cancer immunotherapy. J Clin Invest 2007;117(5): 1167–1174.

[2] Onitilo AA, Nietert PJ, Egede LE. Effect of depression on all-cause mortality in adults with cancer and differential effects by cancer site. Gen Hosp Psychiatry. 2006;28(5): 396–402.

[3] Finn OJ. Cancer immunology. N Engl J Med. 2008;358(25):2704–2715.

[4] Prendergast GC. Immune escape as a fundamental trait of cancer: focus on IDO. Oncogene. 2008;27(28):3889–3900.

[5] Nedospasov SA, Kuprash DV. Oncoimmunology: some fundamental problems of cancer immunotherapy. Mol Biol (Mosk). 2007;41(2):355–368.

[6] Harada Y, Yonemitsu Y. Dramatic improvement of DC-based immunotherapy against various malignancies. Front Biosci. 2011;16:2233–2242.

[7] Hall NR, McGillis JP, Spangelo BL, Goldstein AL. Evidence that thymosins and other biologic response modifiers can function as neuroactive immunotransmitters. J Immunol. 1985;135(2):806s–811s.

[8] Pert CB, Ruff MR, Weber RJ, Herkenham M. Neuropeptides and their receptors: a psychosomatic network. J Immunol. 1985;135(2):820s–826s.

[9] Ader R, Cohen N. The brain and the immune system: conditional responses to commentator stimuli. J Behav Brain Sci. 1985;8(3);413–426.

[10] O'Sullivan C, Lewis CE, Barraclough J. The psychoimmunology of cancer: mind and body in the fight for survival? Oxford: Oxford University Press, 1994.

[11] Dimitroglou E, Zafiropoulou M, Messini-Nikolaki N, Doudounakis S, Tsilimigaki S, Piperakis SM. DNA damage in a human population affected by chronic psychogenic stress. Int J Hyg Environ Health. 2003;206(1):39–44.

[12] Gidron Y, Russ K, Tissarchondou H, Warner J. The relation between psychological factors and DNA-damage: a critical review. Biol Psychol. 2006;72(3):291–304.

[13] Segerstrom SC. Optimism and immunity: do positive thoughts always lead to positive effects? Brain Behav Immun. 2005;19(3):195–200.

[14] Lutgendorf S K, Sood AK, Anderson B. Social support, psychological distress, and natural killer cell activity in ovarian cancer. J Clin Oncol. 2005;23(28):7105–7113.

[15] Cohen S, Janicki-Deverts D, Doyle WJ, Miller GE, Frank E, Rabin BS, Turner RB. Chronic stress, glucocorticoid receptor resistance, inflammation, and disease risk. PNAS. 2012;109(16):5995–5999.

[16] Sood AK, Aparna RB, Kamat AA, Landen CN, Han L, Thaker PH, Li Y, Gershenson DM, Lutgendorf S, Cole SW. Stress hormone-mediated invasion of ovarian cancer cells. Clin Cancer Res. 2006;12(2):369–375.

[17] Thaker PH, Han LY, Kamat AA, Arevalo JM, Takahashi R, Lu Ch, Jennings NB, et al. Chronic stress promotes tumor growthand angiogenesis in a mouse model of ovarian carcinoma. Nat Med. 2006;12(8):939–944.

[18] Reiche EM, Morimoto HK, Nunes SM. Stress and depression-induced immune dysfunction: implications for the development and progression of cancer. Int Rev Psychiatry. 2005;17(6):515–527.

[19] Conrad CD. What is the functional significance of chronic stress-Induced CA3 dendritic retraction within the hippocampus? Behav Cogn Neurosci Rev. 2006;5(1):41–60.

[20] Tsigos C, Chrousos GP. Hypothalamic-pituitary-adrenal axis, neuroendocrine factors and stress. J Psychosom Res. 2002;53(4);865–871.

[21] Simon NM, Smoller JW, McNamara KL, Maser RS, Zalta AK, Pollack MH, Nierenberg AA, Fava M, Wong KK. Telomere shortening and mood disorders: preliminary support for a chronic stress model of accelerated aging. Biol Psychiatry. 2006;60(5): 432–435.

[22] Bukhtoyarov OV, Samarin DM. Psychogenic activation phenomenon of specific antitumor immunity in cancer patients. Int J Med Med Sci. 2013;5(4):198-205.

[23] Tarabrina NV. Workshop on psychology of a post-traumatic stress. St. Petersburg (Russia): Piter, 2001.

[24] Bukhtoyarov OV, Arkhangelskiy AE. Psychogenic cofactor of carcinogenesis: the possibility of using hypnotherapy. Saint-Petersburg (Russia): Aletheia, 2008.

[25] Bukhtoyarov OV, Samarin DM. Psychogenic carcinogenesis. In: Mohan R, ed. Advances in cancer management. Rijeka: InTech, 2012:17–56.

[26] Lockshin A, Giovanella BC,De Ipolyi PD. Exceptional lethality for nude mice of cells derived from a primary human melanoma. Cancer Res. 1985;45(1):345–350.

[27] Wang RF. Tumor antigens discovery: perspectives for cancer therapy. Mol Med. 1997;3(11):716–731.

[28] Habal N, Gupta RK, Bilchik AJ, Yee R, Leopoldo Z, Ye W, Elashoff RM, Morton DL. CancerVax, an allogeneic tumor cell vaccine, induces specific humoral and cellular immune responses in advanced colon cancer. Ann Surg Oncol. 2001;8(5):389–401.

[29] Carroll EW. Cell and tissue functions. In: Porth CM, ed. Essentials of pathophysiology: concepts of altered health states. Philadelphia: Wolters Kluwer/Lippincott Williams & Wilkins, 2011:56–58.

[30] Jacysyn JF, Abrahamsohn IA, Macedo MS. Modulation of delayed-type hypersensitivity during the time course of immune response to a protein antigen. Immunology. 2001;102(3):373–379.

[31] Task Force of the European Society of Cardiology and the North American Society of Pacing and Electrophysiology. Heart rate variability standards of measurement, physiological interpretation, and clinical use. Circulation. 1996;93(5):1043–1065.

[32] Appelhans BM, Luecken LJ. Heart rate variability as an index of regulated emotional responding. Rev Gen Psychol. 2006;10:229–240.

[33] Giese-Davis J, Wilhelm FH, Conrad A, Abercrombie HC, Sephton S, Yutsis M, Neri E, et al. Depression and stress reactivity in metastatic breast cancer. Psychosom Med. 2006;68(5):675–683.

[34] Koocher GP, O'Malley JE. The Damocles syndrome: psychosocial consequences of surviving childhood cancer. New York: McGraw-Hill, 1981.

[35] Montgomery GH, Schnur JB, Kravits K. Hypnosis for cancer care: Over 200 years young. CA Cancer J Clin. 2012;63(1):31-44.

[36] Barrios AA. Hypnotherapy: a reappraisal. Psychother Theor Res Pract. 1970;7(1):2-7.

[37] Bukhtoyarov OV, Arkhangelsky AE, Samarin DM, Senyukov VV, Kozlov VA. [Psychogenic stem cells mobilization phenomenon]. [Article in Russian]. Allergol and Immunol (Moscow). 2006;7(3):369.

[38] Bukhtoyarov OV, Samarin DM, Borisov VI, Senyukov VV, Kozhevnikov VS, Kozlov VA. Immune system re-integration induced by hypnosuggestion in oncological patients. Med Immunol (St. Petersburg). 2008;10(6):527–534.

[39] Biegler KA, Anderson AK, Wenzel LB, Osann K, Nelson EL. Longitudinal change in telomere length and the chronic stress response in a randomized pilot biobehavioral clinical study: implications for cancer prevention. Cancer Prev Res (Phila). 2012;5(10): 1173–1182.

[40] Polak ME, Newell L, Taraban VY, Pickard C, Healy E, Friedmann PS, Al-Shamkhani A, Ardern-Jones MR. CD70-CD27 interaction augments CD8+ T-cell activation by human epidermal Langerhans cells. J Invest Dermatol. 2012;132(6):1636–1644.

[41] Grigioni WF, Errico AD, Biagini G, Mazziotti A, Bolondi L, Liotta LA, Mancini AM, Garbisa S. The capsule surrounding primary liver tumors: wherefrom its prognostic significance? Int J Cancer. 1990;45(4):637–643.

[42] Lunevicius R, Nakanishi H, Ito S, Kozaki K, Kato T, Tatematsu M, Yasui K. Clinicopathological significance of fibrotic capsule formation around liver metastasis from colorectal cancer. J Cancer Res Clin Oncol. 2001;127(3):139–199.

[43] Sherratt JA. Traveling wave solutions of a mathematical model for tumor encapsulation. SIAM J Appl Math. 1999;60(2):392–407.

[44] Mravec B, Gidron Y, Hulin I. Neurobiology of cancer: interactions between nervous, endocrine and immune systems as a base for monitoring and modulating the tumorigenesis by the brain. Semin Cancer Biol. 2008;18(3):150–163.

[45] Sloan EK, Priceman SJ, Cox BF, Yu S, Pimentel MA, Tangkanangnukul V, Arevalo JM, Morizono K, Karanikolas BD, Wu L, Sood AK, Cole SW. The sympathetic nervous system induces a metastatic switch in primary breast cancer. Cancer Res. 2010;70(18):7042–7052.

[46] Weinberg RA. Mechanisms of malignant progression. Carcinogenesis. 2008;29(6): 1092–1095.

[47] Kim R, Emi M, Tanabe K, Arihiro K. Tumor-driven evolution of immunosuppressive networks during malignant progression. Cancer Res. 2006;66(11):5527–5536.

[48] Lutgendorf SK, Sood AK. Biobehavioral factors and cancer progression: physiological pathways and mechanisms. Psychosom Med. 2011;73(9):724–730.

[49] Spiegel D. Mind matters in cancer survival. Psychooncology. 2012;21(6):588–593.

[50] Moreno-Smith M, Lutgendorf SK, Sood AK. Impact of stress on cancer metastasis. Future Oncol. 2010;6(2):1863–1881.

[51] Shumake J, Gonzalez-Lima F. Brain systems underlying susceptibility to helplessness and depression. Behav Cogn Neurosci Rev. 2003;2(3):198–221.

[52] Solinas G, Germano G, Mantovani A, Allavena P. Tumor-associated macrophages (TAM) as major players of the cancer-related inflammation. J Leukoc Biol. 2009;86(5): 1065–1073.

[53] Pollard JW. Tumor-educated macrophages promote tumor progression and metastasis. Nat Rev Cancer. 2004;4(1):71–78.

[54] Gordon S, Martinez FO. Alternative activation of macrophages: mechanism and functions. Immunity. 2010;32(5):593–604.

Chapter 4

Cancer Pain — The Role of an Integrated, Comprehensive Rehabilitation Program in Its Management

Raoul Saggini, Rosa Grazia Bellomo,
Simona Maria Carmignano and Andrea Saggini

Additional information is available at the end of the chapter

http://dx.doi.org/10.5772/60548

1. Introduction

Pain is one of the most frequent and distressing symptoms occurring in cancer patients. Pain is present in 36–61% of cancer patients depending on the histopathological tumor type, on the stage of disease, and patient setting.[1, 3]

Sixty-four percent of patients with advanced cancer are believed to experience substantial pain as a consequence of the neoplastic condition.[4]

Unfortunately, cancer pain is often neglected and undertreated, resulting in a significantly unfavorable impact on the quality of life of the patients and their families. [5]

The National Cancer Institute estimates 1, 660, 290 new patients to be diagnosed with cancer, and about 580, 350 Americans were expected to die from cancer in any sites in 2013. [6]

Cancer pain management relies upon a comprehensive assessment characterized by pain symptoms in terms of phenomenology and pathogenesis, assessing the relation between pain and the causative disease, and clarifying the impact of pain and related co-morbidities on the patient's quality of life.

Despite recent improvements in the cancer management, obstacles to optimal cancer pain management still remain.

Additionally, the lack of psychological and psychiatric support services to support the treatment of cancer pain remains a serious issue.[7]

Hurdles to the treatment of cancer pain have been recognized, including a variety of educational, attitudinal and institutional obstacles. As regards the education in pain management, there appears to be a deficiency in the training of physicians and nurses. Both physicians and nurses indicated that "inability to properly assess the pain" and "inadequate knowledge about pain management" ranked among the most relevant barriers preventing a multidisciplinary approach to pain treatment and adequate cancer pain management. [8]

Despite the increasing availability of pain medications, pain continues to be deemed as moderate-to-severe in more than 50% of cancer patients.

According to a recent population-based study, investigating cancer pain in eleven European countries and Israel, 56% of patients suffered from moderate to severe pain in the previous months, and 69% reported pain-related difficulties hindering everyday activities. [9]

A systematic review completed in 2007 showed that cancer pain is present in 64% of patients with metastatic, advanced disease, in 59% of subjects undergoing cancer-related therapies. Despite effective, curative treatment, a moderate-to-severe pain intensity being reported in more than one third of all cancer patients.

Pain is present in over 50% of cancer patients, reaching higher percentages in patients with cancer at specific sites, such as stomach, uterus, lung, prostate, cervico-facial district, biliary tract, breast, colon, brain, pancreas, cervix, and ovary. [10]

2. Cancer pain

The diagnosis of cancer is typically traumatic and full of uncertainties, due to its prognostic implications and the need for demanding treatment regimens. The word "cancer" still remains synonymous of "pain" and "death". Therefore, both mental and physical pain, in all the aspects and intensity of their clinical expression, characterize every stage of the disease. [11]

Cancer can cause pain at any time during its course, with frequency and intensity of pain tending to increase in the advanced stages. Indeed, roughly 75–95% of patients with metastatic cancer will experience significant amounts of cancer-induced pain.

According to the International Association for the Study of Pain (IASP), pain is defined as "an unpleasant sensory and emotional experience associated with actual or potential tissue damage, or described in terms of such damage." Pain occurring to cancer patients is defined as "total pain" (or "global suffering"), since people with cancer tend to manifest a wide array of functional needs (at a psychological, social, spiritual and existential level) that ought to be recognized and addressed in their complexity.

Relief of pain should, therefore, be seen as part of a comprehensive strategy of care addressing physical, psychological, social, and spiritual aspects of suffering. Physical aspects of pain cannot be treated separately from psychological aspects, whereas patients' anxieties cannot be effectively addressed while patients are physically suffering.

Therefore, all various components of cancer pain should be addressed simultaneously.

Knowledge of the mechanisms of pain has improved considerably over the past few years. We now know that physical injuries, pain pathways, and the emotional processing of this infor-

http://dx.doi.org/10.5772/60548

mation are connected with each other within the nervous system. Anxiety, fear, and insomnia are re-elaborated at the level of the limbic system and the cortex. As a result, the brain responds sending signals back to the spinal cord and, thus, modifies the pain input at spinal levels. The spinal cord sends further impulses back to the brain, establishing in this way a reinforcing loop. [12]

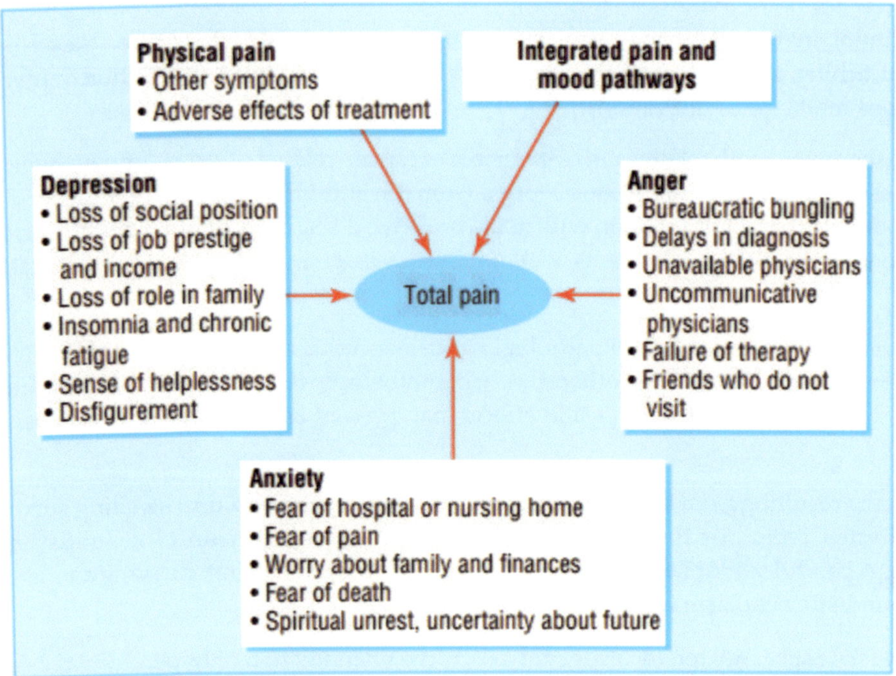

Factors affecting patient's perceptions of pain (adapted from Twycross RG, Lack SA, *Therapeutics in terminal disease*, London: Pitman, 1984)

Figure 1. Factors affecting patient's perceptions of pain (adapted from Waycross RG, Lack SA, Therapeutics in terminal disease, London: Pitman, 1984) from : Principles of control of cancer pain BMJ 2006; 332

Pain is a subjective, heterogeneous experience, affected by patient's genetic background, anamnestic record, mood, expectations, and culture. Cancer pain can be classified according to a number of different features (i.e., etiology or physiopathology).

There is a wide array of potential causes resulting in pain in cancer patients. Indeed, the painful experience involves inflammatory, neuropathic, ischemic, and compression mechanisms occurring in multiple sites. [13]

This section highlights some of the most common causes of pain in cancer patients:

- diagnostic or therapeutic procedures (bone marrow aspiration or biopsy, lumbar puncture) that may result in acute somatic pain, and may require specific premedication protocols as well as analgesic treatments for several days following the mentioned procedures.
- acute postoperative pain or postsurgical syndromes (i.e., following tumor debulking or radical neck dissection) need to be treated with patient-controlled analgesics in selected patients. Such drugs may include cyclooxygenase-2 inhibitors, selective non-steroidal anti-inflammatory drugs (NSAIDs), calcium ligand-gated ion channel anticonvulsants, in addition to pre-procedural local anesthetic nerve blocks.
- direct tumor involvement may cause a painful experience which is often described as constant, aching, gnawing, and well localized (as a result of vascular obstruction or invasion, or mucous membranes ulceration).

Bone metastases are another common responsible of cancer-related physical impairment. Such causes of cancer pain may lead to nociceptive (somatic and visceral), neuropathic, or mixed pain; they may occur in combination with acute or active disease, subacute disease, or chronic disease undergoing palliative care-as well as disease in complete remission with residual effects.

Other sources of pain may include pathologic or osteoporotic stress fractures, and osteonecrosis (following steroids or Radiotherapy). Chemotherapy (CT) side effects may include mucositis, while Radiotherapy (RT) side effects may present as odontophagia, mucositis, or burns.

Lymphedema resulting from RT or surgical excision may result in painful swelling surrounding the affected region or the extremities, eventually leading to painful cellulitis or skin ulceration. A painful scar or keloid may occur following wound healing, carrying an increased risk of wound-site neoplasms.

A controversial aspect related to iatrogenic pain is the phenomenon of hyperalgesia observed during chronic treatment with opioids; although the exact mechanism underlying this phenomenon is still unknown, it seems to be related to tolerance to opioid drugs administered chronically, repetitive stimulation of spinal NMDA receptors, dynorphin activity at the spinal level, specific abnormalities of central processes regulating the neural transmission to the nerve, and a possible action of cholecystokinin at the central nervous system level. [14]

3. Cancer pain: Pathogenetic classification

Onset and assistance of pain during the clinical course of cancer may stem from direct mass effect, relationship between tumor and host, iatrogenic damage; from a physiopathological standpoint, cancer pain may be classified as follows: [15]

- **Nociceptive pain** due to invasion/ulceration of surrounding tissues;
- **Inflammatory pain** through the classical cascade of acute inflammation;

http://dx.doi.org/10.5772/60548

- **Neuropathic pain** due to tumor infiltration / compression of nerves, plexuses, or nerve roots, remote effects of malignant disease on peripheral nerves or side effects of pharmacological treatments. [16]

Cancer pain shares the same neurophysiologic pathways as non-cancer pain. Such nociceptive mechanisms involve activation of sensory afferents by persistent noxious stimuli, signal transduction, transmission, modulation, and, finally, pain perception. [17]

4. Nociceptive pain

Nociceptive pain stems from an acute or persistent injury to somatic or visceral tissues. Somatic nociceptive pain is described by patients as "aching", "stabbing", or "throbbing", and arises from injury to bones, joints or muscles. Visceral nociceptive pain results from injury to viscera. It is poorly localized and is reported as "cramping" or "gnawing", especially when it involves a hollow viscus (e.g. bowel obstruction). Conversely, visceral nociceptive pain may be described as "aching", "stabbing", "sharp", and it is similar to somatic nociceptive pain, whenever it involves other visceral structures (e.g. organ capsules, myocardium). Visceral pain is often referred to somatic sites due to the convergence on somatic afferents within the dorsal root ganglia and dorsal horns. [18]

Stimuli from tissue injury activate primary afferent neurons called nociceptors, located in the skin, muscles, joints, and visceral organs. Nociceptors are high-threshold receptors, i.e. they are silent unless significantly stimulated. [19]

Most nociceptors are polymodal, responding to thermal, physical, and chemical stimuli. Neuron cell bodies are located within the superficial laminae of the dorsal root ganglia and trigeminal ganglia. Once depolarization occurs, transmission advances proximally via thin myelinated A-δ fibers (fast) or reduce unmyelinated C fibers (slow). Interneurons within laminae I and II of the dorsal horn amplify or neurotransmission. Afferent axons end in lamina I or II, and second-order afferent neurons cross the midline and ascend to the brainstem and thalamus through the anterolateral quadrant of the controlateral half of the spinal cord. Together with axons from second-order lamina I neurons, these fibers form the spino-thalamic tract, which is the major ascending pathway with regard to information about pain and temperature. Sensory fibers, associated with affective responses, also ascend in the contro-lateral dorsolateral spinal cord to the medial thalamus or brainstem and, then, to the cingulated cortex and limbic lobe. Downward modulation occurs through the periaqueductal gray (PAG) and rostral ventral medulla (RVM) with axons that run across the dorsal lateral funiculus. The axons just mentioned, modulate pain directly through connections to secondary afferent neurons in the dorsal horn or via connections with interneurons in laminae I and II.

The neurochemistry of these processes involves multiple neurotransmitters including endorphins, prostaglandins, gamma-amino-butyric acid (GABA), cannabinoids, and many others molecules, that are all targets for analgesic medications.[20]

The spine is the most common target of bone metastases, with affected patients experiencing back pain. Direct extension of a vertebral tumor may lead to spinal cord or nerve roots damage, thereby producing substantial neurological compromise. Back pain deriving from vertebral metastases is, therefore, a marker of an increased risk of epidural spinal cord or cauda equina compression.

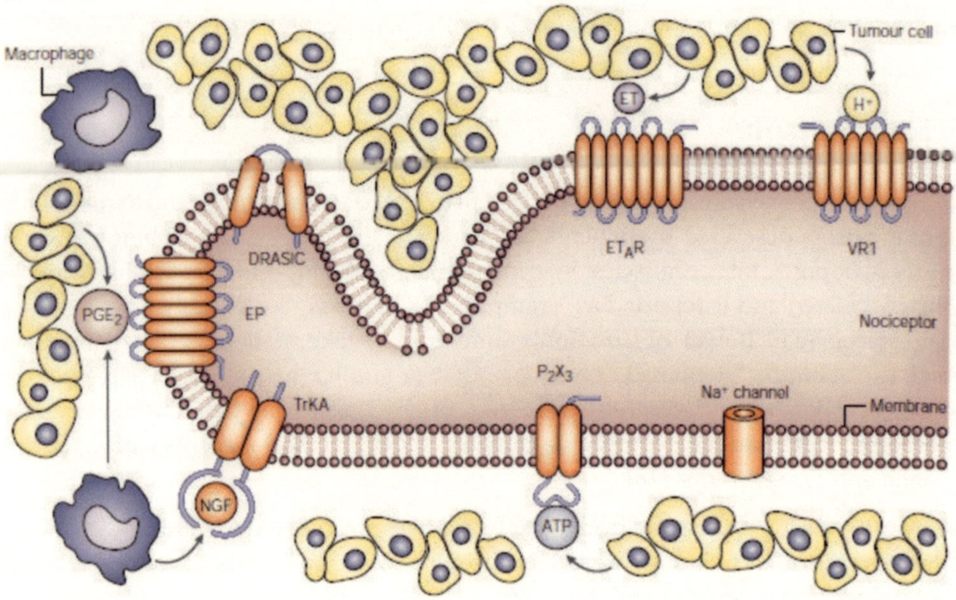

Figure 2. Detection by sensory neurons of noxious stimuli produced by tumours. Figure from Molecular mechanisms of cancer pain. Mantyh PW, Clohisy DR, Koltzenburg M, Steve P. Hunt. Nature reviews I Cancer Volume 2 I March 2002

5. Inflammatory pain

Any given neoplasm harbors several non-cancerous cell types, including immune-system cells such as macrophages, neutrophils, and T cells. These cells may secrete various sensitizing factors, or excite directly primary afferent neurons, such as prostaglandins [21, 22], tumor necrosis factor-α (TNF-α) [23, 24], endothelins [25], interleukin-1 and interleukin-6 [26, 28], epidermal growth factor [29], transforming growth factor-β [30], and platelet derived growth factor. [31, 33] Indeed, specific receptors for these factors are by expressed primary afferent neurons.

Intra- and extracellular pH of solid tumors is lower than that of the surrounding normal tissues. [34]

Local acidosis — secondary to the accumulation of acid metabolites — is a hallmark of tissue injury. [35]

The finding that sensory neurons can be directly excited by protons or acidic compounds has generated sizable interest among basic and clinical researchers. [36]

http://dx.doi.org/10.5772/60548

Studies have shown that several subsets of sensory neurons express different acid-sensing ion channels [37]. The two main classes of acid-sensing ion channels, expressed by nociceptors, are Vanilloid receptor subunit (VR1) [38, 40] and the acid-sensing ion channel-3 receptors (ASIC3). [41]

Both these types of channels are sensitized and excited by a decrease in pH. More specifically, VR1 is activated when the pH falls below the value of 6.0, whereas the pH-induced activation of ASIC3 seems to depend on the co-expression of other ASIC channels by the same nociceptor. [42]

There are several mechanisms by which tumors may induce a decrease in pH. As inflammatory cells invade the neoplastic tissue, they release protons generating local acidosis. The increased frequency of the apoptotic phenomenon within the neoplastic microenvironment contributes to acidosis, as apoptotic cells release intracellular ions in order to create a more acidic pH, thus activating the specific signaling by acid-sensing channels that are expressed by nociceptors. Tumor-induced release of protons and acidosis are thought to be particularly important in the generation of bone cancer pain. Both osteolytic (bone-destroying) and osteoblastic (bone-forming) metastases are characterized by osteoclast proliferation and hypertrophy [43, 45]

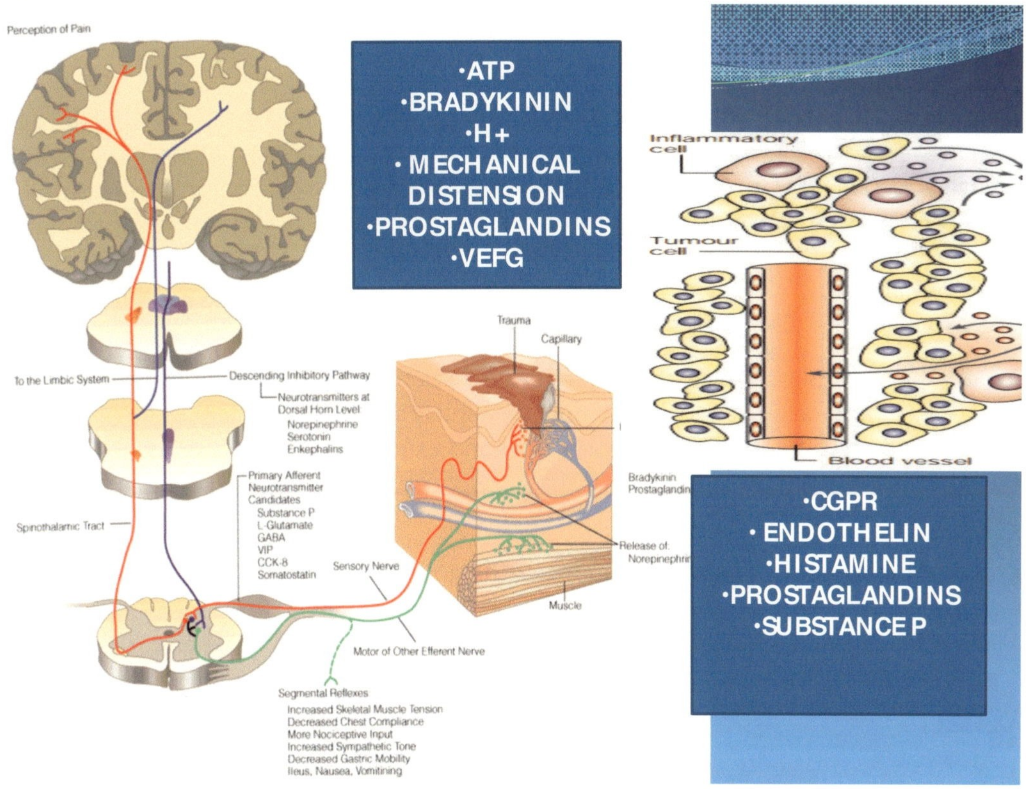

Figure 3. The tumor–nociceptor interface. Figure modified from: Farmaci e Dolore. Di Iorio P. In Saggini R, Buoso S, Pestelli G. (ed) Dolore e Riabilitazione. Minerva Medica 2014. p61

6. Neuropathic pain

Tumors are not densely innervated by sensory neurons. [46, 47] Rapid tumor growth, however, frequently entraps surrounding nerves, causing mechanical injury, compression, ischemia or direct proteolysis.

Proteolytic enzymes that are produced by the tumor cells may cause injury to the sensory and sympathetic fibers, causing neuropathic pain.

Although the mechanisms that generate and keep up neuropathic pain are still not well understood, several therapies have proved to be useful for the control of neuropathic pain in the general population. Recently, the first animal model of cancer pain was developed through the injection of mouse osteolytic sarcoma cells into the intramedullary space of the mouse femur. A crucial component of this model is that the tumor cells are confined to the marrow space of the injected femur, without invading adjacent soft tissues. Once injected, the cancer cells proliferate, and both basal and movement-evoked pain responses increase as the tumor develops. These seem to be produce the same responses of patients with primary or metastatic bone cancer. [48, 50]

Additionally, the therapies aimed at tumor-cell eradication (such as chemotherapeutic agents) may also cause significant nerve fibers damage and lead to ensuing pain.

Potential mechanisms by which chemotherapeutic agents (such as paclitaxel and vincristine) may cause peripheral neuropathy include their ability to disrupt tubulin function. Tubulin polymerization is necessary for axonal transport of trophic factors, and drugs that interfere with this process may cause degeneration of sensory neurons and release of pro-inflammatory cytokines that sensitize directly the primary afferent nociceptors. [51] Chemotherapy-induced polyneuropathy may early develop during the first cycle of treatment but, in most cases, it appears 3-4 months after the first treatment.

Neuropathic pain is associated with dysesthesia, hyperalgesia, hyperpathia, and allodynia; such sensory disturbances occur predominantly at peripheral level, distally and symmetrically, over the upper and lower limbs with a "gloves and socks" distribution; painful disturbances may spontaneously occur or be evoked by tactile or thermal stimuli, with a continuous or intermittent course. [52]

Initially, the symptoms can be insidious and attributable to other conditions, becoming painful in about 25% of patients. Patients with neuropathic pain may also show osteotendinous hyporeflexia, impairment of proprioception, muscle cramps and hypotrophy, reduced muscle tone with reduced muscular endurance, tremor, dystonia, and dyskinesia, resulting in impairment of sensory-motor coordination and sensory ataxia. [53]

The incidence and severity of neuropathic pain are highly dependent on the type of chemotherapy protocol (mono- or poly-therapy with cumulative doses over time), the association with radiotherapy (RT), the age of patient, and co-morbidities such as diabetes, alcoholism, paraneoplastic neuropathies and other diseases affecting the nervous system.

http://dx.doi.org/10.5772/60548

In hormone-producing cancers deriving from endocrine tissues, the use of agents inhibiting the production or the activity of relevant hormones is a common feature, with particular regard to estrogens, progestins, androgens, corticosteroids, and thyroid hormones.

About 40% of women treated with aromatase inhibitors (AI) present joint and muscular pain in a widespread, symmetrical distribution, often associated with morning stiffness that tends to fade with movement, as well as sleep disorders. The onset of pain, usually mild-to-moderate in intensity, typically occurs within the first few months after starting the therapy. Relevant risk factors include: age over 60 years, obesity, recent menopause, rheumatic diseases, previous chemotherapy and hormone replacement therapy, as well as use of anxiolytics and antidepressants. Such symptoms are, most likely, related to the modification of the pain threshold as a direct consequence of the reduction of circulating estrogens, which have a peripheral antinociceptive effect and play an important role in the modulation of central pain. [54]

RT regimens play a synergistic role with CT, surgery, immunotherapy and hormone therapy for the control of primary and secondary tumor lesions, being also potentially useful to reduce the size or vascularization and bleeding of the tumor as well as to relieve the pain. With regard to the use of RT in palliative care, edema and inflammation in the tissues treated with radiotherapy frequently cause recurring pain. Radiodermatitis, whose severity ranges from simple rash to tissue necrosis, may result in skin discoloration with frequent association with hyperpathia.

Lymphedema causes pain because of locoregional tension within soft tissues and joint traction. These painful symptoms may even appear after a considerable time interval, being intensified by the load and the mobilization but, in advanced cases, pain is present even at rest, resulting in hypomobility and reduction of muscle tone.

Post-radiation fibrosis is a serious dose-dependent complication of RT and may involve the lungs and the soft tissues; fibrosis of skin and subcutaneous tissues (mainly in the neck, face and breast) results in hypomobility, compensatory postural defects, muscle and joint contractures and pain.

Radiotherapy can also determine cervical and lumbar pain developing from a few months up to several years after the beginning of the therapy.

A brachial plexus neuropathy (plexopathy) can occur due to radiation treatment for breast cancer, head and neck or pulmonary apex, may represent a difficult differential diagnosis with the possibility of neoplastic infiltration of the plexus.

Post-radiation plexopathies preferentially affect the upper roots (C5-C6), while direct infiltration by neoplastic cells normally involves the lower trunks (C7-C8-T1). The clinical picture may be initially characterized by dull and deep pain referred to the shoulder, armpit and arm, usually of mild-to-moderate intensity, associated with tingling paresthesia in the distribution root C5-C6-C7, followed by motor impairment, heaviness, predominantly proximal weakness, and functional limitations, especially with regard to flexion and abduction. [56]

Coexistence of plexopathy following radiotherapy and postsurgical lymph edema may occur as well, triggering a vicious circle in which limb pain is increased by the weight of the lymphedematous limb determining motor and functional impairment.

The progression of the neurological deficit occurs through multiple steps, with the final result being the flaccid paralysis of the upper limb.

The lumbosacral plexopathy is a rare, adverse effect following irradiation for pelvic, abdominal, uro-gynecological, or bowel tumors. In 50-75% of lumbosacral plexopathy cases, the neuropathy starts at lower limbs level presenting as bilateral deficit affecting the distal surface sensitivity and, to a lesser degree, proprioceptive sensitivity; the motor deficit, mainly involving the districts innervated by the distal roots L5-S1 (55% of patients), presents as a bilateral, asymmetrical lower limbs deficit, resulting in impairment of dorsiflexion of the foot as well as gait and balance disorders. The coexisting pain radiating along the face of the posterolateral thigh and leg increases the risk of falls in association with sensorimotor deficits.

Among patients undergoing RT for prostate cancer, 20% of cases may develop a challenging neuropathy as earlier as after the first 12 months of RT, resulting in chronic pelvic pain often associated with dysuria, dyspareunia, rectal tenesmus, and abdominal pain.

Spine irradiation may cause vascular damage, demyelination, and focal necrosis of the white matter of the spinal cord, resulting in a post-RT myelopathy, which may be classified in acute, sub-acute, and chronic subtypes, depending on the time of onset after RT.

Cancer pain syndromes may be further classified as acute and chronic syndromes.

Acute pain syndromes have a sudden, well-defined onset, present with an identifiable cause (e.g. surgery). They are affected by sympathetic responses (fight or flight response), and are expected to improve with adequate care. The acute form most commonly occurs in head and neck cancers after treatment of the cervical-cephalic district, being characterized by a positive Lehermitte sign, stabbing pains in the neck exacerbated by flexion of the head, and radiation to the column and the limbs, with sensory, motor, and autonomic symptoms.

Chronic pain has a less distinct onset, shows a prolonged and fluctuating course, and is largely driven by central sensitization. [57]

In chronic pain, the algic symptom, referred to the dermatomes at or below the levels treated by RT, precedes the neurological signs and leads to increased difficulties in motor coordination and execution of daily activities. The chronic form may present as transverse myelitis, with tetraparesis or Brown-Sequard syndrome. [58]

A crucial question is whether the spinal cord and forebrain undergo significant neurochemical changes while chronic pain develops. Studies involving the mouse model of bone metastases pain, described above, revealed extensive neuro-chemical reorganization in the spinal cord segments that receive input from primary afferent neurons innervating the tumor-bearing bone.

Such changes include astrocytes hypertrophy, accompanied by decreased expression of glutamate re-uptake transporters. [59, 60]

This results in increased extracellular levels of the excitatory neurotransmitter glutamate and excitotoxicity within the central nervous system. The up-regulation of the proalgesic peptide dynorphin was also observed in the spinal cords of tumor-bearing animals.

http://dx.doi.org/10.5772/60548

Spinal-cord expression of dynorphin — a pro-nociceptive member of the opioid family [61, 62] - has been observed in animal models of neuropathic [63], inflammatory [64, 65], and sarcoma-induced bone cancer pain states. Cancer pain induces, therefore, a state of central sensitization, in which neurochemical changes in the spinal cord and forebrain promote an increased transmission of nociceptive information.

Classically, the main emphasis when examining the ascending conduction of pain has been placed on spino-thalamic tract neurons. This means that the general mood and attitude of the patient might also be a significant factor in determining the intensity and degree of pain.

Clinical studies, however, have resulted in the revision of such thesis, showing that attenuation of some forms of visceral cancer pain can be achieved by disruption of non-spinothalamic-tract axons. [66]

Chronic pain entails adverse effects on various organ systems, as seen with non oncological pain.

An inadequate treatment of pain has negative effects at the psychological, respiratory, cardiovascular, endocrine and metabolic, and gastrointestinal levels. The persistently active proalgesic stimulation affects both somatomotor neurons, generating reflex phenomena such as muscle spasm, and sympathetic neurons, with norepinephrine-mediated activation resulting in peripheral vasoconstriction, cardiac work increase, visceral hypotonia, and gastrointestinal and genito-urinary incontinence.

Indeed, the persistence of pain determines augmented sympathetic nerve activity, with increased release of catecholamines, antidiuretic hormone, (ADH), angiotensin II, aldosterone system, and related cytokines. The activation of the sympathetic-adrenal axis with release of corticotropin releasing hormone (CRH) and ADH activates a subset of processes that the body normally implements when facing emergency situations: in particular, activation of catabolic reactions (ie, those reducing the lean body mass) is accompanied by chronic fatigue and insomnia, as seen when dealing with stressing situations.

Mood disorders (anxiety, apathy, depression) associated with catabolic metabolism are accompanied by an imbalance in the levels of electrolytes, especially potassium. These changes affect the excitable tissues (muscles and nerves) as potassium is a regulator key of the electricity transmission; likewise, it may have effects on the nervous system and transmission of painful signals.

Gastrointestinal disorders (bloating, feelings of fullness, food intolerance, slow digestion) may also occur, as a consequence of the imbalance of electrolytes; indeed, peristalsis is implemented by muscles which, despite not being voluntarily controlled, have similar characteristics to the skeletal.

In addition, the state of catabolism induced by the action of stress factors affects blood regulation and storage of sugars, which are mostly accumulated in muscle tissue. Loss of muscular tissue leads, therefore, to a deregulation of glucose metabolism resulting in loss of appetite or excessive and unjustified sense of hunger (typically during the night). These two symptoms often alternate between each other.

Dysregulation of cortisol release results in peripheral vasoconstriction and limbs muscles catabolism. The inadequate cortisol regulation and the consequent loss of muscle mass can as well affect the amount of adipose tissue, leading to a relative increase of the latter. Chronic pain often predisposes to a complex series of physiological and psychosocial changes, which are an integral part of the chronic pain issue, being added to the existing burdens occurring to those who suffer. [67]

7. Chronic pain syndromes

Causes	Disorders
Nociceptive somatic pain due to bone metastases	Multifocal bone pain, vertebral pain syndrome in epidural spinal cord compression, pain syndrome related to pelvis and hip, base of skull
Nociceptive somatic pain due to soft tissue involvement	Headache and facial pain, ear and eye pain, pleural pain, muscle cramps
Nociceptive visceral pain due to malignancy	Hepatic distention syndrome, chronic bowel obstruction, midline retroperitoneal syndrome, malignant perineal pain, ureteric obstruction
Neuropathic pain due to malignancy	Radiculopathies, mononeuropathies, plexopathies, neuralgias, peripheral neuropathy
Antineoplastic therapies (i.e. chemotherapy, radiation therapy, hormonal treatments, surgery)	Peripheral neuropathy, chronic post-surgical pain (eg.mastectomy, thoracotomy, neck dissection, pelvic surgeries), phantom limb pain, chronic radiation myelopathy, chronic radiation plexopathy, chronic radiation proctitis and enteritis, lymphedema pain, osteoradionecrosis

Table 1. Chronic pain syndrome

8. Breakthrough pain

Breakthrough pain is a common problem in patients with cancer, being associated with significant morbidity. Currently, there is no universally accepted definition of "breakthrough pain". Portenoy et al. have defined breakthrough pain as "a transitory exacerbation of pain experienced by the patient who has relatively stable and adequately controlled baseline (background) pain" (Portenoy et al., 2004).

Breakthrough pain is usually classified into one of two categories:

1. Spontaneous pain ("idiopathic pain") – the episodes are not related to any identifiable precipitant factors.
2. Incident pain ("precipitated pain") – the episodes are related to an identifiable precipitant factor. Incident pain is usually sub-classified into one of three categories:

http://dx.doi.org/10.5772/60548

3. Volitional incident pain – pain is exacerbated by a voluntary act (e.g., walking).
4. Non-volitional incident pain – pain is exacerbated by an involuntary act (e.g., coughing).
5. Procedural pain – pain is related to a therapeutic intervention (e.g., wound dressing).

Breakthrough pain is associated with poor overall pain control (Bruera et al., 1995) as well as decreased patient satisfaction with overall pain management (Zeppetella et al., 2000). In addition, breakthrough pain may result in a number of physical (e.g., immobility), psychological (e.g., insomnia, anxiety, depression) and social (e.g., unemployment, social isolation) complications (Skinner et al., 2006). Indeed, the presence of breakthrough pain may have a significant impact on the quality of life (Skinner et al., 2006).[68]

9. Pain assessment

Clinical practice guidelines developed by the National Comprehensive Cancer Network (NCCN) [69] and American Pain Society (APS) emphasize the essential need of a comprehensive pain assessment. [70]

A careful evaluation of pain should include history, pain description (in particular, establishing whether it worsens during the sleep), precipitating and alleviating factors, functional impairment, psychological associated factors, psychosocial history as well as patient's beliefs, physical examination, and a general knowledge of the different features of cancer-induced and nonmalignant pain; such evaluation will allow a comprehensive assessment of pain. Conversely, an inadequate measurement and assessment of pain poses a significant obstacle to any effective pain management strategy.

Patient interview:

Onset of pain?
Frequency of pain?
Site of pain?
Radiation of pain?
Quality (character) of pain?
Intensity (severity) of pain?
Duration of pain?
Exacerbating factors?
Relieving factors?
Response to analgesics?
Response to other interventions?
Associated symptoms?
Interference with activities of daily living?

Figure 4. Pain assessment: Interview

An adequate pain assessment requires a thorough pain anamnesis as well as physical examination prior to any radiographic study or physiological testing. Failing to collect a comprehensive anamnesis and performing a correct physical examination will result in frequent mistakes, as correspondence between pain severity, as reported by the patient, and presence of underlying pathology, as revealed by imaging studies, is often poor. Location, radiation, quality, intensity and temporal pattern of pain should be ascertained along with provocative and palliative factors associated with pain; afterwards, the physician should map the source of pain and investigate any clues to a possible cause; finally, the following pain features should be identified:

- Type of pain (nociceptive, neuropathic, psychogenic);
- Temporal characteristics (acute, chronic, intense episodic);
- Intensity (mild, moderate, severe).

Physical examination should be focused on the area of pain without overlooking areas of referred pain (such as the right shoulder in case of hepatic metastases).

Physical examination is followed by specific maneuvers in order to provoke or improve pain.

For instance, pain due to bone metastases may be provoked through local palpation and manipulation. Spinal cord compression resulting from epidural tumor extension represents a known challenge. Accordingly, a comprehensive neurologic examination, coupled with manual muscle testing, percussion of point of tenderness, evaluation of joint mobility, and inspection of muscle symmetry are crucial steps of any physical examination.

The assessment of psychiatric and psychosocial co-morbidities is crucial to address factors that may adversely affect pain perception and worsen patient's distress. Radiographic studies should be guided by the anamnesis and the physical examination, as well as stage of disease, patient performance status, therapeutic options, and care endpoints. When dealing with terminally ill patients, or when little would be gained by radiographic procedures, palliative measures should be implemented without putting the patient through painful, unnecessary testing. Whenever appropriate, pain treatment should be started as early as possible so that patients may be comfortable and able to complete the diagnostic procedure. Plain radiographs of painful areas may be of value.

Magnetic resonance imaging (MRI) of the spine and brain and computed tomography (CT) scanning of the chest and abdomen often provide the greatest amount of information. In case of pericardial effusions or biliary or urinary tract obstruction, ultrasonography may be easily accomplished with a portable device, thus avoiding radiation exposure. Electrophysiologic studies may be useful to distinguish mononeuropathies and entrapment neuropathies from plexopathies, as well as ulnar and peroneal entrapment syndromes from brachial and lumbar plexopathies, respectively. Conduction velocities, specific latencies, amplitudes, duration, and configurations of sensory and motor evoked potentials are the keys to identify and locate the neural pathology. Importantly, it should be remembered that results of electrophysiologic studies may be normal even with significantly damaged non-myelinated fibers.

The ability to measure pain implementing valid and standardized approaches has improved in the last years, increasing our ability to quantify the impact of adequate care in terms of outcomes. The use of standardized instruments (scales), both of a specific type (focused on the

http://dx.doi.org/10.5772/60548

pain) and of a generic type (quality measures of life), as well as the implementation of other measures aimed to capture the results in terms of consumption of resources and medical care, has made it possible, when required, to assess the overall impact of pain on the health and life of patient. Initial and ongoing assessment of pain includes the evaluation of pain intensity using a visual or numerical rating scale ranging from 0 (absence of pain) to 10 (presence of the worst imaginable pain). Other relevant factors in pain assessment include ascertaining the quality of pain, onset, and duration as well as any actions that may worsen or relive the pain. Careful patient interviews should also evaluate the extent of patient distress resulting from pain as well as various psychological or social factors.

The Pain Research Group of the WHO Collaborating Centre for Symptom Evaluation in Cancer Care has developed the Brief Pain Inventory (BPI), a pain assessment tool devised for cancer patients. The BPI measures both the intensity of pain (sensory dimension) and the interference of pain with the patient's daily activities (reactive dimension). It also queries the patient about pain relief, pain quality, and patient perception of the cause of pain.

The BPI is a powerful tool and, having demonstrated both reliability and validity across different cultures and populations, it has been adopted in many countries for clinical pain assessment, epidemiological studies, and in studies evaluating the effectiveness of pain treatment.

Key objectives of pain assessment in populations with active cancer

1 To characterise the multiple dimensions of the pain
- Intensity
- Temporal features: onset, course, daily fl uctuation, and breakthrough pains
- Location and radiation
- Quality
- Provocative or relieving factors

2 To formulate an understanding of the nature of the pain
- Cause
- Inferred pathophysiology
- Pain syndrome

3 To characterise the eff ect of the pain on quality-of-life domains
- Eff ect on physical function and wellbeing
- Eff ect on mood, coping, and related aspects of psychological wellbeing
- Eff ect on role functioning and social and familial relationships
- Eff ect on sleep, mood, vitality, and sexual function

4 To clarify the extent of neoplastic disease, planned treatment, and prognosis

5 To clarify the nature and quality of previous testing and past treatments

6 To elucidate medical comorbidities

7 To elucidate psychiatric comorbidities
- Substance-use history
- Depression and anxiety disorders
- Personality disorders

8 To identify other needs for palliative care interventions
- Other symptoms
- Distress related to psychosocial or spiritual concerns
- Caregiver burden and concrete needs
- Problems in communication, care coordination, and goal setting

Figure 5. Pain assessment: Objective

With regard to specific assessment tools, the main validated scales used in oncology are the followings:

- Short-Form McGill Pain Questionnaire 8 (SF) ;
- Brief Pain Inventory (BPI);
- European Organization for Research and Treatment of Cancer Quality of Life Core Questionnaire (EORTC QLQ C309);
- Karnofsky performance status.

10. The management of cancer pain

An adequate control of pain is reached through three basic strategies: modifying the source of the pain, altering the central perception of pain, and blocking the transmission of the pain to the central nervous system. [71]

The optimal use of these strategies in the control of cancer pain requires a thorough assessment of patient's pain, cancer features, concurrent medical problems, and psychosocial status. [72, 73]

An individualized plan of care must be established, implemented, reassessed, and then modified on a regular basis in order to maximize both the quality and duration of life. The pain affecting the vast majority of patients with cancer may be relieved through direct and indirect modifications of the source of pain combined with pharmacologic and non pharmacologic actions aimed at modifying the patients' perception of pain. [74]

The Three-Step Analgesic Ladder of the World Health Organization uses these three categories of pain to guide analgesic-drug therapy. [75]

Patients receiving no analgesic therapy who have mild-to-moderate pain should be treated with nonopioid analgesic drugs (step 1). If a patient has mild-to-moderate pain despite taking a nonopioid analgesic, the dose of the nonopioid analgesic should be maximized and a step 2 opioid analgesic should be added (step 2).

Patients who have moderate- to-severe pain despite being treated with step 2 opioids require an increase in the dose of the opioid or, if that is not feasible, a change to a step 3 opioid. This method has been estimated to effectively relieve pain in 80 to 90 percent of patients.[76, 77]

Many experts recommend a step 2 opioid as initial therapy for patients with moderate pain [78, 80], further suggesting that therapy with a step 3 opioid may be immediately started when pain is severe. Patients who have mild-to-moderate pain while taking a step 3 opioid should have the dose of that opioid increased until an effective level is reached. (Fig 5)

Non-opioid, step 1 analgesic drugs include acetaminophen, aspirin, and other non-steroidal anti-inflammatory drugs (NSAIDs). These drugs are of limited value to patients with pain from advanced cancer because of their relatively low maximal efficacy. [81]

http://dx.doi.org/10.5772/60548

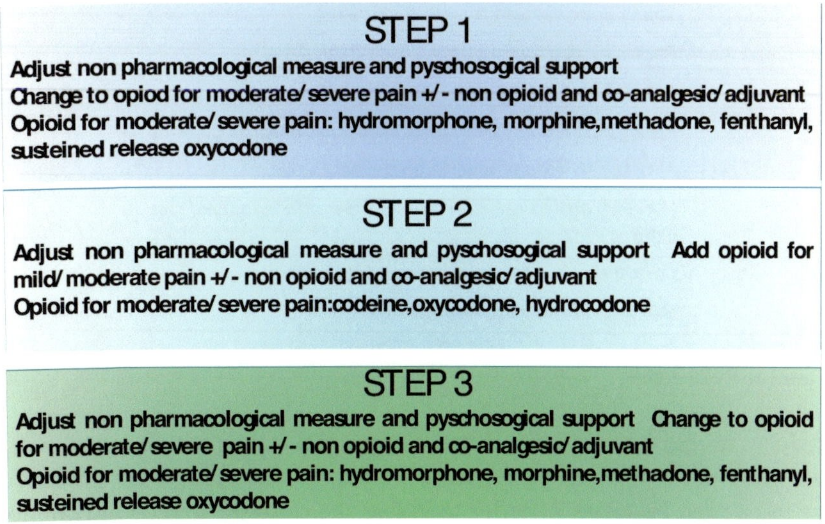

Figure 6. The Three-Step Analgesic Ladder of the World Health Organization uses these three categories of pain to guide analgesic-drug therapy.

The step 2 opioids used to treat moderate pain include codeine, dihydrocodeine, hydrocodone, oxycodone, and propoxyphene. Use of step 2 opioids is limited by dose-limiting side effects or because they are prepared in fixed combinations with non-opioid analgesics.

Step 3 opioids commonly prescribed for the relief of moderate-to-severe cancer pain include morphine, oxycodone, hydromorphone, and fentanyl.

These opioids should be used one at a time to take advantage of possible idiosyncratic differences in patients' responses.

Morphine is the step 3 opioid most commonly used to control severe pain, because of its wide availability, varied formulations, as well as well-characterized pharmacologic properties. [82]

In some patients, switching from one opioid to another can eliminate an unmanageable, idiosyncratic side effect of the initial drug. [83] In patients whose pain is well controlled, the initial dose of the new opioid should be 25 to 50 percent less than the estimated equivalent dose to allow incomplete cross tolerance. [84]

Over the years the above treatment strategy has been undergoing a number of critical changes, as it has been realized that the scale of treatment (i.e. step 1 vs step 2 vs step 3) should not be necessarily gradual, but it should rather comply with the stadium and the clinical phase of pain experienced by each patient.

Accordingly, if pain is already reported as severe from the beginning, then it should be treated with step 3 medications and adequate dosage without the need to follow the steps of sequential scale.

Analgesic drugs, indeed, remain the keys of cancer pain managment. The choice of drug should be based on the severity of the pain, rather than on the stage of disease. Drugs should be given

Select the appropriate analgesic drug

Prescribe the appropriate dose of the drug

Administrer the drug by the appropriate route

Prevent persistent pain and relieve breakthrough pain

Titrate the dose of drug aggressively

Prevent, anticipate,and manage the side effects of the drug

Consider sequential trial of analgesic drugs

Use appropriate adjuvant drugs

Figure 7. Pain assessment: Interview

in standard doses at regular intervals. When a non-opioid drug is to be used with an opioid for moderate pain, patients often prefer to receive fixed combinations of the two analgesic agents. Care must then be taken in order to assess the dose of each drug contained in such formulations; indeed, some combinations of codeine or dihydrocodeine with aspirin or paracetamol (including co-codamol and co-dydramol) contain subtherapeutic doses of the opioid. Likewise, the decision to use an opioid for severe pain should be based on severity of pain rather than on prognosis.

It is also important to emphasize that, at every step, adjuvants drugs may be added to the protocol treatment. Adjuvant drug therapy enhances the analgesic efficacy of opioids, treats concurrent symptoms that may exacerbate pain, and/or results in an independent analgesic effect for specific types of pain. [85]

Early use of adjuvant drugs is warranted in order to optimize patients' comfort and function by preventing or reducing the toxic effects of opioids. Cancer-pain syndromes most amenable to adjuvant therapy are those caused by bone metastases, nerve compression, nerve damage, and visceral distention.

The most commonly used drugs in adjuvant therapy for the treatment of cancer pain are NSAIDs, corticosteroids, tricyclic antidepressant drugs, and anticonvulsant drugs.[86]

Additionally, treatment of pain strategies should allow for two further variables: 1) the possibility to adopt an opioid rotation strategy, and 2) the choice of the correct drug administration route: non invasive or invasive.

The importance of taking care of the cancer patient rehabilitation has been sanctioned also in the Italian Health Plan Oncology 2010-12, with the model "Simultaneous Care" expressing that "Rehabilitation in oncology should start from diagnosis and continue throughout life".

It is, therefore, necessary that the cancer patient is taken care of by a specialist who, through the formulation of Individual Rehabilitation Project, is specifically involved in the prevention, care and clinical monitoring of the pain and disease. [87]

The Cancer Rehabilitation Treatment has the following goals:

- Preventive – to improve function and reduce morbidity and disability;

http://dx.doi.org/10.5772/60548

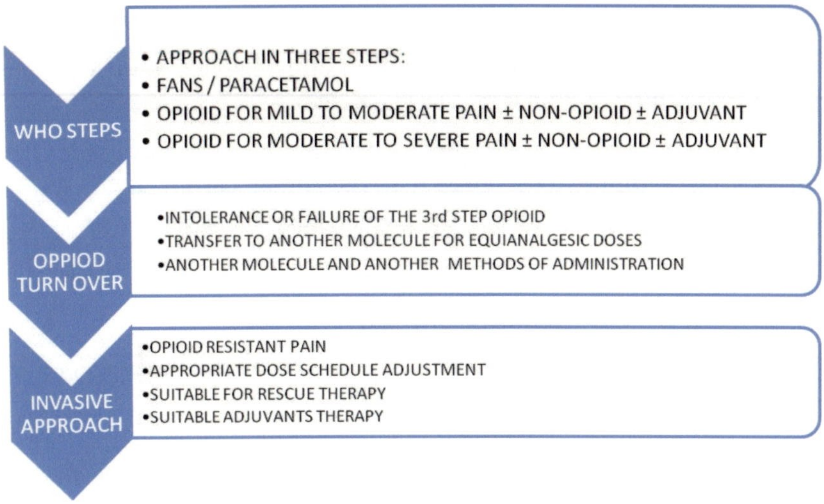

Figure 8. Pharmacologic pain management

- Restorative – for patients with the potential to be completely cured from cancer, to appropriately control, circumvent, or eliminate any residual disabilities;
- Supportive – for patients who are supposed to survive with cancer for a significant time with relative control of disease or remission, to lessen disability, handicap, emotional stress, or discomfort through rehabilitative care;
- Palliative – for patients whose disease is advanced and relentlessly progressive, but whose disability, discomfort, and stress can be mitigated by rehabilitation.

Physiatrists should tailor an individual rehabilitation project depending on the type of tumor, symptoms and signs, presence of complications, stage and evolution, needs and expectations of the patient and his family. [88, 89]

11. Rehabilitation approach to pain

A complex and global rehabilitation program in cancer pain is composed of the following components:

1. Recovery of residual capacity:
    - Educational interventions regarding lifestyle and behavior;
    - Nutritional support;
    - Multimodal Physical Activity;
    - Myofascial manual therapy (relaxation, lymphatic drainage, therapy of the scars);
    - Physical energies;

2. Sensory-motor and functional recovery capacity:

   - Analysis of posture and movement with tridimensional optoelectronics systems, implemented in collaboration with bio-engineers;
   - Therapy in microgravitary environments and Sensorimotor training with swinging platforms in the tridimensional space with the aim of learning again the balance, and postural control through vertebral reeducation and visual feedback;
   - Prescription of prostheses, orthoses;
   - Counseling activities for health and nursing;

3. Quality of life improvement: inclusive approach with home therapy and occupational therapy.

11.1. Recovery of residual capacity

The maintenance of an adequate nutritional status is important because it reduces the risk of recurrence and complications related to cancer therapy by contributing to the general well-being of the patient. Accordingly, nutritional support is an essential part of the treatment of cancer patients.

The need for informed lifestyle choices by cancer survivors becomes particularly important particularly important upon completion of of therapy when trategie self-care improve their long-term results.

Despite being highly variable depending on the type of cancer and stage at diagnosis, cancer may cause several metabolic and physiological alterations affecting the body requirements of macro- and micronutrients.[90]

The American Cancer Society (ACS) convened a group of experts in nutrition, physical activity, and cancer to evaluate and summarize the available scientific evidence and best clinical practices related to nutrition and physical activity after the diagnosis of cancer. Accordingly, it has been highlighted that patients undergoing cancer treatment often experience significant nausea and vomiting, leading to further weight loss. [91]

Because of such clinical evidence, cancer has been considered as a disease associated with weight loss, rather than obesity.

Nonetheless, with growing numbers of overweight or obese patients beginning the cancer treatment protocols, additional weight gain has also been noted as a possible complication of treatment. [92, 94]

Nutritional assessment for survivors should, therefore, begin immediately after diagnosis and should take into consideration treatment goals (curative, control, or palliation), while focusing on both the current nutritional status and the expected nutrition-related symptoms. [95]

During active cancer treatment, the overall goals of nutritional care for survivors should be to prevent or resolve nutrient deficiencies, achieve or maintain a healthy weight, preserve lean body mass, minimize nutrition-related side effects, and maximize the quality of life.

http://dx.doi.org/10.5772/60548

Malnourished patients are less able to tolerate surgical therapy, chemotherapy, radiation therapy, and drug therapy, undergoing pain and related complications such as prolonged bed rest and lymphedema more frequently than subjects in a better nutrition state. For all these reasons, cachexia may threaten the patient's life even more than the local effects of the tumor itself. Cancer cachexia presents clinically with anorexia, altered taste perception, and subsequent weight loss, loss of muscle mass and general malnutrition causing a significant reduction in physical, immune, and mental functions. As a consequence, the body cannot implement adequate defensive strategies.

The causes of anorectic-cachexia syndrome have not been fully clarified yet. The intermediate products of tumor metabolism and the immune response to the tumor itself may be a direct cause of anorexia or early satiety, or produce these same symptoms in a indirect way by an effect on hypothalamic functions.

Macrophage activation products Interleukin-1 and Tumor Necrosis Factor (TNF) thus increasing the release of triglycerides from the adipose tissue and amino acids from the muscular tissue. These cytokines may be important factors in the development of cancer cachexia, but the precise mechanism by which this occurs is not clear. These cancer-dependent metabolites may also be responsible for the anomalies in the sensation of taste and smell that have been observed in cancer patients.

Patients may notice increased or decreased perception of sweet taste. The threshold for salty and sour tastes is often increased, while the one for the bitter taste is usually decreased. A lower threshold for the bitter taste (specific testing substances that can be used include urea) is often responsible for the aversion to meat that is frequently present in these patients. [96]

The psychological stress associated with neoplastic disease may contribute to anorexia. Even in the absence of frank depression, the presence of pain, decreased sense of well-being, depressed mood and anxiety about the treatment regimen or the prognosis, tend to cause a state of emotional stress that antagonizes the sense of gratification from food. Patients complaining of nausea or other disorders, for example as a result of radiation therapy or chemotherapy, may develop food distaste. These aversions tend to persist even after therapy has been completed. Nutritional deficiencies or excesses may occur in patients who decide to avoid certain foods because of misplaced beliefs that they may contribute to the genesis of cancer, or in case of excessive consumption based on the false expectation of beneficial effects.

Although the reduction in nutritional intake seems the main cause of nutritional decay, it cannot entirely explain the progressive loss of weight that often occurs despite an apparently adequate nutritional intake.

Other mechanisms have been suggested, such as the followings: an abnormal adaptation to fasting, with an increase rather than a decrease in catabolism; the cancer invasion of the host tissue during the process of tumoral growth; the alteration of intermediary metabolism.

In general, the tumor is usually considered too small to have a significant effect of metabolic absorption so as to produce the decay of the host; nonetheless, the presence of a tumor may also induce alterations in the metabolism of carbohydrates, fats and proteins increasing, as a consequence, the energy demands.

Depending on the clinical setting, an adequate caloric intake should be 1.2-1.5 times the resting energy consumption (30-35 kcal / kg / day). Lower values should be considered at risk of malnutrition. A caloric intake below 50% of the needs for a period of at least a week poses the need for an artificial nutritional intervention.

Leucine, isoleucine and valine are part of the family of neutral amino acids, and their oral supplementation, at a dosage of about 10-20 g / day, has proved to be effective in improving anorexia (through their ability to reduce the entry of tryptophan in the brain, and therefore the synthesis of serotonin) and, at the same time, promote muscle protein synthesis, at the expense of degradation processes.

The omega-3 fatty acids, in particular eicosapentaenoic acid (EPA), having an anti-inflammatory effect and inhibiting the synthesis of several pro-inflammatory cytokines, have been showed to have, at a dosage of at least 2 g / day, an efficacy equal to that of megestrol acetate in improving the appetite of cancer patients. Such lipid substrates are also able to mitigate the ubiquitin-dependent protein degradation mechanism in a direct way or through an indirect modulation of the action of pro-inflammatory cytokines. Studies dating back to a few years ago seemed to demonstrate that the administration of specific nutritive supplements enriched in proteins and EPA could result in a significant increase of body weight, lean body mass, functional activity and quality of life in patients with pancreas cancer, provided that the daily intake of EPA was not inferior to 2g. A recent meta-analysis conducted on five controlled clinical trials showed that there are insufficient data confirming that supplementation with EPA as a single oral agent is advantageous compared to placebo for therapeutical purposes. However, recent experiences seem to show a significant advantage of EPA supplementation after esophageal surgery.

It seems more appropriate to administer these supplements with a preventive goal, rather than therapeutic, as part of a process of metabolic-nutritional follow-up, supervised by specialists in the field of nutrition.

Carnitine plays a decisive role in the metabolism of long-chain free fatty acids, thus affecting lipid metabolism and energy reserves within the cells. Carnitine is a necessary cofactor for the transport of long-chain fatty acids within the mitochondrial matrix, where they are subjected to oxidation for the production of cellular energy.

A clinical study has shown that administration of 6 g/day of L-carnitine for the duration of 30 days was able to significantly improve the symptom "fatigue", appetite and lean body mass of patients. Therefore, the administration of L-carnitine should be recommended in cachectic patients at a dose of 4-6 g/day orally for a period of time of 3/4 months, being usually well tolerated by the patient. Occasional side effects of L-carnitine include epigastralgia and, more rarely, diarrhea. [97, 100]

After cancer treatment, weight gain or loss should be managed with a combination of diet changes, physical activity, and behavioral strategies. For patients who need to gain weight, this means increasing energy intake to exceed energy expenditure, while for patients who need to lose weight, caloric intake should be reduced while increasing energy expenditure via increased physical activity to exceed energy intake. Reducing the energy density of the diet by recommending low-energy foods (eg, water- and fiber-rich vegetables and fruits) and limiting the intake of foods and beverages rich in fat and added sugars promotes healthy weight control. Likewise, limiting portion sizes of energy-dense foods is an important accompanying strategy. [101]

Two large randomized controlled trials have tested whether a reduction in fat intake following the diagnosis of early stage breast cancer may affect cancer outcomes. The WINS study tested a low-fat diet (aiming for less than 15% of total caloric intake from fat) in 2437 postmenopausal women with early stage breast cancer and found an effect on relapse-free survival that was of borderline statistical significance.[102]

On average, patients in the intervention group decreased their fat intake to 20% of total caloric intake during the first year of the study, and the intervention resulted in a 24% reduction in new breast cancer events, with subset analyses suggesting that this effect was greater among women with ER-negative disease.

As previously described, women assigned to the low-fat diet (intervention group) lost an average of 6 pounds over the course of the study, thus posing the dilemma as to whether the reduction in breast cancer events was due to dietary fat restriction or lower body weight.

The Women's Healthy Eating and Living (WHEL) Study tested the effect of a diet low in fat (aiming for 20% of total caloric intake) and very high in vegetables, fruits, and fiber on cancer outcomes in 3088 pre- and postmenopausal breast cancer survivors who were followed for an average of 7.3 years. After 4 years, women in the intervention group reported a reduction in fat intake (from 31.3% at enrollment to 26.9% of total caloric intake), but recurrence-free survival did not differ between the two groups. [103] Notably, women in the WHEL Study intervention group did not exhibit weight loss, in contrast to the low-fat diet intervention group in WINS. The WHEL Study recorded an improved prognosis in women without hot flashes at time of study enrollment, who were therefore likely to have higher circulating estrogen concentrations, suggesting that there may be a survival benefit in this subgroup. [104]

The maintenance of an adequate body weight is possible in our experience using a special composed Mediterranean food which is precooked and conveniently formulated (Eatarte & Corpo53 Italy) allowing a reduction of body mass index, a reduction in chronic inflammation indices, a decreased risk of lymph edema and a decreased risk of pathological fractures (being thus ultimately associated with an improvement in pain and quality of life).

The general benefits of multimodal physical activity in cancer treatment are numerous and include: improved cardiac output, increased ventilation, improved flexibility and range of motion; increased muscular strength and endurance; decreased resting heart rate; improved stroke volume, vasodilatation, perfusion; improved metabolism; improved blood count parameters; improved psychological attitude and ability to face the cancer disease. The cancer-specific benefits are related to cancer treatment toxicities, with particular regard to muscular degeneration, including 1) fatigue and weakness, 2) neurotoxicity, 3) cardiotoxicity, 4) pulmonary toxicity. [105]

The main goal of exercise is to address inactivity/immobility (specific or general) and fear of movement. The detrimental effects of immobilization are well documented and include muscle wasting/weakness, joint stiffness, reduced motor control, mood changes, decreased self-efficacy, reduced coping capacity and cardiovascular unconditioning. The multimodal exercise program must be tailored to the individual needs of the patient and should start cautiously, building up gradually and being within the patient's tolerance levels.

A recent meta-analysis of 78 exercise intervention trials showed that exercise interventions resulted in clinically meaningful improvements in quality of life that persisted after the completion of the intervention. [106] In another meta-analysis of 44 studies that included over 3000 participants with varying cancer types, cancer survivors randomized to an exercise intervention had significantly reduced cancer related fatigue levels, with evidence of a linear relationship with the intensity of resistance exercise. [107]

Historically, there were concerns that cancer patients with upper extremity lymphedema should not engage in upper extremity resistance training or vigorous aerobic physical activity. There are now multiple trials that have demonstrated that such physical activity is not only safe, but actually reduces the incidence and severity of lymph edema.

There is substantial research on physical activity in breast cancer survivors and multiple systematic reviews focused on its role in these patient subset. [108, 109]

In a meta-analysis of 717 breast cancer survivors participating in 14 randomized controlled trials, physical activity led to statistically significant improvements in quality of life, physical functioning, and peak oxygen consumption, as well as reduction in symptoms of fatigue and pain. [110, 111]

Multimodal physical activity entails instructing patients in strengthening, stretching, and aerobic conditioning. The physical therapists should play a role in providing education on proper body mechanics, lifting techniques, proper posture, benefits of aerobic exercise and discussions of pain behaviors. Importantly, physical measures should be implemented as early as possible to minimize the generalized unconditioning and myofascial pain associated with reduced activity as well as intervals of immobility associated with cancer and its therapy. [112]

The benefits of exercise and increased physical activity among people diagnosed with cancer are numerous, including improved function, quality of life, strength, and endurance, and reduced depression, nausea, and pain. [113] Beaton et al, [114] in their systematic review found strong, high-quality evidence in favor of exercise interventions (aerobic exercises and strength training given alone or as part of a multimodal physical therapy program) in patients with metastatic cancer for improving physical and quality of life measures. McNeely et al, [115] found that a progressive resisted exercise training (PRET) program significantly reduced shoulder pain and disability and improved upper extremity muscular strength and endurance in postsurgical head and neck cancer survivors who had shoulder dysfunction due to spinal accessory nerve damage.

Keays et al [116] found improvements in shoulder range of motion and function in women with breast cancer undergoing radiation therapy, by virtue of a Pilates exercise program involving whole body movements with breath control. Similar improvements in pain and mobility were observed following physiotherapy intervention (exercises, soft tissue massage to surgical scar) in breast cancer patients who underwent axillary dissection. [117]

http://dx.doi.org/10.5772/60548

Graded and regular physical activity as a component of a multimodal physical activity program for the treatment of cancer pain [118] exerts a direct influence on the peripheral musculoskeletal system via the exercising muscles. Importantly, for these programs to be effective, physical activity should be always accompanied by behavioral training and adequate patient education.

Recovery of joint mobility and flexibility and treatment of soft tissue should be achieved through a strategy taking in to account age, sex and underlying disease as well as the intensity of the pain threshold. Additional treatment goals should include increased muscle tone of the healthy fibers as well as re-balancing muscle synergies and reprogramming both static and dynamic posture. Flexibility, one of the physiological parameters involved in almost all forms of human movement, is another trainable fitness parameter in addition to aerobic capacity, strength, and neuromuscular endurance.

Flexibility has been defined as mobility compliance or, alternatively, as the reciprocal counterpart of stiffness. Most of the authors define flexibility as range of motion either at or about a joint. Another definition classifies flexibility as the ability of a joint to move throughout its potential range of motion. Those definitions confuse the property of flexibility with the range of motion, despite the fact that these two terms are not synonymous; range of motion is one of the several variables determining flexibility, so that flexibility cannot be defined based only on range of motion.

We define flexibility like the disposition of body tissues to allow, without injury, excursions at a joint or set of joints. This property is measured through, but is not equivalent to, range of motion. Both joint tissues and the surrounding soft tissues contribute to flexibility, although only the latter should be targeted by specific treatment in order to augment flexibility.

The best method to properly stretch soft tissues involves a series of less than maximal isometric contractions of the agonist muscles in a pre-lengthened state (to set up the stretch), followed by concentric contractions of the antagonist muscle group (to lengthen the agonist) in conjunction with light pressure whenever needed and using an instrumentation like sensitized postural bench system (TecnoBody, Italy). This approach aims to alleviate muscle tension, facilitate healing via increased blood flow, and decrease muscle pain by reducing vasoconstriction. This stretching protocol should be delivered on a daily basis using a specific personalized postural bench like Fleximat postural bench (Posturale.org Italy).

Myofascial therapy improves local circulation and gently stimulates the free nerve endings, also helping draining local tissue edema and inducing local and general relaxation. One of the well-established scientific forms of massage is the manual lymphatic drainage therapy [119] and the complete decongestive therapy (i.e. combination of manual lymphatic drainage, compression garments, adequate skin care, and range of motion exercises). Massage therapy was shown to be very effective to relieve symptoms of cancer-induced pain in numerous studies. Soft tissue mobilization is widely practiced in the management of pain and includes techniques such as scar mobilization/massage, myofascial techniques and connective tissue massage. [120, 121]

Reeves [122] emphasized the relevance of changes in patient positioning, relaxation techniques against insomnia, and energy conservation techniques for chronic fatigue in patients with cancer pain.

Therapeutic modalities such as electrical stimulation (including transcutaneous electrical neurostimulation), heat, or cryotherapy, can be useful adjuncts to standard analgesic therapy in patients with cancer-treatment-related lymphedema and pain. The treatment of lymphedema by use of wraps, pressure stockings, or pneumatic pump devices with Slim Project Physio (General Project Italy) or vibrational technology with EndoSpheres (Fenix group Italy) may both improve function and relieve pain and heaviness. [123]

Physical therapy treatment techniques have also been reported to be effective in cancer-related fatigue by Watson and Mock, in prostate cancer and breast cancer-related lymphedema, cancer therapy-related hyperthermia, and colorectal cancer. [124]

Mufazalov and Gazizov [125] showed that laser therapy enhanced therapeutic efficacy of pain-relieving drug regimens in patients with cancer pain. Cancer treatments like radiation therapy can induce mucositis in patients with oral or head and neck cancer and can cause oral pain due to impaired wound healing. Bensadoun [126] commented on the importance of low-level laser therapy on wound healing and its role in mucositis treatments. Maiya et al, [127] subsequently showed that helium–neon laser therapy was effective to reduce pain and improve healing of radiation-induced mucositis after 6 weeks of therapy in head and neck cancer patients.

Improvement of the uninjured muscle tone and strength may be possible using a focused vibratory acoustic Cancer Treatment - a conventional and innovative approach using stimulation at high intensity with Vissone (Vissman Italy) - followed by anaerobic work with TRX system.

Vibrations are able to induce muscular changes aimed to the recovery of muscle tone through a frequency of 300 Hz, as well as to stimulate the upper motors centers in order to obtain a control of muscle recruitment work.

It has been noted that, using this treatment protocol, it is possible to: 1) activate the aerobic metabolism; 2) determine an analgesic effect; 3) increase local circulation and bone density; 4) finally increase the contractile capacity and elasticity of the treated muscle.

According to the existing literature, mechanic or acoustic vibratory waves at a frequency of 120Hz are a valid therapeutic tool for the treatment of musculoskeletal pain. The focused vibratory acoustic therapy with quadrangle wave shows a muscle relaxing effect, leading to a rapid interruption of the vicious circuit pain-injury-pain as well as a having a high draining, anti-fatigue and stress relieving effect. [128]

Human studies regarding ultra low frequencies and intensity magnetic fields effects have been carried out in several clinical settings over the last 20 years.

They have proven effective for treating bone and joint diseases, neuropathies, spinal cord injury, diabetic neuropathy, immune disorders and cardio myopathy. [129, 134]

Moreover, in addition to the above data, new possible fields of application have been advanced by studies showing possible effect in several specific neurological diseases. Sandik, for example, has published a number of case reports of diseases such as Parkinson's [135]

Alzheimer's disease [136] and Multiple Sclerosis [137], in which a beneficial effect of the fields ELF on cognitive deficits accompanying these morbid conditions has been documented. Another study [138] reported interesting effects on fatigue and quality of life of 117 patients with Multiple Sclerosis. An additional area of research in which there are promising studies is that of analgesia. [139]

The term bio-resonance points to the form of resonance which is established at the level of cell membranes using electromagnetic fields at a very low intensity and at a specific frequency (cyclotron) which is thought to be able to influence and stimulate the metabolism of human cells by adjusting the ordered traffic of selected ions between the internal and external environments of the cell and by stimulating the activity of those ion-dependent enzymes allowing the occurrence of several biological reactions. The above technology generates electromagnetic waves of low intensity and frequency, (Seqex Q.L.. S.i.s.t.e.m.i. Italy) allowing a particular ion current that optimizes the intrinsic ability of maintaining the potential difference between the intra and extracellular environments and which is thought to be indispensable for the proper functioning of metabolism and cellular homeostasis. [140]

One of the most promising fields of application for such technology is undoubtedly the oncological sector; accordingly, it has been observed that a correct use of ELF fields may lead to a reduction of tumor growth and vascularization as well as of the metastatic spread. [141, 142]

The accumulation of lactic acid in cancer tissues is a well-known source of pain. Studying the metabolism of cancer at the cellular level, Otto Warburg demonstrated in 1930 that tumor cells prefer a particular form of metabolism known as anaerobic (non-oxygen-dependent) glycolysis. Indeed, tumor cells are metabolically active and release several waste products. [143]

The ability to modulate the channels of the membrane by the above-mentioned magnetic fields allows the hypothesis that cancer pain, secondary to oxidative stress, may be controlled through the arousal of appropriate currents of cations and anions.

In particular, it is of particular interest the possibility to modulate the water channels, whose opening would allow the efflux of intracellular water. Inflammatory processes in the cells of the muscle or dermis leads to significant water retention (as shown by visible swelling). This water absorption and swelling, which is thought to be linked to associated painful symptoms, may persist over time (as occurs, for example, after the welding of bone fractures). Accordingly, the induction of the opening of membrane channels allowing the leakage of intracellular water might enable rapid resolution of swelling and pain due to excess intracellular water. [144]

11.2. Sensory-motor and functional recovery capacity

The second phase begins with the clinical physiatrist reassessment, aided by specific diagnostic tests and apposite rating scales, analysis of movement and posture through optoelectronic systems in collaboration with bioengineers, gait analysis with pod barometrical examination, body composition assessment through bio-impedenziometry, and evaluation of cardiac and hematological parameters.

To implement an adequate sensory-motor and functional recovery program the patient needs to reach an acceptable walking ability. The ability to walk is the key to any human movement, despite the fact the human movements are not limited to bipedal locomotion; bipedal locomotion is a fundamental part of daily life and is a prominent target of public health physical activity guidelines.

The human gait is a complex combination of concerted movements; objective monitoring of walking evolution, using pedometer and accelerometer technologies, offers an opportunity to formulate guidelines and recommendations for cancer patients.

Available studies in literature have used a variety of objective parameters based on instruments that have been previously validated.

In order to get a better walking performance, two integrate procedures may be implemented:

1. normalization of the foot-ground reaction forces using customized viscoelastic orthotics to control vertical and shear forces on the foot during the stance phase with no need for the obligatory use of athletic shoes;

2. use of the microgravitary system S.P.A.D (Corpo53, Italy) that determine the sensory-motor and functional recovery of the posture during the walking activity in combination to the development of proprioceptive information trasmitted from the periphery to the cortical central system.

After a period of unconditioning typical of the acute phase of cancer, it is necessary to learn again the correct body schema and achieve the complete recovery of postural control through spinal rehabilitation with floating platforms in tridimensional space and visual feedback. It is important to attempt correction of such postural abnormalities early in the rehabilitation process in order to prevent further dysfunctional patterns of movement. [145]

For example, breast cancer patients may develop chronic post-surgical pain following breast cancer treatment (Macrae, 2001) and, thus, adopt specific protective postures resulting in muscle spasm and muscle imbalances (Cheville & Tchou, 2007). Growing evidence is being produced in support for the use of Progressive Resistive Exercise training in head and neck cancer patients, in order to manage shoulder dysfunction and pain secondary to spinal accessory nerve damage. The importance of correcting posture and scapular stability prior to resistance exercise has been documented by McNeely et al (2004).

The system I-Moove is equipped with a balancing platform with helical movement which allow the continuous realignment of the subsystems of the body in order to maintain an optimal posture as well as the use of a traction force. It also provides a real-time visual feedback that allows physicians to monitor the correction. [146]

11.3. Quality of life improvement

The inclusive approach entails therapeutic techniques implemented by physical therapists to improve the quality of life, including: EMG Biofeedback, home therapy-related imagery with Riablo-System (coRehab Italy), music therapy, play therapy, virtual reality- and exercise. The

http://dx.doi.org/10.5772/60548

environment was shown to influence perceived well-being with outdoor exercises being perceived as energizing and indoor exercises being perceived as relaxing; furthermore, Qigong exercises has been shown to have positive effects on mood and anxiety. [147]

Attention-diversion approaches involve redirecting attention to competing external or internal stimuli, with related strategies including relaxation training, diaphragmatic breathing, guided imagery, self-hypnosis, mindfulness meditation and distracting thoughts and activities (Hanson, 1990). Engaging in meaningful and stimulating activities, for example talking to friends, listening to music and going outdoors, may reduce awareness of pain. Using methods deriving from cognitive therapy, patients are taught how to identify and change unhelpful or negative thoughts (cognitive restructuring) that contribute to psychological distress, while facilitating coping thoughts that reduce distress and enhance other coping efforts. Occupational therapists can help patient to maintain or resume their previous social role despite cancer-related pain. Occupational or Physiotherapists' role in this context encompasses active listening, education, prevention, problem solving, and provision of experiential learning.

A controversial aspect is the role of rehabilitation in patients with pain from bone metastases.

Patients with skeletal metastases may have a relatively long clinical course. Coleman and Rubens determined that the median duration of survival for 498 patients with metastatic breast cancer with first relapse in bone was 20 months.

In 253 of these patients, where disease spread was confined to the bone, the median duration of survival was even longer (24 months).

Rehabilitative intervention to optimize the functional capacity of patients with smoldering bone metastases is often needed. Such intervention is frequently aimed at preventing patients from becoming bed-bound and helping them to maintain as much autonomy as possible.

Treatment sessions commonly focus on training the patient to use residual function or to develop compensatory techniques, training in the use of assistive equipment, and educating both patient and family to help them adjust to an altered way of life. [148]

12. Conclusion

The management of cancer pain with a planning of a complex rehabilitation program, in the context of a comprehensive treatment, encompasses nutritional support, multimodal training, correction of lifestyle, as well as use of advanced physical energies. Therefore, for the purposes of the optimal management of cancer pain, it is essential to identify the pathogenetic features and the clinical characteristics of pain, in order to tailor the different treatment modalities in rehabilitation. Terminal patients should have access to rehabilitation services and be encouraged to remain functional and independent.

Clinical experience suggests that the application of the fundamental principles of rehabilitation medicine is likely to improve the care of patients with cancer.

A specialist in the identification, evaluation, and rehabilitation of neuromuscular, musculoskeletal, and functional disorders associated with cancer and its treatment should aim to the restoration and maintenance of function and quality of life.

Too often physicians tend to limit the treatment of pain in cancer patients to a pharmacological approach, tailored according to the severity of the symptoms as per the guidelines of the OMS.

A global and complex rehabilitation program may decrease the need for pharmacological medications and the occurrence of related side effects.

While oncologists are responsible for prolonging survival and nurses and counselors for optimizing comfort, the physical therapists play a major role in optimizing functions in patients suffering from cancer pain.

Physiatrist and physical therapists should thus be part of the team taking care of the integrated cancer management in primary, secondary and tertiary care, with a particular role being played with regard to cancer pain.

Molecular mechanisms in pain perception will direct mechanism-based drug therapy prescription in palliative care, whereas understanding of pain pathogenesis will direct physical therapy treatment, allowing proper decision-making and efficient treatment delivery in patients with cancer pain.

Despite being unquestionable that the primary goal in cancer patients management should be to prolong the overall survival, treatment of cancer pain is important in order to preserve daily functions and quality of life.

The development of an evidence-based body of knowledge will ensure that patients receive appropriate rehabilitation interventions in cancer pain.

Future research should, thus, focus on a better understanding of the role of rehabilitation and on defining appropriate interventions for this patient population.

Author details

Raoul Saggini[1*], Rosa Grazia Bellomo[2], Simona Maria Carmignano[3] and Andrea Saggini[4,5]

*Address all correspondence to: saggini@unich.it

1 Department of Neuroscience and Imaging, "G. d'Annunzio" University, Chieti, Italy

2 Department of Medicine and Science of Aging, "G. d'Annunzio" University, Chieti, Italy

3 School of Specialties in PRM, "G. d'Annunzio" University, Chieti, Italy

4 Pathology, University of California San Francisco, San Francisco, California, USA

5 Department of Dermatology, University of Rome Tor Vergata, Rome, Italy

References

[1] Rustoen T, Fossa SD, Skarstein J, Moum T. The impact of demographic and disease-specific variables on pain in cancer patients. J Pain Symptom Manage 2003;26(2):696–704.

[2] Beck SL, Falkson G. Prevalence and management of cancer pain in South Africa. Pain 2001;94(1):75–84.

[3] Strohbuecker B, Mayer H, Evers GC, Sabatowski R. Pain prevalence in hospitalized patients in a German university teaching hospital. J Pain Symptom Manage 2005;29(5):498–506.

[4] van den Beuken-van, Everdingen MH, de Rijke JM, Kessels AG, Schouten HC, van Kleef M, Patijn J. Prevalence of pain in patients with cancer: a systematic review of the past 40 years. Ann Oncol 2007;18(9):1437–49.

[5] Goldberg DS, McGee SJ. Pain as a global public health priority. BMC Public Health 2011;11:770.

[6] Siegel R, Naishadham D, Ahmedin J. Cancer statistics, 2013. CA CANCER J CLIN 2013;63:11–30.

[7] Pargeon KL, Hailey B Jo. Barriers to Effective Cancer Pain Management: A Review of the Literature. Journal of Pain and Symptom Management 1999; Pages 358–368.

[8] Oldenmengera WH, Sillevis Smittc PAE, van Doorena S, Stotera G, van der Rijta CCD. A systematic review on barriers hindering adequate cancer pain management and interventions to reduce them: A critical appraisal. European Journal of Cancer 2009; 1370 – 1380.

[9] Brescia FJ, Portenoy RK, Ryan M, Krasnoff L, Gray G. Pain, opioid use, and survival in hospitalized patients with advanced cancer. J Clin Oncol 1992; 10:149–155.

[10] Maltoni M, Caraceni A. et al. Terapia del dolore in oncologia- linee guida AIOM, Milano, 2009.

[11] Schieroni MP, Merli P. Dolore Oncologico in Dolore e Riabilitazione. Edition Minerva Medica 2014.

[12] Fallon M, Hanks G, Cherny N. Principles of control of cancer pain BMJ 2006; 332 http://dx.doi.org/10.1136/bmj.332.7548.1022 (accessed 27 April 2006).

[13] Pathophysiology of cancer pain and opioid tolerance. In: The British Pain Society's Cancer Pain Management. The British Pain Society website. www.britishpainsociety.org. (accessed 29 January 2013).

[14] Hjermasted MJ, Gibbins J. Pain assessment tools in palliative care: an urgent need for consensus. Palliative med 2008;22:895 -580.

[15] Turk DC, Dworkin RH, Allen RR, Bellamy N, Brandenburg N, Carr DB, Cleland C, Dionne R, Farrar JT, Galer BS, Hewitt DJ, Jadad AR, Katz NP, Kramer LD, Manning DC, McCormick CG, McDermott MP, McGrath P, Quessy S, Rappaport BA, Robinson JP, Royal MA, Simon L, Stauffer JW, Stein W, Tollett J, Witter J. Core outcome domains for chronic pain clinical trials: IMMPACT recommendations. Pain 2003;106:337-345.

[16] Maiello E. Italian Oncology Guidelines 2013-2014.

[17] Portenoy RK. Treatment of cancer pain. Lancet 2011;377:2236–47.

[18] Module 1 pain management. pathophysiology of pain and pain management. American Medical Association website. www.ama-cmeonline.com (accessed 29 January 2013).

[19] Davis MP. Drug management of visceral pain: concepts from basic research. Pain Res Treat 2012; 2012:265605.

[20] Julius D, Basbaum AI. Molecular mechanisms of nociception. Nature 2001; 413:203–210.

[21] Sabato F. Dolore nocicettivo, neuropatico e infiammatorio in:Dolore e Riabilitazione. Edition Minerva Medica 2014.

[22] Galasko, CS. Diagnosis of skeletal metastases and assessment of response to treatment. Clin Orthop. 1995; 312, 64–75.

[23] Nadler, RB et al. IL-1β and TNF-α in prostatic secretions are indicators in the evaluation of men with chronic prostatitis. J.Urol 2000;164:214–218.

[24] Nielsen OS, Munro AJ, Tannock IF. Bone metastases: pathophysiology and management policy. J. Clin. Oncol 1991;9:509–24.

[25] Davar G. Endothelin-1 and metastatic cancer pain. Pain Med 2001; 2, 24–27.

[26] Nelson JB, Carducci MA. The role of endothelin-1 and endothelin receptor antagonists in prostate cancer. BJU Intern 2000; 85:45–48.

[27] De Leo JA, Yezierski RP. The role of neuroinflammation and neuroimmune activation in persistent pain. Pain 2001;1:90(1-2):1-6.

[28] Kawasaki Y, Zhang L, Cheng JK, Ji R.R. Cytokine Mechanisms of Central Sensitization: Distinct and Overlapping Role of Interleukin-1β, Interleukin-6, and Tumor Necrosis Factor-α in Regulating Synaptic and Neuronal Activity in the Superficial Spinal Cord. J Neurosci. 2008; 28(20): 5189–5194.

[29] Watkins LR, Goehler LE, Relton, J, Brewer, MT, Maier SF. Mechanisms of tumor necrosis factor-α (TNF-α) hyperalgesia. Brain Res. 1995; 692, 244–250.

[30] Christa M, Stoscheck Lloyd E, King Jr. Role of epidermal growth factor in carcinogenesis. Cancer Res. 1986;46:1030–1037.

[31] Poon RTP, Fan ST, Wong J. Clinical implications of circulating angiogenic factors in cancer patients. J. Clin. Oncol. 2001;19:1207–1225.

[32] Roman C, Saha DR, Beauchamp D.TGF-β and colorectal carcinogenesis. Microsc. Res. Tech. 2001; 52:450–457.

[33] Silver BJ. Platelet-derived growth factor in human malignancy. Biofactors 1992;3:217–227.

[34] Sameer A, John D, Lesley A, Judith A, Lindsay G, Nicola A, Xiao X, Robert C, Leah J, Timothy Adams E. Biochemical Characterization of Individual Human Glycosylated pro-Insulin-like Growth Factor (IGF)-II and big-IGF-II Isoforms Associated with Cancer J Biol Chem 2013;288(1): 59-68.

[35] Griffiths JR. Are cancer cells acidic? Br. J. Cancer 1991;64:425–427.

[36] Julius D, Basbaum AI. Molecular mechanisms of nociception. Nature 2001;413:203–210.

[37] Stephani P, Sean P, Edwin W. Chemical mediators of pain due to tissue damage and ischemia. Prog. Brain Res. 2000;129:21–38.

[38] Timothy H, Maureen S, Xilma, Robert R. An acid sensing ion channel (ASIC) localizes to small primary afferent neurons in rats. Neuroreport 1998; 9:1109–1113.

[39] Caterina MJ, Schumacher MA, Tominaga M, Rosen TA, Levine JD, Julius D. The capsaicin receptor: a heat-activated ion channel in the pain. Nature 1997;389: 816–824.

[40] Tominaga M, Caterina MJ, Malmberg AB, Rosen TA, Gilbert H, Skinner K, Raumann BE, Basbaum AI, Julius D. The cloned capsaicin receptor integrates multiple pain-producing stimuli. Neuron 1998; 21:531–543.

[41] Stephani P, Sean P, Edwin W. Chemical mediators of pain due to tissue damage and ischemia. Prog. Brain Res. 2000;129:21–38.

[42] Lingueglia E, de Weille JR, Bassilana F, Heurteaux C, Sakai H, Waldmann R, Lazdunski M. A modulatory subunit of acid sensing ion channels in brain and dorsal root ganglion cells. J. Biol. Chem. 1997; 272:29778–29783.

[43] Clohisy DR, Perkins SL, Ramnaraine ML. Review of cellular mechanisms of tumor osteolysis. Clin. Orthop. 2000; 373:104–114.

[44] Clohisy DR, Ramnaraine ML, Scully S, Qi M, Van G, Hong Lin T. Lacey DL. Osteoprotegerin inhibits tumor-induced osteoclastogenesis and bone growth in osteopetrotic mice. J. Orthop. 2000;18:967–976.

[45] Clohisy DR, Patrick F, Ramnaraine ML. Pamidronate decreases tumor-induced osteoclastogenesis in mice. J. Orthop. Res. 2001;19:554–558.

[46] Terada T, Matsunaga YS-100-positive nerve fibers in hepatocellular carcinoma and intrahepatic cholangiocarcinoma: an immunohistochemical study. Pathol. Int. 2001; 51:89–93.

[47] O'Connell JX, Nanthakumar SS, Nielsen GP, Rosenberg AE. Osteoid osteoma: the uniquely innervated bone tumor. Modern Pathol. 1998;11:175–180.

[48] Patrick W, Clohisy DR, Koltzenburg M, Hunt SP. Molecular mechanisms of cancer pain Nature Reviews Cancer 2002; 2:201-209.

[49] Peters CM, Ghilardi JR, Keyser CP, Kubota K, Lindsay TH, Luger NM, Mach DB, Schwei MJ, Sevcik MA, Mantyh PW Tumor-induced injury of primary afferent sensory nerve fibers in bone cancer pain. Exp Neurol. 2005;193(1):85-100.

[50] Lipton RB, Apfel SC, Dutcher JP, Rosenberg R, Kaplan J, Berger A, Einzig AI, Wiernik P, Schaumburg HH. Taxol produces a predominantly sensory neuropathy. Neurology 1989;39:368–373.

[51] Terada T, Matsunaga, Y.S-100-positive nerve fibers in hepatocellular carcinoma and intrahepatic cholangiocarcinoma: an immunohistochemical study. Pathol. Int. 2001;51:89–93.

[52] Polomano RC, Mannes AJ, Clark US, Bennett GJ. A painful peripheral neuropathy in the rat produced by the chemotherapeutic drug, paclitaxel. Pain 2001;94:293–304.

[53] van den Beuken-van Everdingen MH, de Rijke JM, Kessels AG, Schouten HC, van Kleef M, Patijn J. Prevalence of pain in patients with cancer: a systematic review of the past 40 years. Ann Oncol 2007;18:1437-49.

[54] Bertoldo F, Ripamonti C, Del Mastro L. Gestione dei sintomi artromialgici indotti dagli inibitori dell'aromatasi. In: Therapy Perspectives in Science Communications (Anno XIII, N.14). Roma 2010.

[55] Robustelli della Cuna G. Sindromi paraneoplastiche. In: Bonadonna G, Robustelli della Cuna G, Valagussa P. (ed.) Medicina oncologica. Milano: Elsevier-Masson; 2009. p1635.

[56] FAVO, Fondazione IRCCS, Health Organization of Cancer Units for Rehabilitation Activities. Libro bianco sulla riabilitazione oncologica. Napoli; 2008.

[57] Fornasari D. Pain mechanisms in patients with chronic pain. Clin Drug Investig 2012;32(1):45–52.

[58] Scott Fishman, Jane Ballantyne, James P. Rathmell. Bonica's Management of Pain. Lippincott Williams & Wilkins;2010.

[59] Fukamachi S, Furuta A, Ikeda T, Ikenoue T, Kaneoka T, Rothstein JD, Iwaki T. Altered expressions of glutamate transporter subtypes in rat model of neonatal cerebral hypoxia-ischemia. Brain Res. Dev. 2001;132:131–139.

[60] Rothstein JD, Martin LJ, Kuncl RW. Decreased glutamate transport by the brain and spinal cord in amyotrophic lateral sclerosis. N. Engl. J. Med. 1992;326:1464–1468.

[61] Laughlin TM, Todd WV, Lashbrook J, Nichols ML, Ossipov M, Porreca F, Wilcox GL. Spinally administered dynorphin. A produces long-lasting allodynia: involvement of NMDA but not opioid receptors. Pain 1997;72:253–260.

[62] Vanderah TW, Ossipov MH, Lai J, Malan TP, Porreca F. Mechanisms of opioid-induced pain and antinociceptive tolerance: descending facilitation and spinal dynorphin. Pain 2001;92:5–9.

[63] Kajander KC, SaharaY, Iadarola MJ, Bennett GJ. Dynorphin increases in the dorsal spinal cord in rats with a painful peripheral neuropathy. Peptides 1990;11:719–728.

[64] Iadarola MJ, Douglass J, Civelli O, Naranjo JR. Differential activation of spinal cord dynorphin and enkephalin neurons during hyperalgesia: evidence using cDNA hybridization. Brain Res.1988;455: 205–212.

[65] Portenoy RK, Dhingra LK. Assessment of cancer pain. In: Drews RE, ed. UpToDate. Waltham, MA: UpToDate; 2013.

[66] Bellomo RG. Il significato del dolore:il dolore acuto e cronico. In Saggini R, Buoso S, Pestelli G. (ed) Dolore e Riabilitazione. Minerva Medica; 2014.p29-41.

[67] National Comprehensive Cancer Network. Clinical Practice Guidelines in Oncology for Adult Cancer Pain. Fort Washington, PA: National Comprehensive Cancer Network; 2010. www.nccn. org. (accessed 1 November 2010).

[68] Davies AN, Dickman A, Reid C, Stevens AM, Zeppetella G. The management of cancer-related breakthrough pain: Recommendations of a task group of the Science Committee of the Association for Palliative Medicine of Great Britain and Ireland European Journal of Pain 2009;331–338.

[69] Gordon DB, Dahl JL, Miaskowski C, McCarberg B, Todd KH, Judith A. Paice, Lipman AG, Bookbinder M, Sanders SH. Turk DC., Carr DB. American Pain Society Recommendations for Improving the Quality of Acute and Cancer Pain Management Arch Intern Med. 2005;165(14):1574-1580.

[70] Ferrer-Brechner T. The management of pain associated with malignancy. Semin Anesth 1985;4:313-22.

[71] Levy MH. Integration of pain management into comprehensive cancer care. Cancer 1989;63:Suppl:2328-35.

[72] Jacox A, Carr DB, Payne R. Management of cancer pain: clinical practice guideline. Rockville, Md.: Agency for Health Care Policy and Research. AHCPR 1994;94-0592.

[73] Cherny NI, Portenoy RK. The management of cancer pain. CA Cancer J Clin. 1994;44:263-303.

[74] World Health Organization. Cancer pain relief and palliative care: report of a WHO expert committee. WHO Tech Rep Ser. 1990;804:1-73..

[75] Schug SA, Zech D, Dorr U. Cancer pain management according to WHO analgesic guidelines. J Pain Symptom Manage 1990;5:27-32.

[76] Ventafridda V, Caraceni A, Gamba A. Field-testing of the WHO guidelines for cancer pain relief: summary report of demonstration projects. In: Foley KM, Bonica JJ, Ventafridda V, eds. Proceedings of the Second International Congress of Cancer Pain. Vol. 16 of Advances in pain research and therapy. New York: Raven Press, 1990:451-64.

[77] Jacox A, Carr DB, Payne R, et al. Management of cancer pain: clinical practice guideline. Rockville, Md.: Agency for Health Care Policy and Research. AHCPR 1994;94-0592.

[78] Cherny NI, Portenoy RK: The management of cancer pain. CA Cancer J Clin Review 1994;44:263-303.

[79] Jadad AR, Browman GP. The WHO Analgesic Ladder for Cancer Pain Management Stepping Up the Quality of Its Evaluation JAMA. 1995;274(23):1870-1873.

[80] American Pain Society. Principles of analgesic use in the treatment of acute pain and chronic cancer pain. ed. Skokie, American Pain Society Ill;1999.

[81] Galer BS, Coyle N, Pasternak GW, Portenoy RK. Individual variability in the response to different opioids: report of five cases. Pain 1992;49:87-91.

[82] de Stoutz ND, Bruera E, Suarez-Almazor M. Opioid rotation for toxicity reduction in terminal cancer patients. J Pain Symptom Manage 1995; 10:378-84.

[83] Levy MH. Pharmacologic management of cancer pain. Semin Oncol 1994;21:718-39.

[84] Harden, R Norman MD. Chronic Neuropathic Pain: Mechanisms, Diagnosis, and Treatment. Neurologist: 2005 journals.lww.com.

[85] Jacox A, Carr DB, Payne R, et al. Management of cancer pain: clinical practice guideline. Rockville, Md.: Agency for Health Care Policy and Research. AHCPR 1994;94-0592.

[86] Armento G, Tonin G. Palliative care and models for integrated medicine. The National Cancer Institute of Milan and the Campus Bio-Medico University of Rome: a comparison MEDIC 2014; 22(1): 32-36.

[87] Black JF, Kishner S. Cancer and Rehabilitation. http://emedicine.medscape.com/article/320261-overview.

[88] Paice JA, Ferrell B. The Management of Cancer Pain CA CANCER J CLIN 2011;61:157–182.

[89] Schattner M, Shike M. Nutrition support of the patient with cancer. In: Shils ME, Shike M, Ross AC, Cabellero B, Cousins RJ, eds. Modern Nutrition in Health and Disease. 10th ed. Philadelphia, PA:Lippincott Williams & Wilkins; 2006:1290-1313.

[90] Rock CL, Colleen Doyle MS, Demark-Wahnefried W, Meyerhardt J, Courneya KS.Schwartz AL, Bandera Elisa V, Hamilton KK, Grant B, McCullough M, Byers T, Gansler T. Nutrition and Physical Activity Guidelines for Cancer Survivors CA CANCER J CLIN 2012;62:242-274.

[91] Pekmezi DW, Demark-Wahnefried W. Updated evidence in support of diet and exercise interventions in cancer survivors. Acta Oncol. 2011;50:167-178.

[92] Chlebowski RT, Aiello E, McTiernan A. Weight loss in breast cancer patient management. J Clin Oncol. 2002;20:1128-1143.

[93] Schattner M, Shike M. Nutrition support of the patient with cancer. In: Shils ME, Shike M, Ross AC, Cabellero B, Cousins RJ, eds. Modern Nutrition in Health and Disease. 10th ed. Philadelphia, PA: Lippincott 2006:1290-1313.

[94] McMahon K, Brown JK. Nutritional screening and assessment. Semin Oncol Nurs. 2000;16:106-112.

[95] Inui A. Cancer anorexia-cachexia syndrome: current issues in research and management. CA Cancer J Clin. 2002;52:72-91.

[96] Ravasco P, Monteiro-Grillo I, Vidal PM. Dietary counseling improves patient outcomes: a prospective, randomized, controlled trial in colorectal cancer patients undergoing radiotherapy. J Clin Oncol. 2005;23:1431-8.

[97] Muscaritoli M, Costelli P, Aversa Z. New strategies to overcome cancer cachexia: from molecular mechanisms to the 'Parallel Pathway' Asia Pac J Clin Nutr 2008;17 (S1):387-390 387.

[98] Dewey A, Baughan C, Dean T, Higgins B, Johnson I. Eicosapentaenoic acid (EPA, an omega-3 fatty acid from fish oils) for the treatment of cancer cachexia. Cochrane Database Syst Rev. 2007;(1):CD004597.

[99] Silvério R, Laviano A, Rossi Fanelli F, Seelaender M. L-carnitine and cancer cachexia: Clinical and experimental aspects Cachexia Sarcopenia Muscle. 2011; 2(1): 37–44.

[100] W. C. Willett. Diet and cancer. Oncologist. 2000;.5:393–404.

[101] Saggini R, Calvani M. The Treatment of Cancer: A Comprehensive Therapeutic Model Entailing a Complex of Interaction Modalities. http://dx.doi.org/10.5772/55696 (accesed from Dicember 2013).

[102] Ibrahim EM, Al-Homaidh A. Physical activity and survival after breast cancer diagnosis: meta-analysis of published studies. Med Oncol. 2011;28:753-765.

[103] Ferrer RA, Huedo-Medina TB, Johnson BT, Ryan S, Pescatello LS. Exercise interventions for cancer survivors: a meta-analysis of quality of life outcomes. Ann Behav Med. 2011;41:32-47.

[104] John P. Diet and Breast Cancer Prognosis: Making Sense of the WHEL and WINS Trials.Curr Opin Obstet Gynecol. 2009; 21(1): 86–91.

[105] Saggini R, Calvani M. The Treatment of Cancer: A Comprehensive Therapeutic Model Entailing a Complex of Interaction Modalities. http://dx.doi.org/10.5772/55696 (accesed from Dicember 2013).

[106] Ibrahim EM, Al-Homaidh A. Physical activity and survival after breast cancer diagnosis: meta-analysis of published studies. Med Oncol. 2011;28:753-765.

[107] Brown JC, Huedo-Medina TB, Pescatello LS, Pescatello SM, Ferrer RA, Johnson BT. Efficacy of exercise interventions in modulating cancer-related fatigue among adult cancer survivors: a meta-analysis. Cancer Epidemiol Biomarkers Prev. 2011;20:123-133

[108] McNeely ML, Campbell KL, Rowe BH, Klassen TP, Mackey JR, Courneya KS. Effects of exercise on breast cancer patients and survivors: a systematic review and metaanalysis.CMA J. 2006;175:34-41.

[109] Chlebowski RT, Blackburn GL, Thomson CA, et al. Dietary fat reduction and breast cancer outcome: interim efficacy results from the Women's Intervention Nutrition Study. J Natl Cancer Inst. 2006;98:1767-1776.

[110] Pierce JP, Natarajan L, Caan BJ, et al. Influence of a diet very high in vegetables, fruit, and fiber and low in fat on prognosis following treatment for breast cancer: the Women's Healthy Eating and Living (WHEL) randomized trial. JAMA. 2007;298:289-298.

[111] Gold EB, Pierce JP, Natarajan L, et al. Dietary pattern influences breast cancer prognosis in women without hot flashes: the women's healthy eating and living trial. J Clin Oncol. 2009;27:352-359.

[112] Hooten WM, Timming R, Belgrade M, Gaul J, Goertz M, Haake B, Myers C, Noonan MP, Owens J, Saeger L, Schweim K, Shteyman G, Walker N. Institute for Clinical Systems Improvement. Assessment and Management of Chronic Pain. Updated November 2013.

[113] Barbaric M, Brooks E, Moore L, Cheifetz O. Effects of physical activity on cancer survival: A systematic review. Physiother Can. 2010;62:25–34

[114] Beaton R, Pagdin-Friesen W, Robertson C, Vigar C, Watson H, Harris SR. Effects of exercise intervention on persons with metastatic cancer: A systematic review. Physiother Can. 2009;61:141–53.

[115] McNeely ML, Parliament MB, Seikaly H, Jha N, Magee DJ, Haykowsky MJ, et al. Effect of exercise on upper extremity pain and dysfunction in head and neck cancer survivors: A randomized controlled trial. Cancer. 2008;113:214–22.

[116] Keays KS, Harris SR, Lucyshyn JM, MacIntyre DL. Effects of Pilates exercises on shoulder range of motion, pain, mood, and upper extremity function in women living with breast cancer: A pilot study. Phys Ther. 2008;88:494–510.

[117] Beaton R, Pagdin-Friesen W, Robertson C, Vigar C, Watson H, Harris SR. Effects of exercise intervention on persons with metastatic cancer: A systematic review. Physiother Can. 2009;61:141–53.

[118] Beurskens CH, van Uden CJ, Strobbe LJ, Oostendorp RA, Wobbes T. The efficacy of physiotherapy upon shoulder function following axillary dissection in breast cancer, a randomized controlled study. BMC Cancer. 2007;7:166.

[119] Guilherme-Soares L, Chan VW. The rationale for a multimodal approach in the management of breakthrough cancer pain: A review. Am J Hosp Palliat Care. 2007;24:430–9.

[120] Osaka I, Kurihara Y, Tanaka K, Nishizaki H, Aoki S, Adachi I. Endocrinological evaluations of brief hand massages in palliative care. J Altern Complement Med. 2009;15:981–5.

[121] Puthusseril V. Special foot massage as a complimentary therapy in palliative care. Indian J Palliat Care.2006;12:71–7.

[122] Reeves K. A cancer pain primer. Medsurg Nurs 2006;17:413-9.

[123] Hughes D, Ladas E, Rooney D, Kelly K. Massage Therapy as a Supportive Care Intervention for Children With Cancer Oncology Nursing 2008; 35(3): 431-442.

[124] Cherny NI, Portenoy RK. The management of cancer pain. CA Cancer J Clin 1994;44:262-303.

[125] Mufazalov FF, Gazizov AA. Laser therapy for chronic pain in cancer patients. Vopr Onkol.2002;48:91–4.

[126] Kumar SP, Anand J. Physical Therapy in Palliative Care: From Symptom Control to Quality of Life: A Critical Review. Indian J Palliative Care 201;16(3)-138-146

[127] Maiya GA, Sagar MS, Fernandes D. Effect of low level helium-neon (He-Ne) laser therapy in the prevention and treatment of radiation induced mucositis in head and neck cancer patients. Indian J Med Res.2006;124:399–402.

[128] Saggini R, Carmignano SM. La Meccano-trasduzione In Saggini R, Buoso S, Pestelli G. (ed) Dolore e Riabilitazione. Minerva Medica; p77-95.

[129] Markov MS. Magnetic Field Therapy: A Review., Electromagnetic Biology and Medicine, 26: 1–23, 2007.

[130] Pieber K, Herceg M, Paternostro-Sluga T. Electrotherapy for the treatment of painful diabetic peripheral neuropathy: a review. J Rehabil Med. 2010 Apr;42(4):289-95.

[131] Ganesan K, Gengadharan AC, Balachandran C, Manohar BM, Puvanakrishnan R Low frequency pulsed electromagnetic field - A viable alternative therapy for arthritis. Indian Exp Biol. 2009

[132] Effectiveness of pulsed electromagnetic field therapy in the management of osteoarthritis of the knee: a meta-analysis of randomized controlled trials. - Vavken P, Arrich F, Schuhfried O, Dorotka R. - J Rehabil Med. 2009 May;41(6):406-11.

[133] Strauch B, Herman C, Dabb R, Ignarro LJ, Pilla AA. -. Evidence-based use of pulsed electromagnetic field therapy in clinical plastic surgery. - Aesthet Surg J. 2009;29(2): 135-43.

[134] 134. Saggini R, Bellomo RG, Saggini A, Iodice P, Toniato E. Rehabilitative treatment for low back pain with external pulsed electromagnetic fields. International journal of immunopathology and pharmacology.2009; 25-28.

[135] Sandyk R. Improvement in word-fluency performance in Parkinson's disease by administration of electromagnetic fields. Int J Neurosci. 1994;77(1-2):23-46.

[136] Sandyk R.Alzheimer's disease: improvement of visual memory and visuoconstructive performance by treatment with picotesla range magnetic fields. Int J Neurosci.; 76(3-4):185-225.

[137] Sandyk R.Improvement in word-fluency performance in patients with multiple sclerosis by electromagnetic fields. Int J Neurosci. 1994 Nov;79(1-2):75-90.

[138] Ganesan K, Gengadharan AC, Balachandran C, Manohar BM, Puvanakrishnan R. Low frequency pulsed electromagnetic field - A viable alternative therapy for arthritis. Indian Exp Biol. 2009.

[139] Vavken P, Arrich F, Schuhfried O, Dorotka R. Effectiveness of pulsed electromagnetic field therapy in the management of osteoarthritis of the knee: a meta-analysis of randomized controlled trials. - J Rehabil Med. 2009 May;41(6):406-11.

[140] Lappin MS, Lawrie FW, Richards TL, Kramer ED. Effects of a pulsed electromagnetic therapy on multiple sclerosis fatigue and quality of life: a double-blind, placebo controlled trial. Altern Ther Health Med.. 2003;9(4):38-48.

[141] Weintraub MI, Cole SP. Pulsed magnetic field therapy inrefractory neuropathic pain secondary to peripheral neuropathy: electro diagnostic parameters - pilot study. - Neurorehabil Neural Repair. 2004;18(1):42-6.

[142] Markov MS. Magnetic Field Therapy: A Review, Electromagnetic Biology and Medicine 2007; 26: 1–23, .

[143] Jiménez-García MN, Arellanes-Robledo J, Aparicio-Bautista DI, Rodríguez-Segura MA, Villa-Treviño S, Godina-Nava JJ. Anti-proliferative effect of extremely low fre-

http://dx.doi.org/10.5772/60548

quency electromagnetic field on preneoplastic lesions formation in the rat liver. - BMC Cancer. 2010 ; 24;10:15

[144] Saggini R, Giuliani L. Campi Magnetici e Dolore. In Saggini R, Buoso S, Pestelli G. (ed) Dolore e Riabilitazione. Minerva Medica; 2014.p129-148

[145] Di Pancrazio L, Bellomo RG, Franciotti R, Iodice P, Galati V, D'Andreagiovanni A, Bifolchetti S, Thomas A, Onofrj M, Bonanni L, Saggini R. Combined rehabilitation program for postural instability in progressive supranuclear palsy.NeuroRehabilitation. 2013;32(4):855-60.

[146] Bellomo RG, Iodice P, Savoia V, Saggini A, Vermiglio G, Saggini R. Balance and posture in the elderly: an analysis of a sensorimotor rehabilitation protocol. International journal of Immunopathology and pharmacology 2009;37-44.

[147] Ernst E. Complementary therapies in palliative cancer care. Cancer. 2001;91:2181–5.

[148] Robert W. Bunting, She B. Bone Metastasis and Rehabilitation. Cancer Rehabilitation in the New Millennium supplement to Cancer 2001; 1020–102815.

Chapter 5

Chemotherapy for Gastric Cancer — What Comes Next?

Shouji Shimoyama

Additional information is available at the end of the chapter

http://dx.doi.org/10.5772/60420

1. Introduction

Gastric cancer (GC) is the fourth (in men) and fifth (in women) most commonly newly diagnosed cancer worldwide and the third (in men) and fifth (in women) leading cause of cancer death [1]. Radical resection remains the only way cure, but cure rates following surgery for resectable GC in the West lag behind those in Japan. In addition, many GC patients will suffer recurrence even after curative resection in approximately 50% of cases [2], which eventually results in a still poor 5-year survival rate of <30% both in the USA [3] and in Europe [4]. Although the 5-year survival rate in Japan is much better than that in the West, there is a global consensus that advanced GC patients need further anticancer therapy.

Currently, five classes of cytotoxic agents (fluoropyrimidines, platinums, taxanes, topoisomerase inhibitors, and anthracyclines) and new molecular targeting agents have been used in GC. Recent randomized controlled trials (RCTs) in the field of treatment for advanced GC have established first-line chemotherapy, although the approach and management for advanced GC varies from region to region so that there is no worldwide consensus on this matter. The most promising regimens are ECF (epirubicin, cisplatin, and 5-fluorouracil) in Europe [5], DCF (docetaxel, cisplatin, and 5-fluorouracil) in the USA (V325 trial) [6], and SP (S-1 and cisplatin) in Japan (SPIRITS trial) [7]. Strikingly, however, the global RCT conducted in the USA (FLAGS trial) failed to exhibit any survival advantage of the SP regimen over the FP (5-fluorouracil plus cisplatin) regimen [8]. Very recently, trastuzumab combined with cisplatin and fluoropyrimidines has been found to be active for human epidermal growth factor receptor-2 (HER2 or ERBB2)-positive GC (ToGA trial) [9]. Although these regimens are active, the treatment progress is painfully slow [4]. The median time to progression (TTP) or progression free survival (PFS) was 7.4 months by ECF [5], 5.6 months by DCF [6], 6.0 months by Japanese style SP [7], 4.8 months by global style SP [8], and 6.7 months even by adding trastuzumab [9], suggesting that many advanced GC patients experience failure after first-line chemotherapy.

Interestingly, the median TTP or PFS of these regimens are almost equivalent (5.6-7.4 months) [5-7] while median overall survival times (OS) differ between the studies (Figure 1). The 13 months of median OS by the Japanese SP regimen [7] was apparently longer than those (8.7-9.2 months) by ECF and DCF regimens [5,6] (Figure 1). In addition, even by the use of the SP regimen, the post-progression survival –the survival length difference between median PFS and median OS– differed considerably, being 7 months in the SPIRITS trial [7] and 3.8 months in the FLAGS trial [8] (Figure 1). Such inter-trial differences in post-progression survival are partly attributable to different proportions of subsequent second-line therapy after the failure of first-line chemotherapy, being over 70% in the SPIRITS trial while 30-45% in other trials [6, 8,9]. In this regard, patients who retain good performance status at the time of first-line treatment failure are candidates for second-line therapy. Currently, however, no standard regimens for any second-line therapy hitherto determined suggest an urgent need for the establishment of second-line therapy. Reflecting this urgency, clinical research concerning second-line therapy has been recently commenced. In the era of post first-line chemotherapy, this chapter reviews the next research issues deserving of focus in the field of advanced GC treatment.

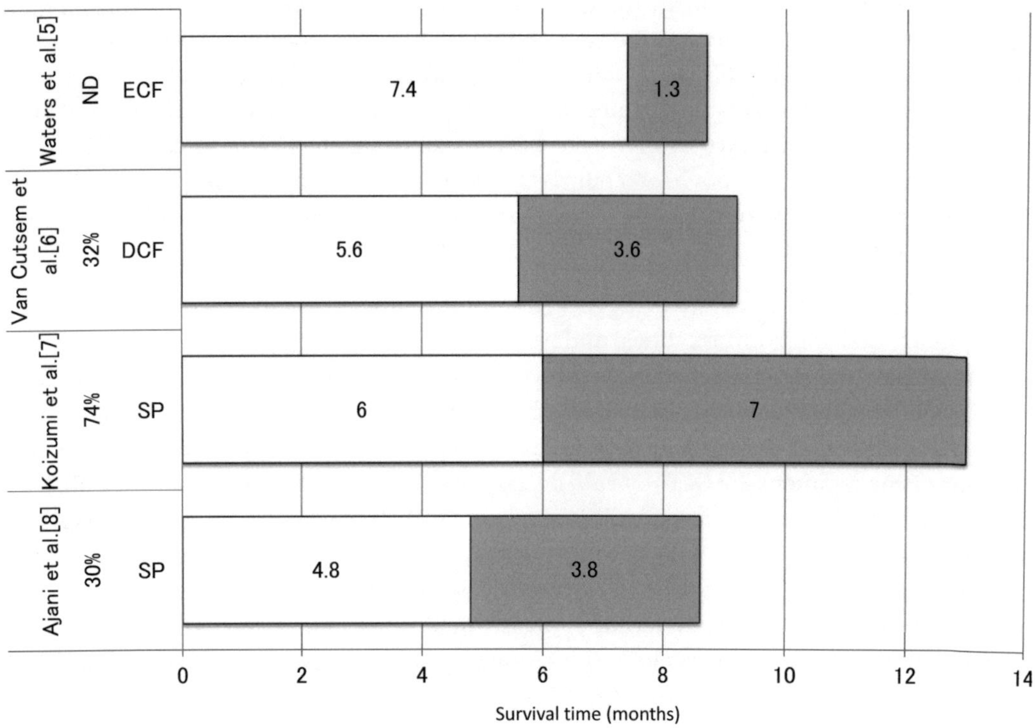

Figure 1. Median TTP or PFS (white bar) and post-progression free survivals (gray bar) of the previous first-line RCTs. The sum of the white and gray bars indicates median OS. Percentages indicate the proportion of patients receiving further therapy. The reference numbers are expressed in brackets. ECF; epirubicin, cisplatin, and 5-fluorouracil, DCF; docetaxel, cisplatin, and 5-fluorouracil, SP; S-1 and cisplatin. ND; not described.

2. Rationale for second-line therapy

The significance of second-line therapy after disease progression by first-line chemotherapy has been evaluated by several randomized comparisons of survival times between second-line therapy and best supportive care (BSC) or placebos. Various kinds of agents have been investigated in the RCTs of second-line therapy, such as chemotherapy drugs [10-12] and molecular targeting agents [13-15]. Some of these trials have demonstrated significantly improved survival times by second-line therapies as compared with BSC or a placebo (Table 1).

The AIO conducted a RCT to compare irinotecan (21 patients) with BSC (19 patients) [10]. Although this study was closed prematurely due to poor patient accrual, irinotecan could significantly (p=0.012) prolong median OS (4.0 months) as compared to those by BSC (2.4 months). The second RCT conducted in Korea [11] assigned patients in a ratio of 2:1 to chemotherapy (docetaxel or irinotecan) plus BSC (133 patients) or BSC alone (69 patients). Choice of chemotherapy drugs was left to the discretion of the investigators. Median OS of the chemotherapy arm (5.3 months) was significantly (p=0.007) longer than those of the BSC arm (3.8 months). This survival difference may be partly ascribed to the significantly (p=0.02) greater number of patients receiving further chemotherapy (third-line chemotherapy) in the chemotherapy arm (40%) than in the BSC arm (22%) because median OS was longer (8.0 months) for patients who received subsequent treatment than those who did not (3.76 months), regardless of treatment arm. Of note, the lack of any difference in median OS between docetaxel use (5.2 months) and irinotecan use (6.5 months) implies that both agents are equally active, although bias for patient allocation can not be denied. In the third RCT conducted in the UK [12], 168 patients were allocated to either docetaxel plus active symptom control or active symptom control alone (84 patients each). The median OS in the docetaxel group (5.2 months) was significantly longer (p=0.01) than that in the active symptom control alone group (3.6 months). Measurements of disease specific quality of life showed benefits for docetaxel in reducing dysphagia and abdominal pain.

The efficacy of molecular targeting agents as a second-line setting has been investigated by three other RCTs [13-15]. First, a GRANITE-1 trial [13] randomly assigned 656 patients at a 2:1 schedule either to everolimus (n=439) or a matching placebo (n=217). Significantly longer median PFS by everolimus (1.7 months, p<0.0001) than that by placebo (1.4 months) did not reflect a difference in median OS (5.4 months in the everolimus arm versus 4.3 months in the placebo arm, p=0.12). Such a discrepancy, namely a significant PFS difference and nonsignificant OS difference, could be ascribed to the fact of the similar or even longer median OS (4.3 months) in the placebo arm in this study as compared to those (2.4-3.8 months) of BSC arms in other second-line RCTs [10-12]. Therefore, one should remember that the longer survival length in the control arm might diminish any statistical significance even when the experimental regimen is effective. Subsequently, a global REGARD trial [14] was able for the first time to demonstrate that ramucirumab, a monoclonal antibody of vascular endothelial growth factor receptor (VEGFR)-2, was significantly superior to placebo with regard to median OS (5.2 months versus 3.8 months, p=0.047) and median PFS (2.1 months versus 1.3 months, p<0.0001), respectively. In addition, more patients receiving ramucirumab experienced stable or improved QOL than those in the placebo arm. Finally, apatinib, a tyrosine-inhibitor agent targeting VEGFR with an anticipated anti-angiogenesis effect, has been now tested in a clinical trial (NCT 01512745) [15]. This study aims to determine whether apatinib can improve PFS or OS compared to placebos.

Subsequently, a metaanalysis has very recently elucidated a 36% reduction in the risk of death ($p<0.0001$) by second-line therapy [16], suggesting that second-line therapy is effective and should be considered in some segments of GC patients refractory to first-line therapy.

3. Seeking the best regimen of second line therapy

Several randomized trials have been released to explore the optimal combination and doses for second-line therapy using the currently active agents or those deemed active. The agents investigated by these trials include chemotherapeutic drugs [17-20], a molecular targeting agent [21], and their combinations [22-26].

The efficacy of chemotherapy as a second-line setting has been investigated in several RCTs. In the TCOG GI-0801 trial [17], median PFS was significantly longer (3.8 months, n=64) by biweekly irinotecan plus cisplatin than by irinotecan alone (2.8 months, n=63), but median OS did not differ between the arms (10.7 months versus 10.1 months). Notably, the proportion of patients receiving third-line therapy was the same (75%) in both groups. The results of another randomized trial (ECRIN) have been reported in the abstract form [18], in which irinotecan plus cisplatin (n=84) was compared with irinotecan alone (n=84) in patients refractory to an S-1 containing regimen. WJOG 4007 [19] is a RCT comparing weekly paclitaxel (n=108) with biweekly irinotecan (n=111) in GC patients refractory to fluoropyrimidines plus cisplatin. Although there are no statistically significant differences between weekly paclitaxel and biweekly irinotecan for median OS (9.5 months vs 8.4 months, p=0.38), median PFS (3.6 months vs 2.3 months, p=0.33), or response rate (20.9% vs 13.6%, p=0.24), the median OS of both arms are equally longer than those of the previous second-line studies (Table 1, Figure 2). Several explanations are possible for the longer median OS in this study. One explanation is the lower proportion of patients with severe peritoneal metastasis in this study (25.6%) as compared with those in the AIO [10] (45%) and Kang [11] (45%) studies. Another explanation is that the proportion of patients receiving third-line therapy in this study was substantial, being 89.8% in the paclitaxel arm and 72.1% in the irinotecan arm. Interestingly, the third-line therapy was an irinotecan-containing regimen in 75% of patients of the paclitaxel arm and a taxane-containing regimen in 60% of the irinotecan arm. Including later lines, 81% patients in the paclitaxel arm received irinotecan and 68% of patients in the irinotecan arm received paclitaxel. The more prolonged median OS in both arms of the WJOG 4007 than those of the previous studies implies that both irinotecan and paclitaxel in second- and further-line settings could potentially contribute to prolonged survival. The ongoing fourth RCT (JACCRO GC05) [20] has been comparing irinotecan plus S-1 with irinotecan alone to GC patients refractory to S-1. Since the standard regimen in adjuvant and advanced settings in Japan is respectively S-1 and S-1 plus cisplatin, this study will provide one answer to the clinically important question of whether the prolonged use of S-1 is effective even to the S-1 resistant patients whom the clinicians face.

	Study drug	Dose and schedule	Number of patients Study arm	Control arm	median OS Study arm	Control arm	median PFS Study arm	Control arm
Thuss-Patience [10]	Iriontecan	250-350mg/m2, q3w	21	19	4 p=0.012	2.4	2.5	ND
Kang [11]	Iriontecan or Docetaxel	150mg/m2, q2w or 60mg/m2, q3w	133	69	5.3 p=0.007	3.8	ND	ND
COUGAR-02 [12]	Docetaxel	75mg/m2, q3w	84	84	5.2 p=0.01	3.6	ND	ND
GRANITE-1 [13]	Evelorimus	10mg/day	439	217	5.4 p=0.12	4.3	1.7 p<0.001	1.4
REGARD [14]	Ramucirumab	8mg/kg, q2w	238	117	5.2 p=0.047	3.8	2.1 p<0.0001	1.3

OS; overall survival, PFS; progression free survival, ND; not described

Table 1. Published results of randomized controlled trials of second-line therapy versus best supportive care or placebo.

The RCT comparing a molecular targeting agent with a chemotherapeutic agent has been ongoing. HER2-positive advanced GC patients have been allocated to either trastuzumab emtansine or taxane (GATSBY, NCT01641939) [21].

A combination of molecular targeting agents and chemotherapy agents has been investigated in several RCTs. First, paclitaxel with or without lapatinib, which binds to the intracellular tyrosine kinase domains of ERBB1 and ERBB2 (HER2), was compared in HER2-positive advanced GC (TYTAN) [22]. Neither median OS nor median PFS were prolonged by lapatinib plus paclitaxel (n=132) as compared to paclitaxel alone (n=129). Second, the results of the RAINBOW trial [23,24], which compared ramucirumab plus paclitaxel with placebo plus paclitaxel, have been very recently reported in the abstract form. Sixty hundred and sixty-five GC patients, who were refractory to cisplatin and fluoropyrimidine-containing regimens, were randomized in a 1:1 ratio to receive paclitaxel plus ramucirumab or paclitaxel plus a placebo. The paclitaxel and ramucirumab arm showed a significant benefit in median OS (HR=0.807, p=0.0169) and median PFS (HR=0.635, p<0.0001). The subsequent geographical region-stratified analysis elucidated that the advantage of median PFS and median OS was more evident in Western patients than in Japanese patients (Figure 2). Such a regional difference could partly explained by a higher use of post-discontinuation treatment in Japan (75% of patients) than in Western countries (36-38% of patients), which may eventually mask any potential OS benefit of ramucirumab plus paclitaxel in Japan. Two other RCT trials [25,26] are now ongoing. Paclitaxel with or without everolimus has been compared in patients with advanced GC refractory to fluoropyrimidine containing regimens [25]. Patients will be randomized in a 1:1 ratio for a total of 240 patients per treatment arm. Nimotuzumab plus irinotecan versus irinotecan monotherapy as second-line therapy has been investigated in

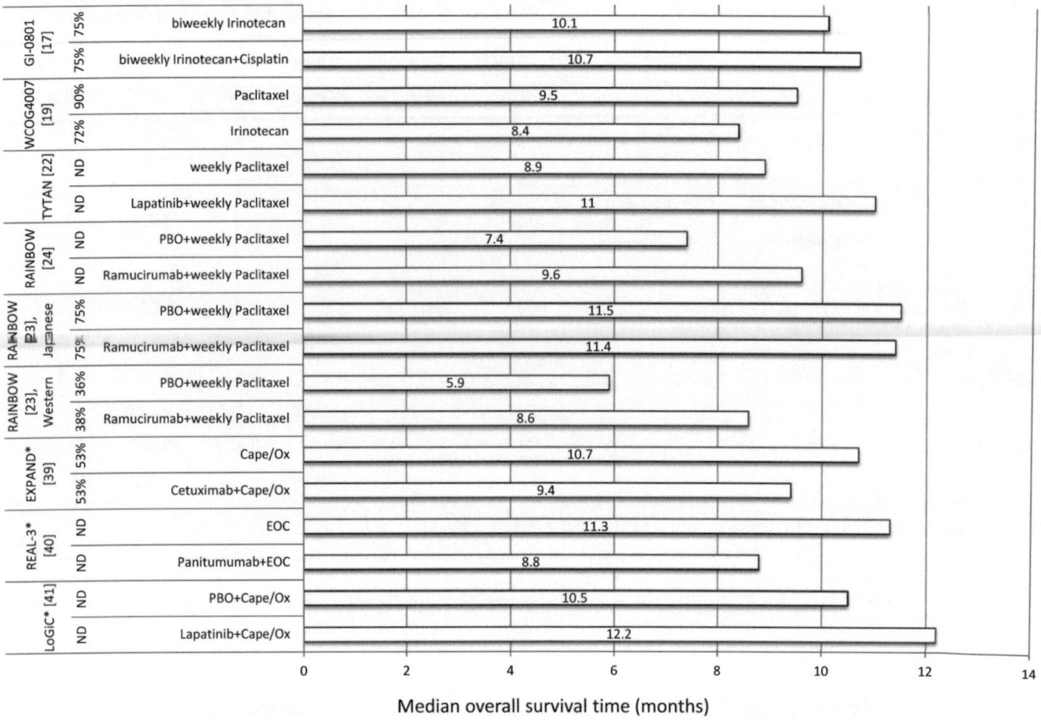

Figure 2. Comparisons of median OS between the previous RCTs. The percentage indicates the proportion of patients receiving further therapy in each trial. The reference numbers are expressed in brackets. *; first-line trials, BSC; best supportive care, PBO; placebo, Cape; capecitabine, Ox; oxaliplatin, EOC; epirubicin, oxaliplatin, and capecitabine, ND; not described.

patients with ERBB1 overexpressed advanced GC [26]. This is a Japan and Korea collaborative RCT allocating patients at 1:1 ratio for a total of approximately 400 patients per arm.

The results of some trials have been published; however, at present, trials in which the primary endpoint has been met have been unfortunately very limited. The positive results hitherto obtained include a prolonged PFS by a combination of irinotecan and cisplatin after the failure of S-1 based first-line chemotherapy, and prolonged PFS and OS by ramucirumab in combination with weekly paclitaxel. The results of other studies, especially using molecular targeting agents, are awaited.

4. Consideration of adverse events

When considering second-line therapy, clinicians must be aware that, by definition, patients receiving second-line therapy are not chemonaive and experience treatment failure; thus, they are more likely to be resistant to therapy than first-line treatment. Furthermore, patient performance status is more likely to deteriorate due to a recurrent cancer burden and treatment

against it. Indeed, widely ranging grades of gastrointestinal symptoms-related adverse events occurred in a substantial proportion of patients in the BSC arms of clinical trials, suggesting a poor quality of life even by the BSC. In addition, a more intensive regimen aiming at a prolonged OS may cause a higher likelihood of severe adverse events that may result in treatment discontinuation and limitation. For example, the DCF regimen caused 82% of grade 3-4 neutropenia and 29% of febrile neutropenia. Therefore, balancing efficacy and adverse events should be taken into account when developing second-line therapy. The development of more intensive while less toxic second-line regimens could be positioned as a breakthrough marker of GC treatment, which can then ultimately achieve further survival prolongation without treatment withdrawal.

In this context, another direction for research is to establish less toxic regimens with preserved anticancer activity. As described earlier, the conventional first-line treatment comprises 5-fluorouracil and emetogenic/nephrotoxic cisplatin. Therefore, the challenges for a less toxic regimen are the substitution of oxaliplatin for nephrotoxic cisplatin [27,28] or substitution of oral capecitabine for intravenous 5-fluorouracil [29]. Such substitutions aim to reduce toxicity and maintain organ function, thus avoiding treatment withdrawal and prolonged treatment duration.

Fluorouracil, leucovorin, and oxaliplatin (FLO) were associated with significantly less anemia, nausea, vomiting, fatigue, renal toxicity, and serious adverse events related to the treatment as compared with fluorouracil, leucovorin, and cisplatin (FLP) [27]. In addition, there was a better trend toward improved median PFS by FLO than FLP. Similarly, as compared to SP, S-1 plus oxaliplatin (SOX) resulted in a reduced risk of grade 3/4 neutropenia (41.5% vs 19.5%) and febrile neutropenia (6.9% vs 0.9%) while median PFS was similar between the two regimens (5.4 months versus 5.5 months) [28]. These findings further support the possibility that the substitution of oxaliplatin for cisplatin reduced toxicity while maintaining efficacy. Accordingly, length of hospital stay per cycle of SOX regimen (0.85 day) was significantly shorter than that for the SP regimen (6 days) [28]. Furthermore, capecitabine and cisplatin (XP) versus 5-fluorouracil and cisplatin (FP) proved similar median OS (10.5 months versus 9.3 months), suggesting that the inconvenience of infusional 5-fluorouracil could be replaced by oral capecitabine, thus realizing a more simplified dosing schedule [29]. Whether this concept can be applied to second-line therapy warrants further investigation.

5. Future perspectives

With the development of a new generation of cytotoxic agents and molecular targeting agents, the research field of GC treatment appears to be transitioning into a new era with a focus on the targetable molecules in GC. Several molecular targeting agents are currently being evaluated both in first- and second-line settings. The pending results of ongoing clinical trials motivates researchers to continue the challenge of establishing the best second-line regimens or less toxic combinations for the treatment of advanced GC.

a. Clarifying the genetic alterations of targeted molecules and their interactions.

Unfortunately, in sharp contrast to colorectal cancer in which there has been a significant achievement in treatment by the use of molecular targeting agents, only one agent (ramucirumab) has been currently proved to be an agent for second-line therapy presumably due to the genetic complexity and molecular heterogeneity of the disease.

Recent findings have highlighted the mechanisms of the actions of molecular targeting agents or patterns of expression of targetable molecules in several tumors. For example, genetic alterations that are critical for cell growth occur with considerably different frequencies, being 60%, 33%, and 32% in cancers of the pancreas, biliary tract, and colon, respectively [30]. Furthermore, certain combinations of targets are expressed in a mutually exclusive or co-occurring manner in the same tumor. A mutually exclusive fashion would be a case being KRAS and BRAF in colorectal cancer, or ERBB1 and KRAS in lung cancer [31]. The co-occurring expression of targets is a case of being ERBB2 and PIK3CA in breast cancer [32]. With regard to GC, although KRAS mutations are initially recognized as an infrequent phenomenon in GC [33], the alterations and amplifications of other genes --both known or previously unreported-- have been subsequently found in a substantial number of GC patients in a mutually exclusive manner [34,35] or co-amplified manner [36]. These findings create a challenge in the treatment regimen with either a use of each blockade of each targetable molecule or a use of dual- or pan-inhibitors of kinases [37]. In addition, elucidation of the roles of each domain in ERBB2 that plays a role in resistance to anti-HER2 therapy further provides the theoretical basis to modify therapeutic strategies to circumvent this resistance [38]. These advances may expand therapeutic options, thereby making larger proportions of GC patients possible candidates for molecular targeting therapies than previously appreciated. Accordingly, there may be a desperate need for multiple gene profiling which could help establish rational molecular criteria for patient inclusion and exclusion in clinical trials. Patient selection by gene profiling may allow better patient recruitment for those most likely to respond to targeted therapies.

b. Positive and negative interactions between chemotherapy and molecular targeting therapies.

It should be noted that the recent clinical trials of first-line molecular targeting therapies regrettably resulted in some negative results [39-41] (Figure 2). The addition of cetuximab to cisplatin plus capecitabine had a similar median PFS (4.4 months) and median OS (9.4 months) compared to cisplatin plus capecitabine alone (5.6 months and 10.7 months, respectively) [39] (EXPAND). Surprisingly, the addition of panitumumab to epirubicin, oxaliplatin, and capecitabine (EOC) resulted in a significantly shorter (p=0.013) median OS (8.8 months) compared to EOC (11.3 months) (REAL-3) [40]. Furthermore, lapatinib in combination with capecitabine and oxaliplatin could not show any significant survival benefit (LoGiC) [41]. These negative results lead to speculation that there may be ideal combinations or compatibility between chemotherapy and molecular targeting therapy. In addition, even the addition of panitumumab to EOC achieved only similar median OS to those of the WCOG 4007 trial (Figure 2) [19,40]. Therefore, a certain combination, such as anti-EGFR antibody and capeci-

http://dx.doi.org/10.5772/60420

tabine or oxaliplatin, may be ineffective or even interfere with the other. This speculation can be supported by the observation that addition of cetuximab to oxaliplatin plus fluoropyrimidine-based chemotherapy failed to demonstrate survival benefits for advanced colorectal cancer [42].

c. Need to evaluate the updated molecular profile.

Another obstacle for the progression of second-line treatment lies in the possibility that the molecular profile of GC is likely to change under the stress of treatment. Generally, lower response rates and shorter survival times in patients receiving second-line therapy than chemonaive patients may partly be explained by such molecular changes that lead to a resistance to therapy. Ideally, the on-demand tissue samples from tumor sites currently of interest are needed to assess the updated genetic and molecular patterns and to predict whether the planned second-line therapy is really effective. However, direct tumor tissue sampling and subsequent gene analysis are often hampered by virtually inaccesible tumor localization and by overly small sample volumes to perform gene analysis. It is necessary to discover novel markers which can be alternatives for those obtained only by direct tumor tissue sampling as well as to improvise new methods to assess them in order to select the right patients for the right second-line regimen.

Motivated by the first promising results of trastuzumab use in the ToGA trial, several molecular targeting therapies have been challenged in clinical trials. Continuous efforts should be necessary to clarify the mutation and amplification of targeted molecules, and novel methods for their genetic profiling should probably become part of clinical routines. Ultimately, GC patients harboring unique genetic profiles of targeted molecules should be allocated into specific, suitable trials. Targeted therapies tailored to individual genetic profiles maximize treatment efficacy because this allows the recruitment of selected, most suitable patients rather than unselected ones [43].

6. Conclusions

Against the background of survival advantages of second-line therapy over BSC in GC patients refractory to first-line treatment, efforts to establish the most effective regimens have been just begun. Parallel to the development of molecular targeting agents, the investigated regimens comprise doublet or triplet chemotherapeutic agents, molecular targeting agents, and their combinations. In addition, the minimization of adverse events should be taken into account to avoid treatment discontinuation. There is a desperate need to explore genetic mutations of targeted molecules and the interactions between them, to establish novel methods to assess them, to clarify the positive or negative interactions between chemotherapy and molecular targeting agents, and to find regimens in which adverse events are least likely to occur for avoiding treatment discontinuation. These could help determine rational molecular criteria for patient inclusion and exclusion in clinical trials, realize the most efficient patient recruitment for those most likely to respond to therapies, and accelerate the establishment of the most effective second-line therapy that could achieve greater survival prolongation.

Author details

Shouji Shimoyama

Address all correspondence to: shimoyama@apost.plala.or.jp

Gastrointestinal Unit, Settlement Clinic, Towa, Adachi-ku, Tokyo, Japan

References

[1] Jemal A, Bray F, Center MM, Ferlay J, Ward E, Forman D. Global cancer statistics. CA Cancer J Clin. 2011; 61(2): 69-90.

[2] Buzzoni R, Bajetta E, Di Bartolomeo M, Miceli R, Beretta E, Ferrario E, Mariani L. Pathological features as predictors of recurrence after radical resection of gastric cancer. Br J Surg. 2006; 93(2): 205-9.

[3] Siegel R, Ma J, Zou Z, Jemal A. Cancer statistics, 2014. CA Cancer J Clin. 2014; 64(1): 9-29. doi: 10.3322/caac.21208.

[4] De Angelis R, Sant M, Coleman MP, Francisci S, Baili P, Pierannunzio D, Trama A, Visser O, Brenner H, Ardanaz E, Bielska-Lasota M, Engholm G, Nennecke A, Siesling S, Berrino F, Capocaccia R; EUROCARE-5 Working Group. Cancer survival in Europe 1999-2007 by country and age: results of EUROCARE--5-a population-based study. Lancet Oncol. 2014; 15(1): 23-34. doi: 10.1016/S1470-2045(13)70546-1.

[5] Waters JS, Norman A, Cunningham D, Scarffe JH, Webb A, Harper P, Joffe JK, Mackean M, Mansi J, Leahy M, Hill A, Oates J, Rao S, Nicolson M, Hickish T. Long-term survival after epirubicin, cisplatin and fluorouracil for gastric cancer: results of a randomized trial. Br J Cancer. 1999; 80: 269-72.

[6] Van Cutsem E, Moiseyenko VM, Tjulandin S, Majlis A, Constenla M, Boni C, Rodrigues A, Fodor M, Chao Y, Voznyi E, Risse ML, Ajani JA; V325 Study Group. Phase III study of docetaxel and cisplatin plus fluorouracil compared with cisplatin and fluorouracil as first-line therapy for advanced gastric cancer: a report of the V325 Study Group. J Clin Oncol. 2006; 24: 4991-7.

[7] Koizumi W, Narahara H, Hara T, Takagane A, Akiya T, Takagi M, Miyashita K, Nishizaki T, Kobayashi O, Takiyama W, Toh Y, Nagaie T, Takagi S, Yamamura Y, Yanaoka K, Orita H, Takeuchi M. S-1 plus cisplatin versus S-1 alone for first-line treatment of advanced gastric cancer (SPIRITS trial): a phase III trial. Lancet Oncol. 2008; 9(3): 215-21. doi: 10.1016/S1470-2045(08)70035-4.

[8] Ajani JA, Rodriguez W, Bodoky G, Moiseyenko V, Lichinitser M, Gorbunova V, Vynychenko I, Garin A, Lang I, Falcon S. Multicenter phase III comparison of cisplatin/S-1 with cisplatin/infusional fluorouracil in advanced gastric or gastroeso-

phageal adenocarcinoma study: the FLAGS trial. J Clin Oncol. 2010; 28(9): 1547-53. doi: 10.1200/JCO.2009.25.4706.

[9] Bang YJ, Van Cutsem E, Feyereislova A, Chung HC, Shen L, Sawaki A, Lordick F, Ohtsu A, Omuro Y, Satoh T, Aprile G, Kulikov E, Hill J, Lehle M, Rüschoff J, Kang YK; ToGA Trial Investigators. Trastuzumab in combination with chemotherapy versus chemotherapy alone for treatment of HER2-positive advanced gastric or gastro-oesophageal junction cancer (ToGA): a phase 3, open-label, randomised controlled trial. Lancet. 2010; 376(9742): 687-97. doi: 10.1016/S0140-6736(10)61121-X.

[10] Thuss-Patience PC, Kretzschmar A, Bichev D, Deist T, Hinke A, Breithaupt K, Dogan Y, Gebauer B, Schumacher G, Reichardt P. Survival advantage for irinotecan versus best supportive care as second-line chemotherapy in gastric cancer--a randomised phase III study of the Arbeitsgemeinschaft Internistische Onkologie (AIO). Eur J Cancer. 2011; 47(15): 2306-14. doi: 10.1016/j.ejca.2011.06.002.

[11] Kang JH, Lee SI, Lim do H, Park KW, Oh SY, Kwon HC, Hwang IG, Lee SC, Nam E, Shin DB, Lee J, Park JO, Park YS, Lim HY, Kang WK, Park SH. Salvage chemotherapy for pretreated gastric cancer: a randomized phase III trial comparing chemotherapy plus best supportive care with best supportive care alone. J Clin Oncol. 2012; 30(13): 1513-8. doi: 10.1200/JCO.2011.39.4585.

[12] Ford HE, Marshall A, Bridgewater JA, Janowitz T, Coxon FY, Wadsley J, Mansoor W, Fyfe D, Madhusudan S, Middleton GW, Swinson D, Falk S, Chau I, Cunningham D, Kareclas P, Cook N, Blazeby JM, Dunn JA; COUGAR-02 Investigators. Docetaxel versus active symptom control for refractory oesophagogastric adenocarcinoma (COUGAR-02): an open-label, phase 3 randomised controlled trial. Lancet Oncol. 2014; 15(1): 78-86. doi: 10.1016/S1470-2045(13)70549-7.

[13] Ohtsu A, Ajani JA, Bai YX, Bang YJ, Chung HC, Pan HM, Sahmoud T, Shen L, Yeh KH, Chin K, Muro K, Kim YH, Ferry D, Tebbutt NC, Al-Batran SE, Smith H, Costantini C, Rizvi S, Lebwohl D, Van Cutsem E. Everolimus for previously treated advanced gastric cancer: results of the randomized, double-blind, phase III GRANITE-1 study. J Clin Oncol. 2013; 31(31): 3935-43. doi: 10.1200/JCO.2012.48.3552.

[14] Fuchs CS, Tomasek J, Yong CJ, Dumitru F, Passalacqua R, Goswami C, Safran H, dos Santos LV, Aprile G, Ferry DR, Melichar B, Tehfe M, Topuzov E, Zalcberg JR, Chau I, Campbell W, Sivanandan C, Pikiel J, Koshiji M, Hsu Y, Liepa AM, Gao L, Schwartz JD, Tabernero J; REGARD Trial Investigators. Ramucirumab monotherapy for previously treated advanced gastric or gastro-oesophageal junction adenocarcinoma (REGARD): an international, randomised, multicentre, placebo-controlled, phase 3 trial. Lancet. 2014; 383(9911): 31-9. doi: 10.1016/S0140-6736(13)61719-5.

[15] http://www.ClinicalTrial.gov. NCT 01512745

[16] Kim HS, Kim HJ, Kim SY, Kim TY, Lee KW, Baek SK, Kim TY, Ryu MH, Nam BH, Zang DY. Second-line chemotherapy versus supportive cancer treatment in ad-

vanced gastric cancer: a meta-analysis. Ann Oncol. 2013; 24(11): 2850-4. doi: 10.1093/annonc/mdt351.

[17] Higuchi K, Tanabe S, Shimada K, Hosaka H, Sasaki E, Nakayama N, Takeda Y, Moriwaki T, Amagai K, Sekikawa T, Sakuyama T, Kanda T, Sasaki T, Azuma M, Takahashi F, Takeuchi M, Koizumi W; Tokyo Cooperative Oncology Group, Tokyo, Japan. Biweekly irinotecan plus cisplatin versus irinotecan alone as second-line treatment for advanced gastric cancer: a randomised phase III trial (TCOG GI-0801/BIRIP trial). Eur J Cancer. 2014; 50(8): 1437-45. doi: 10.1016/j.ejca.2014.01.020.

[18] Inagaki H, Nishikawa K, Fujitani K, Sugimoto N, Shigematsu T, Ishiguro T, Tsuburaya A, Nakamura M, Nashimoto A, Yamane T, Yamada M, Imano M, Iijima S, Oka Y, Kataoka M, Hironaka S, Andoh H, Morita S, Sakamoto J, Tsujinaka T. Efficacy analyses of a randomized phase III clinical trial of combined therapy with CPT-11/CDDP versus CPT-11 alone in patients with advanced or recurrent gastric cancer refractory to prior S-1 chemotherapy. Proc ASCO 2013; abstr 69.

[19] Hironaka S, Ueda S, Yasui H, Nishina T, Tsuda M, Tsumura T, Sugimoto N, Shimodaira H, Tokunaga S, Moriwaki T, Esaki T, Nagase M, Fujitani K, Yamaguchi K, Ura T, Hamamoto Y, Morita S, Okamoto I, Boku N, Hyodo I. Randomized, open-label, phase III study comparing irinotecan with paclitaxel in patients with advanced gastric cancer without severe peritoneal metastasis after failure of prior combination chemotherapy using fluoropyrimidine plus platinum: WJOG 4007 trial. J Clin Oncol. 2013; 31(35): 4438-44. doi: 10.1200/JCO.2012.48.5805.

[20] http://www.ClinicalTrial.gov. NCT 00639327

[21] http://www.ClinicalTrial.gov. NCT 01641939

[22] Satoh T, Xu RH, Chung HC, Sun GP, Doi T, Xu JM, Tsuji A, Omuro Y, Li J, Wang JW, Miwa H, Qin SK, Chung IJ, Yeh KH, Feng JF, Mukaiyama A, Kobayashi M, Ohtsu A, Bang YJ. Lapatinib plus paclitaxel versus paclitaxel alone in the second-line treatment of HER2-amplified advanced gastric cancer in Asian populations: TyTAN--a randomized, phase III study. J Clin Oncol. 2014; 32(19): 2039-49. doi: 10.1200/JCO.2013.53.6136.

[23] Hironaka S, Shimada Y, Sugimoto N, Komatsu Y, Nishina T, Yamaguchi K, Segawa Y, Omuro Y, Tamura T, Doi T, Yukisawa S, Yasui H, Nagashima F, Gotoh M, Esaki T, Emig M, Chandrawansa K, Muro K, Wilke H, Ohtsu A. RAINBOW: A global, phase III, randomized, double-blind study of ramucirumab (RAM) plus paclitaxel (PTX) versus placebo (PL) plus PTX in the treatment of metastatic gastroesophageal junction and gastric adenocarcinoma (mGC) following disease progression on first-line platinum- and fluoropyrimidine-containing combination therapy—Efficacy analysis in Japanese and Western patients. Proc ASCO 2014; abstr 4005

[24] Wilke H, Van Cutsem E, Oh SC, Bodoky G, Shimada Y, Hironaka S, Sugimoto N, Lipatov ON, Kim T-Y, Cunningham D, Ohtsu A, Rougier P, Emig M, Carlesi R, Chandrawansa K, Muro K. RAINBOW: A global, phase III, randomized, double-blind

study of ramucirumab plus paclitaxel versus placebo plus paclitaxel in the treatment of metastatic gastroesophageal junction (GEJ) and gastric adenocarcinoma following disease progression on first-line platinum- and fluoropyrimidine-containing combination therapy rainbow IMCL CP12-0922 (I4T-IE-JVBE). Proc ASCO 2014; abstr LBA7

[25] http://www.ClinicalTrial.gov. NCT 01248403

[26] http://www.ClinicalTrial.gov. NCT 01813253

[27] Al-Batran SE, Hartmann JT, Probst S, Schmalenberg H, Hollerbach S, Hofheinz R, Rethwisch V, Seipelt G, Homann N, Wilhelm G, Schuch G, Stoehlmacher J, Derigs HG, Hegewisch-Becker S, Grossmann J, Pauligk C, Atmaca A, Bokemeyer C, Knuth A, Jäger E; Arbeitsgemeinschaft Internistische Onkologie. Phase III trial in metastatic gastroesophageal adenocarcinoma with fluorouracil, leucovorin plus either oxaliplatin or cisplatin: a study of the Arbeitsgemeinschaft Internistische Onkologie. J Clin Oncol. 2008; 26(9): 1435-42. doi: 10.1200/JCO.2007.13.9378.

[28] Higuchi K, Koizumi W, Yamada Y, Nishikawa K, Gotoh M, Fuse N, Sugimoto N, Nishina T, Amagai K, Chin K, Niwa Y, Negoro Y, Imamura H, Tsuda M, Yasui H, Fujii H, Yamaguchi K, Yasui H, Hamada C, Hyodo I. Randomized phase III study of S-1 plus oxaliplatin versus S-1 plus cisplatin for first-line treatment of advanced gastric cancer. Proc ASCO 2013; abstr 60

[29] Kang YK, Kang WK, Shin DB, Chen J, Xiong J, Wang J, Lichinitser M, Guan Z, Khasanov R, Zheng L, Philco-Salas M, Suarez T, Santamaria J, Forster G, McCloud PI. Capecitabine/cisplatin versus 5-fluorouracil/cisplatin as first-line therapy in patients with advanced gastric cancer: a randomised phase III noninferiority trial. Ann Oncol. 2009; 20(4): 666-73. doi: 10.1093/annonc/mdn717.

[30] Schubbert S, Shannon K, Bollag G. Hyperactive Ras in developmental disorders and cancer. Nat Rev Cancer. 2007; 7(4): 295-308.

[31] Ding L, Getz G, Wheeler DA, Mardis ER, McLellan MD, Cibulskis K, Sougnez C, Greulich H, Muzny DM, Morgan MB, Fulton L, Fulton RS, Zhang Q, Wendl MC, Lawrence MS, Larson DE, Chen K, Dooling DJ, Sabo A, Hawes AC, Shen H, Jhangiani SN, Lewis LR, Hall O, Zhu Y, Mathew T, Ren Y, Yao J, Scherer SE, Clerc K, Metcalf GA, Ng B, Milosavljevic A, Gonzalez-Garay ML, Osborne JR, Meyer R, Shi X, Tang Y, Koboldt DC, Lin L, Abbott R, Miner TL, Pohl C, Fewell G, Haipek C, Schmidt H, Dunford-Shore BH, Kraja A, Crosby SD, Sawyer CS, Vickery T, Sander S, Robinson J, Winckler W, Baldwin J, Chirieac LR, Dutt A, Fennell T, Hanna M, Johnson BE, Onofrio RC, Thomas RK, Tonon G, Weir BA, Zhao X, Ziaugra L, Zody MC, Giordano T, Orringer MB, Roth JA, Spitz MR, Wistuba II, Ozenberger B, Good PJ, Chang AC, Beer DG, Watson MA, Ladanyi M, Broderick S, Yoshizawa A, Travis WD, Pao W, Province MA, Weinstock GM, Varmus HE, Gabriel SB, Lander ES, Gibbs RA, Meyerson M, Wilson RK. Somatic mutations affect key pathways in lung adenocarcinoma. Nature. 2008; 455(7216): 1069-75. doi: 10.1038/nature07423.

[32] Saal LH, Holm K, Maurer M, Memeo L, Su T, Wang X, Yu JS, Malmström PO, Mansukhani M, Enoksson J, Hibshoosh H, Borg A, Parsons R. PIK3CA mutations correlate with hormone receptors, node metastasis, and ERBB2, and are mutually exclusive with PTEN loss in human breast carcinoma. Cancer Res. 2005; 65(7): 2554-9.

[33] Lee SH, Lee JW, Soung YH, Kim HS, Park WS, Kim SY, Lee JH, Park JY, Cho YG, Kim CJ, Nam SW, Kim SH, Lee JY, Yoo NJ. BRAF and KRAS mutations in stomach cancer. Oncogene. 2003; 22(44): 6942-5.

[34] Shimoyama S. BRAF mutations and their implications in molecular targeting therapies for gastrointestinal cancers. J Pharmacogenom Pharmacoproteomics 2011; 2: e102. doi: 10.4172/2153-0645.1000e102

[35] Deng N, Goh LK, Wang H, Das K, Tao J, Tan IB, Zhang S, Lee M, Wu J, Lim KH, Lei Z, Goh G, Lim QY, Tan AL, Sin Poh DY, Riahi S, Bell S, Shi MM, Linnartz R, Zhu F, Yeoh KG, Toh HC, Yong WP, Cheong HC, Rha SY, Boussioutas A, Grabsch H, Rozen S, Tan P. A comprehensive survey of genomic alterations in gastric cancer reveals systematic patterns of molecular exclusivity and co-occurrence among distinct therapeutic targets. Gut. 2012; 61(5): 673-84. doi: 10.1136/gutjnl-2011-301839.

[36] Kiyose S, Nagura K, Tao H, Igarashi H, Yamada H, Goto M, Maeda M, Kurabe N, Suzuki M, Tsuboi M, Kahyo T, Shinmura K, Hattori N, Sugimura H. Detection of kinase amplifications in gastric cancer archives using fluorescence in situ hybridization. Pathol Int. 2012; 62(7): 477-84. doi: 10.1111/j.1440-1827.2012.02832.x.

[37] Prahallad A, Sun C, Huang S, Di Nicolantonio F, Salazar R, Zecchin D, Beijersbergen RL, Bardelli A, Bernards R. Unresponsiveness of colon cancer to BRAF(V600E) inhibition through feedback activation of EGFR. Nature. 2012; 483(7387): 100-3. doi: 10.1038/nature10868.

[38] Shimoyama S. Unraveling trastuzumab and lapatinib in gastric cancer. Future steps. Mol Clin Oncol 2014; 2 (2): 175-181. DOI: 10.3892/mco.2013.218

[39] Lordick F, Kang YK, Chung HC, Salman P, Oh SC, Bodoky G, Kurteva G, Volovat C, Moiseyenko VM, Gorbunova V, Park JO, Sawaki A, Celik I, Götte H, Melezínková H, Moehler M; Arbeitsgemeinschaft Internistische Onkologie and EXPAND Investigators. Capecitabine and cisplatin with or without cetuximab for patients with previously untreated advanced gastric cancer (EXPAND): a randomised, open-label phase 3 trial. Lancet Oncol. 2013; 14(6): 490-9. doi: 10.1016/S1470-2045(13)70102-5.

[40] Waddell TS, Chau I, Barbachano Y, de Castro DG, Wotherspoon A, Saffery C, Middleton GW, Wadsley J, Ferry DR, Mansoor W, Crosby TDL, Coxon FY, Smith D, Waters JS, Iveson T, Falk S, Slater S, Okines AFC, Cunningham D. A randomized multicenter trial of epirubicin, oxaliplatin, and capecitabine (EOC) plus panitumumab in advanced esophagogastric cancer (REAL3). Proc ASCO 2012; abstr LBA4000

[41] Hecht JR, Bang Y-J, Qin S, Chung H-C, Xu J-M, Park JO, Jeziorski K, Shparyk Y, Hoff PM, Sobrero AF, Salman P, Li J, Protsenko S, Buyse ME, Afenjar K, Kaneko T, Kemn-

er A, Santillana S, Press MF, Slamon DJ. Lapatinib in combination with capecitabine plus oxaliplatin (CapeOx) in HER2-positive advanced or metastatic gastric, esophageal, or gastroesophageal adenocarcinoma (AC): The TRIO-013/LOGiC Trial. Proc ASCO, 2013; abstr LBA4001

[42] Maughan TS, Adams RA, Smith CG, Meade AM, Seymour MT, Wilson RH, Idziaszczyk S, Harris R, Fisher D, Kenny SL, Kay E, Mitchell JK, Madi A, Jasani B, James MD, Bridgewater J, Kennedy MJ, Claes B, Lambrechts D, Kaplan R, Cheadle JP; MRC COIN Trial Investigators. Addition of cetuximab to oxaliplatin-based first-line combination chemotherapy for treatment of advanced colorectal cancer: results of the randomised phase 3 MRC COIN trial. Lancet. 2011; 377(9783): 2103-14. doi: 10.1016/S0140-6736(11)60613-2.

[43] Asaoka Y, Ikenoue T, Koike K. New targeted therapies for gastric cancer. Expert Opin Investig Drugs. 2011; 20(5): 595-604. doi: 10.1517/13543784.2011.566863.

Chapter 6

A Comprehensive Fitness and Nutrition Plan for Cancer Survivors

Karen Y. Wonders

Additional information is available at the end of the chapter

http://dx.doi.org/10.5772/60268

1. Introduction

The American Cancer Society recommends that exercise serve as an important part of an individual's cancer care plan, asserting that exercise will decrease feelings of fatigue both during and after treatment, and improve an individual's feeling of control and hope [5]. This is in light of more than two decades of research [6-9, 11, 19, 22], which support a link between a physically active lifestyle and positive physiological changes in cancer survivors. These include improvements in $VO_{2max,}$ blood volume, and gas exchange [13], improvements in muscular strength and endurance [14], fatigue reduction [15 – 19], and improvements in quality of life [19; 20; 23], anxiety [21, 22] depression [21; 24] body image [25], immune function [26], and emotional well-being [22].

According to ACSM (Schmitz et al., 2010), the general objectives for exercise training among cancer survivors are as follows:

1. To regain and improve physical function, aerobic capacity, strength, and flexibility.
2. To improve body image and QOL.
3. To improve body composition.
4. To improve cardiorespiratory, endocrine, neurological, muscular, cognitive, and psychosocial outcomes.
5. Potentially, to reduce or delay recurrence or a second primary tumor.
6. To improve the ability to physically and psychologically withstand the on-going anxiety regarding recurrence or a second primary cancer.
7. To reduce, attenuate, and prevent long-term and late effects of cancer treatment.

8. To improve the physiologic and psychological ability to withstand any current or future cancer treatments.

With the right program, remaining physically active during and after cancer treatment will have a favorable effect on symptom management and quality of life. As such, we wish to present a step-by-step guide intended to assist an exercise trainer when working with a client who has been diagnosed with cancer. This guide will begin with pre-participation paperwork and will cover all pertinent information through exercise program development. Presented are guidelines for both facility-based settings and a home-based setting. These techniques have been employed by Maple Tree Cancer Alliance, a non-profit organization in southwest Ohio whose mission is to improve the physical and spiritual well-being of individuals battling cancer.

It is important to mention, however, that "cancer" is a broad term. No two cancer diagnoses are alike. Similarly, no two patients are alike. With so many different forms of cancer existing, each with its own treatment regimen, it is vital for the exercise trainer to remain in communication with the patient's physician. Equally important, is the need to personalize each exercise program to the ever-changing needs of the patient. Therefore, the guidelines described in this book are just that – guidelines. Adjustments can and should be made accordingly, where appropriate.

2. Pre-participation paperwork

Obtaining information about the patient is vital to ensuring a safe and effective exercise program. Before any exercise is conducted, the exercise trainer must learn all they can about the patient's medical and cancer history, treatment regimen, psychological well-being, exercise history, as well as any pertinent negative side effects related to cancer treatment. The exercise trainer will also want to have the patient's physician sign a release form, and the patient sign a waiver prior to beginning any exercise program.

3. Fitness assessment procedures

After all necessary paperwork is complete and the physician's clearance has been signed and returned, the exercise trainer may begin the exercise program development process. The first step in this process a comprehensive fitness assessment. The purpose of the fitness assessment is to determine the patient's current level of fitness. This will assist in goal setting and exercise program development. It is important to note, however, that cancer-specific norm charts have yet to be developed. Thus, any score received on the fitness assessment will be compared to a norm chart representative of a healthy population. Therefore, it would be wise to set goals that are relatively modest, particularly when working with a patient who is currently in treatment.

At Maple Tree Cancer Alliance, we recommend conducting one test for each component of fitness. To measure VO2, we utilize the Bruce Treadmill Protocol, and have each patient

http://dx.doi.org/10.5772/60268

exercise to 75% of their estimated HRmax, or volitional fatigue. To measure body composition, we conduct the 7-site skinfold assessment. Muscular endurance is measured via the partial curl-up test. Muscular Strength is assessed via hand-grip dynamometer, and finally, flexibility is measured with the modified sit-and-reach. For patients who undergo breast cancer surgery, we also measure upperbody (flexion/extension) using the goniometer, and do upper extremity circumference measurements to check for lymphedema.

4. Exercise prescription

Once the fitness assessment has been completed and reviewed, the cancer exercise trainer designs an individualized exercise prescription for the patient, where recommendations pertaining to the frequency, intensity, duration, mode, and progression of exercise are addressed. Ideally, for an individual undergoing cancer treatment, the prescription will include a whole-body workout that targets all the major muscle groups. The overall goal of the exercise program should be to minimize the general de-conditioning that often results from cancer treatment so that the cancer treatments are better tolerated. In general, the exercise prescription should include a slow progression and demonstrate adaptability to changes in the patient's health status, which frequently will change from day-to-day during treatment.

At present, the optimal frequency, duration, and time course of adaptation to aerobic and resistance exercise training in cancer patients are not known, although research indicates that individuals undergoing cancer therapy benefit from low-to-moderate intensity aerobic and resistance exercise [13]. Based on available data, Table 1 presents some general guidelines a fitness professional may follow when designing an exercise program (Schmitz et al., 2010; Physical Activities Guidelines Advisory Committee, 2008; Haskell et al., 2007; Schneider & Carter, 2003).

	Aerobic Training	Strength Training	Flexibility Training
Frequency	3-5 days/wk	2-3 days/wk	2-7 days/wk
Intensity	40-60% HRR*	40-60% HRR*	Stretch to the point of mild discomfort
Duration	20-60 min/session	1-3 sets, 8-12 reps per exercise	10-30 seconds per stretch
Mode	Walking, cycling, cross trainers, swimming	Free weights, machines, resistance bands, resistance balls	Static stretching

Table 1. Guidelines for Designing an Exercise Prescription for Individuals Undergoing Cancer Treatment.

Initially, intensity will depend on the patient's functional status and exercise history prior to cancer diagnosis. Typically, previously active cancer patients may continue their exercise regimen, although intensity may need to be decreased during treatment. Progression should consist of increases in frequency and duration rather than in intensity (Physical Activities Guidelines Committee, 2008; Schneider & Carter, 2003).

5. Exercise program

5.1. Pre-exercise guidelines

Prior to each exercise session, the cancer exercise trainer must assess the patient's readiness to exercise. Resting heart rate and blood pressure should be measured, and general information regarding the patient's overall health status should be obtained. Contraindications to exercise are listed in Table 2. Depending on the information attained from the patient, the exercise intervention may need to be adjusted for that day.

Onset of nausea following exercise initiation
Vomiting within the last 24 hours
Leg pain
Decreased heart rate and blood pressure with increased workload
Chest pain
Difficult or shallow breathing
Unusual muscle weakness
Numbness in the extremities
Chemotherapy treatment within the last 24-hours
Irregular pulse during exertion
Disorientation and confusion
Dizziness

Table 2. Contraindications to exercise in cancer patients.

5.2. Supervised exercise training session

- **Warm up:** Each session should begin with a 5- to 10-minute warm-up that stimulates blood flow to the working muscles. The warm-up should involve some mild stretching and light aerobic activity.

- **Aerobic Component:** During the aerobic component of exercise, it is important to frequently monitor blood pressure and heart rate. If the patient is on a medication that affects heart rate, the Borg Scale of Exertion (Borg, 1973) (Figure 1) may be used to monitor intensity. Based on this scale, a light-to-moderate intensity (RPE of 11 to 14) should be encouraged. If

http://dx.doi.org/10.5772/60268

dizziness, nausea, or chest pain occurs, all exercise should be stopped. Frequent short breaks are sometimes encouraged to accommodate therapy-related fatigue.

- **Resistance Training:** The type of resistance exercise performed will depend on the patient's range of motion, tissue removal, and wound healing. ACSM recommends at least 48 hours of rest between each resistance training session (Schneider & Carter, 2003). Therefore, it may be advisable to plan a whole body approach to resistance training, where all major muscle groups are targeted in one day. If the patient is unwilling or unable to participate in traditional modes of strength training, Yoga, or Pilates may serve as an alternative form of strength exercise.

- **Cool Down:** Aerobic exercise should be followed up by static stretching and range of motion exercises for all major muscle groups.

The Borg Scale

6	No exertion at all
7	Extremely light
8	
9	Very light
10	
11	Light
12	
13	Somewhat hard
14	
15	Hard (heavy)
16	
17	Very hard
18	
19	Extremely hard
20	Maximal exertion

Figure 1. The Borg Scale Rating Perception of Effort (RPE).

6. Follow up

To assist in progression, patients should be reassessed approximately every 6 months (Schneider & Carter, 2003). In addition, it is advisable to maintain communication with the patient's primary oncologist. The following form, used by Maple Tree Cancer Alliance, is sent to the physician every 3-6 months, and is a simple way to keep the doctor abreast of the patient's progress.

7. Nutrition guidelines during cancer

Nutritional guidance during cancer treatments is very important, since cancer treatments typically result in side effects that lead to eating problems. Such side effects include trouble swallowing, sore mouth, dry mouth, thick saliva, altered taste and smell, nausea and vomiting, decreased appetite and constipation. Nutritional interventions specific to these side effects have been shown to contribute shorter hospital stays, decreased healthcare costs, faster healing, increased tolerance to treatment duration and higher treatment dosages, as well as decreased complications during their cancer treatment.

A registered dietitian may provide nutritional counseling, develop meal plans, and monitor the body weight, caloric, and dietary needs of a person diagnosed with and being treated for cancer. Ideally, each individual would be given a personalized dietary plan according to their specific needs and goals. Dietary plans should be closely monitored and changed according to the client's changing nutritional health requirements throughout their battle with cancer. The purpose of nutritional guidance is to help the patient:

- Improve quality of life
- Maintain a healthy weight
- Improve treatment tolerance
- Manage treatment-related side effects
- Improve eating habits

Sound nutrition practices include eating a variety of foods that will give the body the nutrients needed to help fight cancer. Included in these nutrients are protein, fats, and carbohydrates, as well as water, vitamins, and minerals.

Proteins are important for growth, immune system function, and building and repairing body tissue. When protein is lacking in the diet, the body breaks down its muscle, which lowers resistance to infection and makes it harder for the body to recover from illness. Good sources of protein include lean meats, fish, poultry, eggs, dairy, nuts, beans, peas, and lentils.

Carbohydrates are a major source of energy for the body, giving it the energy it needs for activity and proper function. Most of all carbohydrates turn into glucose after it is digested. Glucose is used by the body to create adenosine triphosphate, the energy currency of the cells. Glucose can also be stored, in the form of glycogen, in the liver and skeletal muscle. During times of starvation or exercise, glycogen is broken down into glucose to be used to make energy.

When selecting dietary sources of carbohydrates, it is important to choose foods that don't have a dramatic effect on blood sugar. This can be done by examining the glycemic index of

http://dx.doi.org/10.5772/60268

the food. Glycemic index is a number between 50-100 associated with food, that indicates its effect on blood sugar. A lower glycemic index suggests slower rates of digestion and absorption of the foods' carbohydrates, and may also indicate greater extraction from the liver and periphery of the products of carbohydrate digestion. A lower glycemic response usually equates to a lower insulin demand but not always, and may improve long-term blood glucose control. Therefore, the best sources of carbohydrates are those that have a low glycemic index (whole grains, peaches, strawberries, mushrooms, chillis, most vegetables, and seeds), compared to high glycemic index foods (white breads and pastas, most commercial cereals, bagels, white rice, and white potatoes).

Fats are a rich source of energy for the body. There are different types of dietary fat, and some are better for the cancer patient than others. In general, monounsaturated and polyunsaturated fats are better choices than saturated or trans fats. Monounsaturated fats are mainly in vegetables, including olive, canola, and peanut oils. Polyunsaturated fats are the main fats found in seafood, as well as safflower, sunflower, corn, and flaxseed oils. Saturated fats are primarily found in animal sources, like meat, poultry, milk, cheese, and butter. Because saturated fats can raise cholesterol, the American Cancer Society recommends that less than 10% of an individual's calories come from saturated fat. (ACS, 2006). Trans fats are found in foods made with partially hydrogenated vegetable oils, margarine, or shortening. They have a negative effect on cholesterol and are not recommended in the diet.

8. Sound nutrition during treatment

Sound nutrition practices are very important during cancer treatment to help the body maintain strength, prevent tissue break down, manage side effects, and maintain immunity. The healthier an individual's diet, the better they can tolerate treatments and the more effective cancer treatments are in their body.

In general, a plant-based diet is ideal. At least 5 servings of fruits and vegetables are recommended each day, in a variety of colors. Colorful fruits and vegetables contain phytochemicals, which have preventative or disease-protective properties. High-fat foods, especially those from animal sources, should be avoided, as well as salt-cured, smoked, and pickled foods. Small snacks may be ingested during the day, as caloric needs often increase during cancer treatment. It may be helpful to keep a variety of protein-rich snacks on hand, including yogurt, soup, cheese, and crackers.

It is also very important to ensure that the patient is getting enough fluids each day. These can be in the form of water, juices, or other clear liquids that are sipped throughout the day. Fluids are lost through vomiting or diarrhea, and may lead to dehydration if not replenished.

During treatment, there will most likely be days when side effects make eating difficult or undesirable. On those days, it might be helpful to eat several small snacks throughout the day, rather than three large meals. Liquid supplements or high-protein beverages might be helpful to increase calories. Also, the patient should not be limited to food choices. In other words, if they want to eat breakfast for dinner, or vice versa, it is okay. When eating is difficult, it is more important to get calories in so that the patient can maintain strength. Then, on days when appetite is good, the patient should be encouraged to eat as healthy as possible.

9. Food safety

Because cancer and its associated treatments can weaken the immune system, food safety is essential. It is very important to avoid being exposed to germs when food is not handled or prepared properly. Hand washing is very important anytime food is going to be handled or eaten. Keeping food at the proper temperature and defrosting frozen foods correctly is also very important. Fruits and vegetables should be washed thoroughly under running water before peeling or cutting. Food that has been cut at the grocery store (i.e. melon or squash) should be avoided. Use a clean knife and cutting board to cut different foods, and clean counter tops with hot, soapy water. Foods should be cooked well, but not charred.

Once treatment ends, most eating-related side effects of cancer treatments go away. It is still very important for the patient to continue to eat a healthy diet, in order to regain strength, build tissue, and improve quality of life. Patients will want to continue to eat at least 5-7 fruits and vegetables each day, especially those that are dark-green, deep-yellow, and citrus fruits. Foods high in fiber, including whole-grain breads, should also be consumed. Red meat intake should be limited to no more than 3-4 servings each week. Alcohol consumption should also be limited. Salt-cured, smoked, and pickled foods, such as bacon, sausage, and deli meats, should be avoided. Low-fat milk and dairy products should be selected, and food should be prepared in such a way to reduce the total amount of fat (i.e. bake or broil over fry).

Author details

Karen Y. Wonders[1,2*]

Address all correspondence to: karen.wonders@wright.edu

1 Wright State University, 301 Nutter Center, Dayton, OH, USA

2 Maple Tree Cancer Alliance, Dayton OH, USA

References

[1] Rowland JH. Cancer survivorship: rethinking the cancer control continuum. Semin Oncol Nurs 2008; 24 145-152.

[2] Surveillance, Epidemiology, and End Results (SEER) Program. Prevalence database: US Estimated Complete Prevalence Counts on 1/1/2004. National Cancer Institute, DCCPS, Surveillance Research Program, Statistical Research and Applications Branch, released April 2007, based on the November 2006 SEER data submission.

[3] Hewitt M, Rowland JH, Yancik R. Cancer survivors in the United States: age, health, and disability. J Gerontol A Biol Sci Med Sci 2003; 58 82-91.

[4] Hewitt M, Rowland JH. Mental health service use among adult cancer survivors: analyses of the National Health Interview Survey. J Clin Oncol 2002; 20: 4581-4590.

[5] American Cancer Society. (2011). Stay Healthy. Healthy living information to help you stay well. Date of access: March 24, 2011. Available from: http://www.cancer.org/Healthy/EatHealthyGetActive/GetActive/index

[6] Douglas E. Exercise in cancer patients. The Physical Therapy Review 2005; 10 71-88.

[7] Wiggins MS. & Simonavice EM. Quality of life benefits: A 12-month exercise cancer recovery case study. KAHPERD Journal. 2008; 44 16-9.

[8] Kruk J. Physical activity in the prevention of the most frequent chronic diseases: An analysis of the recent evidence. Asian Pacific Journal of Cancer Prevention 2007; 8 325-38.

[9] Miles L. Physical activity and the prevention of cancer: A review of recent findings. Nutrition Bulletin 2007; 32 250-82.

[10] Courneya KS. & Friedenreich CM. Physical activity and cancer control. Seminars in Oncology Nursing 2007; 23 242-52.

[11] Friedenreich CM Orenstein MR. Physical activity and cancer prevention: Etiologic evidence and biological mechanisms. The Journal of Nutrition 2002; 132 5456-64.

[12] Wiggins MS. & Simonavice EM. Cancer prevention, aerobic capacity, and physical functioning in survivors related to physical activity: A recent review. Cancer Management and Research 2010; 2 157-64.

[13] Swartz AL. Cancer, In: ACSM's Exercise Management for Persons with Chronic Diseases and Disabilities (3rd ed.). Durstine, J.L., Moore, G.E., Painter, P.L., Roberts, S.O., (Eds.). 2009; 211-218, Human Kinetics, ISBN-10: 0736074333, Champaign, IL.

[14] Quist M, Rorth M, Zacho M, Andersen C, Moeller T, Midtgaard J, Adamsen L. High-intensity resistance and cardiovascular training improve physical capacity in cancer patients undergoing chemotherapy. Scandinavian Journal of Medicine & Science in Sports 2006; 16(5) 349-57.

[15] Dimeo F, Bertz H, Finde J, Fetscher S, Mertelsmann R, & Kuel J. An aerobic exercise program for patients with haematological malignancies after bone marrow transplantation. Bone Marrow Transplantation 1996; 18 (6) 1157-60.

[16] Mock V, Dow KH, Meares CJ, Grimm PM, Dienemann JA, Haisfield-Wolfe ME, Quitasol W, Mitchell S, Chakravorthy A, Gage I. Effects of exercise on fatigue, physical functioning, and emotional distress during radiation therapy for breast cancer. Oncology Nursing Forum 2007; 24 (6) 991-1000.

[17] Schwartz AI, Mori M, Gao R, Nail LM, King ME. Exercise reduced daily fatigue in women with breast cancer receiving chemotherapy. Medicine and Science in Sports and Exercise 2001; 33 (5) 718-23.

[18] Segal R, Evans W, Johnson D, Smith J, Colletta S, Gayton J, Woodard S, Walls G, Reid R. Structured exercise improves physical functioning in women with stages I and II breast cancer: Results of a randomized controlled trial. Journal of Clinical Oncology 2001;19 (3) 657-65.

[19] Wiggins MS. Simonavice EM. Quality of life benefits: A 12-month exercise cancer recovery case study. KAHPERD Journal 2008; 44 16-9.

[20] Wiggins MS Simonavice EM. Quality of life benefits in cancer survivorship with supervised exercise. Physiological Reports, 2009; 104 (2) 421-24.

[21] Courneya KS. Keats MR, Turner AR. Physical exercise and quality of life in cancer patients following a high dose chemotherapy and autologous bone marrow transplatation. Psycho-oncology 2000; 9 (2) 127-36.

[22] Courneya KS, Friedenreich CM, Quinney HA, Fields ALA, Jones LW, Fairey AS. A randomized trial of exercise and quality of life in colorectal cancer survivors. European Journal of Pharmacology 2003; 12 347-57.

[23] Courneya KS, Friedenreich, CM, Quinney HA, Fields ALA, Jones LW, Fairey AS. A randomized trial of exercise and quality of life in colorectal cancer survivors. European Journal of Pharmacology 2003; 12 347-57.

[24] Pirl WF Roth AJ. Diagnosis and treatment of depression in cancer patients. Oncology 1999; 13 (9) 1293-1301.

[25] Galvo DA. Newton RU. Review of exercise intervention studies in cancer patients. Journal of Clinical Oncology 2005; 23 (4) 899-909.

[26] Doyle C, Kushi L, Byers T, Courneya KS, Denmark-Wahnefried W, Grant B, McTiernan A, Rock CL, Thompson C, Gansler T, Andrews KS. Nutrition and physical activity during and after cancer treatment: an American Cancer Society guide for informed choices. Cancer Journal for Clinicians 2006; 56(6) 323-53.

[27] American Cancer Society. Nutrition for the person with cancer during treatment. A guide for patients and families. American Cancer Society, Inc. 2006.

Chapter 7

Targeting the PI3K/AKT/mTOR Pathway in Cancer Cells

Isabella S. Guimarães, Nayara G. Tessarollo, Paulo C.M. Lyra-Júnior, Diandra Z. dos Santos, Roger C. Zampier, Laura F.R.L. de Oliveira, Krislayne V. Siqueira, Ian V. Silva and Leticia B.A. Rangel

Additional information is available at the end of the chapter

http://dx.doi.org/10.5772/61676

1. Introduction

The phosphoinositide 3-kinase (PI3K)/protein kinase B (AKT)/mammalian target of rapamycin (mTOR) pathway is a critical regulator of many essential physiological processes, but it also plays a key role in the malignant transformation of human tumors and their subsequent growth, metabolism, proliferation, and metastasis [1]. Previous studies have demonstrated that the PI3K/AKT/mTOR pathway is frequently activated in human cancers due to the somatic mutation and amplification of genes encoding key components [2,3]. In addition, aberrant PI3K/AKT/mTOR signaling activation also confers resistance to conventional therapies and is a poor prognostic factor for many types of cancers [4,5]. Several agents that target the PI3K/AKT/mTOR cascade elements are undergoing evaluation in preclinical and clinical studies. These include PI3K inhibitors, AKT inhibitors, mTOR catalytic site inhibitors, and dual PI3K-mTOR inhibitors. This chapter focuses on recent preclinical and clinical data on the efficacy of PI3K/AKT/mTOR pathway inhibitors either as monotherapy or in combination with conventional chemotherapy or others target drugs. Herein, we review four different classes of PI3K pathway inhibitors: PI3K inhibitors, AKT inhibitors, mTOR catalytic site inhibitors, and dual PI3K-mTOR inhibitors.

2. The PI3K/AKT/mTOR pathway

The PI3K/AKT/mTOR constitutes an important pathway downstream of growth factor tyrosine kinase receptors, thus regulating a plethora of biological processes as angiogenesis, proliferation, metabolism, survival, and differentiation [3]. Accumulating evidences indicate, therefore, that alterations in the PI3K/AKT/mTOR axis play critical and multifaceted role in cancer pathogenesis and progression. Indeed, systematic analysis performed in 3.281 tumors from 12 cancer types of the Cancer Genome Atlas Pan-Cancer effort has revealed that elements of the PI3K/AKT/mTOR signaling pathway are among the highest frequently mutated genes in cancer, such as uterine corpus endometrioid, breast, colon, lung, head and neck, and ovarian carcinomas [4,5].

Subunit	Protein	Gene name (human)
Class I		
Class IA		
Catalytic	p110α	PIK3CA
	p110β	PIK3CB
	p110δ	PIK3CD
Regulatory	p50α, p55α, p85α	PIK3R1
	p85β	PIK3R2
	p55γ	PIK3R3
Class IB		
Catalytic	p110γ	PIK3CG
Regulatory	p101	PIK3R5
	p84, p87	PIK3R6
Class II		
Catalytic	PI3KC2α	PIK3C2A
	PI3KC2β	PIK3C2B
	PI3KC2γ	PIK3C2G
Class III		
Catalytic	Vps34	PIK3C3
Regulatory	Vps15	PIK3R4

Table 1. The PI3K proteins family

PI3K is a heterodimer of its catalytic and regulatory subunits and has been classified as class I, II, and III. Class I PI3K is constituted by four 110-kDa catalytic subunits and two main regulatory domains, which is subdivide in class IA and IB. Class IA PI3K (PI3K α, β, and δ) is activated by receptors with tyrosine kinase activity, and class IB PI3K (PI3K γ) is activated by G protein-coupled receptors. The class IA enzymes are dimers of p110α, p110β, or p110δ catalytic subunits and the regulatory subunits p85α (or its splice variants p55a and p50a), p85β, p55γ, p101, or p84 [6,7]. In turn, class IB enzymes are dimers of p110γ catalytic subunit and either p101 or p84 (also known as p87PIKAP) regulatory subunits [8]. The four class I catalytic isoforms share overlapping but distinct functions. Although the expression of p110c and p110d isoforms seems to be confined to immune cells, p110a and p110b are ubiquitously expressed but exhibit isoform-specific cell-type- and context-dependent requirements, thus being involved in a wide range of cellular effects [9–13]. Class II PI3K (PI3KC2) subfamily has additional domains in both N- and C-terminal extensions and exists as 3 isoforms, PI3K-C2α, PI3K-C2β, and PI3K-Cγ [14]. On the other hand, class III PI3K occurs as a single isoform constituted by the catalytic subunit Vps34p and regulatory subunit Vps15 [14] (Table 1).

The PI3K family recruits effector proteins, altering their localization, activity, and conformation. There are some binding proteins domains that mediate such events [14]. The best-characterized domains among them are FYVE (Fab 1, YOTB, Vac 1, EEA1) [15–17], PH (pleckstrin homology) [18], and PX (Phox) [19-23]. Nonetheless, the peculiar composition of the three PI3K subfamilies results in the activation of distinct cellular functions.

In brief, after activation by receptor tyrosine kinases, including members of platelet-derived growth factor receptor, the insulin and insulin-like growth factor 1 (IGF-1) receptors and human epidermal growth factor receptor family (EGFR and HER2), PI3K phosphorylates phosphatidylinositol 4,5-trisphosphate (PIP_2) to generate phosphatidylinositol 3,4,5-trisphosphate (PIP_3) [24]. In physiological conditions, the level of PIP3 is strictly regulated by PTEN (phosphatase and tensin homolog), a phosphatase that specifically catalyzes the dephosphorylation of PIP3, converting PIP3 back to PIP2, thus constituting an important endogenous-negative feedback loop of the PI3K signaling pathway [25,26]. The lipid product of PI3K, PIP_3, recruits a subset of signaling proteins with PH domains to the membrane, including 3-phosphoinositide-dependent protein kinase (PDK1) and AKT, resulting in its phosphorylation at threonine-308 and activation [24].

In both physiological and pathological conditions, AKT exists in three isoforms in mammals: AKT1, AKT 2, and AKT 3 [27,28]. AKT phosphorylates tuberous sclerosis complex 2 (TSC2), thereby inhibiting the GTPase activity of the TSC1/TSC2 complex and enabling mTOR activation by RAS homologue enriched in brain (RHEB), thus allowing signal propagation [26,29]. mTOR exists in two different structural protein complex: mTORC1 and mTORC2, each of which is expressed in different subcellular compartments, therefore affecting their activation and function. mTORC1 complex is composed of a catalytic subunit mTOR, regulatory-associated protein of mTOR (RAPTOR), mammalian lethal with SEC13 protein 8 (MLST8), and the noncore components PRAS40 and DEP domain-containing mTOR-interacting protein (DEPTOR). Once activated, mTORC1 leads to increased protein synthesis via its effectors, named translation-regulating factors ribosomal S6 kinase-1 (S6K-1) and eukaryote translation initiation factor 4E binding protein-1 (4EBP-1). S6K-1 and 4EBP1 are major regulators of protein translation [30]. On the other hand, mTORC2 is composed by rapamycin-insensitive companion of mTOR (RICTOR), MLST8, and mammalian stress-activated protein kinase interacting protein 1 (SIN1). The function of mTORC2 remains not fully understood, but it is required to phosphorylate AKT at serine-473, thus resulting in its maximal activation [31]. Of clinical relevance, differently from mTORC1, mTORC2 is insensitive to rapamycin inhibition, opening an avenue for drug discovery in face of the development of resistance by cancer cells against first-generation mTOR inhibitors (rapalogs) that particularly target mTORC1 [32] (Figure 1).

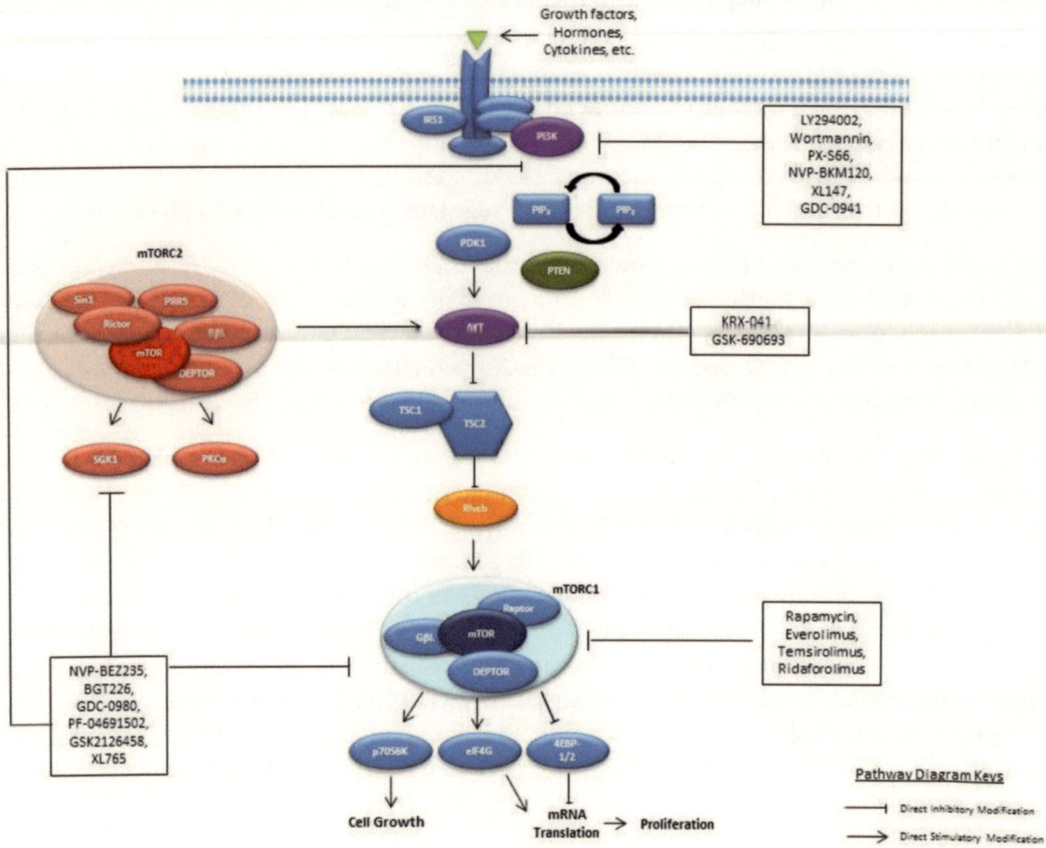

Figure 1. Overview of PI3K/AKT/mTOR signaling pathway and some inhibitors of this pathway in clinical studies. The activation of the PI3K by receptor tyrosine kinases promotes conversion of PIP_2 to PIP_3. PTEN dephosphorylates PIP_3, negatively regulating the PI3K signaling. The phosphorylation and activation of AKT impacts many downstream effectors, such as mTORCI, and finally leads to multiple cellular processes.

3. The role of PI3K/AKT/mTOR in cancer

Somatic mutations and/or gains and losses of genes are possible genetic alterations affecting the PI3K/AKT/mTOR pathway in different solid and hematological tumors [33,34]. Indeed, PI3K pathway can be activated by direct upstream signs and can be intrinsically activated due to gain of functional mutations or amplifications in PIK3CA (p110 subunit), mutations in PIK3R (p85 subunit), and mutations or amplifications in one of the AKT isoforms or loss of PTEN [35]. Loss of PTEN via inactivating mutations, due to either copy number loss or homozygous deletions, is associated with both resistance to chemotherapy and reduced survival of human patients [3].

PIK3CA mutations in primary breast tumors have been associated with lymph node metastases and overexpression of ER, PR, and HER2 [36]. Furthermore, the presence of activating

http://dx.doi.org/10.5772/61676

PI3KCA mutations and loss of PTEN in HER2-overexpressing cancers is correlated with a lower response to trastuzumab and lapatinib [37]. In non-small cell lung cancer, the downregulation of PTEN is also related with poor prognosis [38,39]. In ovarian cancer, PI3K/AKT/mTOR molecular alteration appears to be histological subtype specific. Studies have described amplifications in PIK3CA, amplifications of one of the AKT isoforms, and PTEN deletions in 20%, 15%, and 5% of the high grade serous ovarian cancer (HGSOC) cases, respectively [40,41]. The individual mutations, rare events in HGSOC, are prevalent in low grade serous, mucinous, endometrioid, and clear cell ovarian cancer; 20% of endometrioid and 35% of clear cell ovarian tumors display these PIK3CA mutations [42,43]. Besides, copy number changes in the genes encoding PIK3CA and PIK3CB subunits have been associated with a poor prognosis, and the inhibition of PI3K/mTOR was found to delay tumor growth and prolong survival [44,45].

Moreover, mutations of mTOR itself and/or in components of mTOR-related signaling pathways have frequently been described in human malignant diseases [46-48]. Different genetic lesions that mediate mTORC1 activation have diverse consequences: PTEN loss uncouples mTORC1 activation from growth factor signaling; liver kinase B1/serine/threonine kinase 11 (LKB1/STK11) mutations allow mTORC1 activation despite nutrient deprivation in poorly vascularized tumors; P53 mutations uncouple DNA damage from the inhibition of bioenergetic processes and cell cycle arrest [49]; and hyperactivation of S6K-1, 4EBP1 and eIF4E, and cancer growth by activating the lipid and protein biosynthesis. Furthermore, the increased phosphorylation of mTOR is associated with acquired cisplatin resistance, and AKT signaling has been implicated in primary platinum resistance [50]. In fact, AKT or mTOR inhibitors likely restore chemosensitivity to platinum derivates *in vitro* and in xenograft models [51,52].

These molecular alterations, in addition to the druggability of the components of the PI3K/AKT/mTOR signaling cascade, suggest that targeting the pathway might represent a useful treatment strategy in the fight against cancer.

4. PI3K inhibitors in cancer therapy

As aforementioned, PI3K/AKT/mTOR pathway has been implicated in tumorigenesis, promotion of cell survival, angiogenesis, cellular invasion, tumor growth, and the acquisition of chemoresistant phenotype by cancer cells [1]. Currently, more than fifty PI3K/AKT/mTOR axis inhibitors are in different stages of development, with a great number of such inhibitors reaching clinical trials [53]. Analogs of rapamycin (inhibitors of mTORC1), temsirolimus and everolimus, are currently in the lead, having already been approved by the Food and Drug Administration (FDA) as anticancer agents [54-56]. The PI3K/AKT/mTOR pathway inhibitors are summarized in Table 2.

4.1. PI3K inhibitors

PI3K inhibitors can be divided in isoform-specific inhibitors or pan-PI3K inhibitors. pan-PI3K inhibitors target all class IA PI3Ks in tumor cells, whereas isoform-specific inhibitors were developed to decrease toxicity and might be particularly effective in cancers with PIK3CA mutations, for example.

The first-generation of PI3K inhibitors include wortmannin, a fungal metabolite isolated from *Penicillium wortimannin* that irreversibly inhibits p110 by reacting covalently with the catalytic site [57], and LY294002, a synthetic, competitive, and reversible inhibitor of the ATP binding site of PI3K [58]. Both agents achieve significant antiproliferative and pro-apoptotic effects in preclinical *in vitro* and *in vivo* studies. However, unfavorable pharmacokinetic properties, insolubility in water, high levels of toxicity, and lack of selectivity for oncogenic isoforms of Class I PI3K limit its use in clinical trials [59,60]. Although this limiting features for their clinical use, wortmannin and LY294002 have served as important research tool for elucidating diverse signal transduction processes involving PI3K pathway and has spawned a new generation of PI3K inhibitors [61] (Table 2).

Currently, water-soluble wortmannin conjugates are being developed to overcome this issue. PX-866 is a semisynthetic analog of wortmannin with potent, irreversible, pan-class I PI3K inhibitory property against p110-α, p110-δ, and p110-γ enzymes in biochemical assays [62]. In preclinical studies, the compound alone or in combination with chemotherapy (cisplatin), radiotherapy, and targeted cancer drugs (gefitinib) exhibited *in vivo* antitumor activity against numerous mouse xenograft models of human cancers [62,63]. In addition, a phase I study in eighty-four patients with advanced solid tumors showed that PX-866 is well tolerated. The most frequent study drug-related adverse events were gastrointestinal disorders, with diarrhea being the most common [64]. PX-866 is being currently tested in a combination phase I/II studies with cetuximab (NCT01252628) in squamous cell carcinoma of the head and neck (SCCHN) and in metastatic colorectal carcinoma. Furthermore, more two phase I/II studies with PX866 are ongoing: with docetaxel (NCT01204099) in non-small cell lung cancer and SCCHN and in combination with vemurafenib in patients with advanced melanoma (NCT01616199).

Buparlisib (NVP-BKM120) is an oral highly specific pan-class I PI3K inhibitor with inhibitory property against p110-α, p110-β, p110-δ, and p110-γ enzymes [65]. The compound is also active against activating p110α somatic mutations but does not significantly inhibit the related class III and class IV PI3K kinases. In preclinical cancer studies, buparlisib has shown antiproliferative and proapoptotic activity against a panel of 353 cell lines that display different genetic abnormalities that promote PI3K pathway activation [66]. *In vivo* studies have also shown that buparlisib potently inhibits the growth of human xenografts models and behaves synergistically when combined with cytotoxic agents such as temozolomide, alkylating agent, and docetaxel, antimitotic drug, or with targeted agents such as HER2 and mitogen-activated protein kinase kinase (MEK) inhibitors [66].

A phase I dose-escalation study in thirty-five patients with advanced-stage solid tumors showed that buparlisib is a safe and well-tolerated drug with favorable pharmacokinetic properties. The major treatment-related adverse events included rash, hyperglycemia, diarrhea, anorexia, mood alteration, nausea, fatigue, pruritus, and mucositis [67]. Importantly, hyperglycemia was more common at higher doses and represents a class effect of the inhibition of PI3K signaling, commonly observed with other PI3K/AKT/mTOR pathway inhibitors [67].

http://dx.doi.org/10.5772/61676

Later, phase I dose-escalation and expansion study of buparlisib was performed in eighty-three patients with advanced solid tumors demonstrating that buparlisib was well tolerated up to 100 mg/day and showed preliminary activity in patients with advanced cancers [68]. This subsequently led to the initiation of several clinical trials in multiple cancer types, such as non-small cell lung cancer, prostate cancer, breast cancer, colon cancer, and glioblastoma multiform (GBM).

BASALT-1, an ongoing phase II trial (NCT01297491), is investigating the efficacy of single-agent buparlisib in patients with metastatic non-small cell lung cancer with PI3K pathway activation. Furthermore, phase Ib/II is under evaluation in patients with advanced non-small cell lung cancer of different histotype, testing buparlisib in combination with other targeted agents such as everolimus (NCT01470209), erlotinib (NCT01487265), MEK inhibitor (NCT01363232), or in combination with standard chemotherapeutic drugs, such as docetaxel (NCT01911325), gemcitabine, and cisplatin (NCT01971489) and carboplatin and paclitaxel (NCT01820325).

At present, several active, not recruiting, and recruiting clinical trials are being conducted in all the biological subsets of breast cancer, including combinations with endocrine therapy, anti-HER2 agents, poly (ADP-ribose) polymerase (PARP) inhibitors, and chemotherapy with buparlisib. Two large phase III studies (BELLE-2 and BELLE-3) (NCT01610284, NCT01633060) are investigating the combination of buparlisib plus fulvestrant in postmenopausal women with hormone receptor-positive/HER2-negative breast cancer after failure of aromatase inhibitor alone or aromatase inhibitor plus mTOR inhibitor treatment, respectively. Another ongoing clinical study is BELLE-4, a placebo-controlled phase II trial of buparlisib with paclitaxel in the first-line treatment of HER2-negative metastatic breast cancer (NCT01572727). Buparlisib has also been evaluated in a phase II study of paclitaxel plus trastuzumab in HER2-overexpressing breast cancer (NCT01816594).

Pilaralisib (XL147) is an oral pan-class I PI3K inhibitor (α, β, γ, and δ) through reversible, competitive inhibition with ATP for p110-α, -δ, -γ, and -β enzymes [69]. *In vitro* tests revealed that pilaralisib inhibits the formation of PIP_3 in the membrane and phosphorylation of AKT and S6K-1 in multiple tumor cell lines with diverse genetic alterations in PI3K pathway [70]. Moreover, in mouse xenograft models, oral administration of pilaralisib results in significant tumor growth inhibition and combination with chemotherapeutic agents improved the growth-inhibitory effect observed with the single agents [71]. Based on this preclinical rationale, pilaralisib has been evaluated in phase I/II clinical trials.

In a phase I dose-escalation trial of sixty-nine patients with advanced solid tumors, pilaralisib was tolerable at doses associated with PI3K pathway inhibition, and the most frequent drug-related adverse events included dermatologic toxicities, diarrhea, nausea, and decreased appetite [72]. However, a phase I dose-escalation study of pilaralisib with erlotinib in patients with solid tumors showed that combination had limited antitumor activity with moderate inhibition of PI3K, MAPK and EGFR pathways [73]. Moreover, phase I/II study of pilaralisib in combination with trastuzumab or trastuzumab plus paclitaxel in trastuzumab-refractory HER2-positive metastatic breast cancer related that no responses were observed in patients treated with pilaralisib plus trastuzumab while clinical activity was observed in paclitaxel arm

[74]. Additional clinical evaluation of this PI3K inhibitor is ongoing in phase I/II studies (NCT01587040).

Pictilisib (GDC-0941) is another potent, selective, and orally bioavailable inhibitor of pan-class I PI3K. In biochemical assays, pictilisib demonstrates selectivity over a large panel of protein kinases and PI3K family kinases, including mTOR and DNA-dependent protein kinase (DNA-PK) [75]. Interestingly, pictilisib induces apoptosis in a subset of human tumor cell lines and potently inhibited tumor growth in xenograft models, including those with mutations in PI3K, PTEN, and K-Ras [76]. Significant *in vivo* antitumor activity has also been observed when administered orally in combination with other anticancer drugs, for example, docetaxel and MEK inhibitor U0126 [77-80].

In a first-in-human phase I study of pictilisib in sixty patients with advanced solid tumors, the most frequently reported drug-related adverse events were nausea, fatigue, and rash [81]. Importantly, one patient with V600E BRAF-mutant melanoma and another with platinum-refractory ovarian cancer exhibiting PTEN loss and PIK3CA amplification demonstrated partial response [81]. Pictilisib is currently under evaluation in several phase I/II clinical trials, mainly in non-small cell lung cancer and breast cancer (NCT01918306, NCT01740336, NCT01493843, and NCT00974584).

One strategy to achieve significant pathway inhibition clinically with tolerable adverse effect profile is the use of isoform-specific PI3K inhibitors. As aforementioned, each isoform has distinct role in normal physiological processes and disease (Table 1). PI3K catalytic subunit p110α is predominantly responsible for mediating growth factor signaling from receptor tyrosine kinases and is a frequent genetic driver (*PIK3CA* mutations) in several cancers [82]. However, p110α is dispensable for PI3K pathway activation in tumors lacking PTEN. Thus, these cells depend largely on p110β to activate the pathway [82,83]. Preclinical tests showed that p110β-selective inhibitors had a significantly greater activity in cell lines with PTEN null than in those with PTEN intact, although, some PTEN-intact cell lines were sensitive and a number of cells lines lacking PTEN were resistant [84]. GSK-2636771 is a PI3K p110β-selective inhibitor currently in phase I studies in subjects with advanced solid tumors with PTEN deficiency (NCT01458067). Moreover, PI3Kδ is predominantly expressed in leukocytes and control immune responses [85]. Idelalisib (CAL-101), a highly specific PI3Kδ inhibitor, was the first isoform-specific PI3K inhibitors approved for cancer treatment [86].

Alpelisib (NVP-BYL719) is an oral inhibitor that selectively targets PI3K p110α equipotent against the wild type and the most common somatic mutations of p110α [87]. NVP-BYL719 has been the first PI3Kα-selective inhibitor to enter in clinical trials after positive preclinical investigations. *In vivo* studies have demonstrated dose-dependent antitumor activity of NVP-BYL719 in PIK3CA-mutant or PIK3CA-amplified tumor xenograft models, such as ovarian, breast, and head and neck cancers [88, 89]. Preliminary results of phase I study performed in patients with advanced solid tumors carrying *PIK3CA* gene alterations demonstrated that NVP-BYL719 has a favorable safety profile with manageable toxicities, as hyperglycemia, nausea, diarrhea, decreased appetite, vomiting, and fatigue [90]. To date, more than fifteen clinical trial is ongoing in order to evaluate the combination of NVP-BYL719 with several agents, such conventional cytotoxic drugs (paclitaxel, cisplatin, and irinotecan) and target drugs (cetuximab, olaparib, and trastuzumab) in a subset of cancers (NCT02051751, NCT01822613, NCT01602315, NCT01623349, and NCT02167854)

Taselisib (GDC-0032) is a PI3K inhibitor with higher affinity for mutated PI3Kα with reduced inhibitory activity against PI3Kβ [91]. Preclinical studies show that taselisib has enhanced activity against PI3Kα isoform mutant cancer cell lines [92]. In an ongoing phase I study, taselisib has been well tolerated with hyperglycemia and fatigue being the dose-limiting toxicities [93]. This selectivity profile and excellent pharmacokinetic properties allowed fewer clinical studies with GDC-0032. Currently, several clinical studies are ongoing to evaluate the combination of taselisib with endocrine therapy, trastuzumab, and conventional chemotherapy in breast cancer (NCT02285179, NCT02390427, and NCT01862081). In addition, a phase I study is currently ongoing in taselisib with CDK4/6 inhibitor, palbociclib, in advanced solid tumors and breast cancer (NCT02389842).

Idelalisib was approved in 2014 in the United States and European Union for the treatment of three indolent B-cell neoplasms: relapsed chronic lymphocytic leukemia, in combination with rituximab, relapsed follicular B-cell non-Hodgkin's lymphoma, and relapsed small lymphocytic lymphoma (as monotherapy) [94]. In lymphoid cell lines and primary patient samples, idelalisib abrogates PI3K/AKT/mTOR signaling and promotes apoptosis [95,96]. The first phase I trial in healthy volunteers established the bioavailability and safety of idelalisib [97]. Another phase I study in patients with relapsed/refractory mantle cell lymphoma reported the most common adverse events, which includes diarrhea, nausea, pyrexia, fatigue, rash, upper respiratory infection, pneumonia and alanine transaminase, or aspartate transaminase elevations [98]. To date, about twenty-five clinical trials are ongoing with idelalisib. A phase I/II trial studies aimed evaluated idelalisib in combination with lenalidomide and rituximab in patients with relapsed or refractory mantle cell lymphoma (NCT01838434). In addition, idelalisib is being evaluated in combination with rituximab in adults with previously treated indolent non-Hodgkin lymphoma (NCT01732913).

5. AKT inhibitors in cancer therapy

AKT inhibitors constitute another class of drugs that has gained recent interest. As discussed previously, AKT is involved in the regulation of various signaling downstream pathways involved in cell survival, growth, proliferation, metabolism, and angiogenesis. AKT inhibition promotes decreasing cancer cell survival by preventing signal transduction through its downstream effectors. In addition, targeting AKT is an interesting pharmacological approach due to the AKT activation in consequence of the feedback loop release when mTOR is inhibited.

AKT inhibitors can be grouped into three classes, including lipid-based phosphatidylinositol (PI) analogs, ATP-competitive inhibitors (catalytic inhibitors), and allosteric inhibitors. To date, the most developed inhibitor of AKT is perifosine (KRX-0401), a lipid-based inhibitor. Perifosine is an allosteric inhibitor that targets the PH domain of AKT, thereby preventing its translocation to the plasma membrane required for pathway activation [99]. Perifosine has demonstrated great efficacy *in vitro* and *in vivo* against several human cancers such as breast, osteosarcoma, ovarian, multiple myeloma, leukemia, and glioma [100,101]. Additional *in vitro* data demonstrate synergistic effects of perifosine and traditional chemotherapeutic agents such as paclitaxel and cisplatin in ovarian cancer [102,103], etoposide in leukemia cells [104], doxorubicin in multiple myeloma cells [105], and gemcitabine in pancreatic cells [106].

Despite these encouraging preclinical studies, results from phase I/II clinical trials of perifosine as single agent in a various tumor types (metastatic breast cancer, metastatic head and neck cancer, locally advanced soft tissue sarcoma, prostate cancer, and metastatic

In behalf of the poor efficacy of perifosine as a single agent observed in most tumor types evaluated thus far, efforts have been made to combine this drug with target agents and chemotherapy. Phase I studies have now confirmed the safety of these combinations with different agents, including sorafenib in patients with Hodgkin lymphoma and taxanes in high-grade epithelial ovarian cancer [112,113]. Currently, one clinical trial with perifosine is recruiting patients, a phase II study with perifosine and temsirolimus in patients with malignant gliomas (NCT02238496).

GSK-690693 is a potent ATP-competitive AKT inhibitor selective for all three AKT isoforms versus the majority of kinases assessed by biochemical tests [114]. GSK690693 displayed antiproliferative activity *in vitro* and *in vivo* models of ovarian, breast, and prostate cancer [114]. The compound has entered phase I trials for refractory hematologic malignancies but was withdrawn prior to enrolment (NCT00666081).

6. mTOR inhibitors in cancer therapy

6.1. Rapamycin and its derivatives

As discussed previously, mTOR is involved in many cell signaling pathways, and clinical trials for cancer treatment showed that tumor cells with mutations in p53 or PTEN are susceptible to mTOR inhibitors [115]. mTOR inhibitors are categorized in first- and second-generation presenting a wide variety of target and mechanism. The first-generation mTOR inhibitors include rapamycin and its analogs that employ allosteric mechanism to block, whereas the second-generation mTOR inhibitors (AZD8055, Torin1, PP242, and PP30) have as target ATP binding site to impede kinase activity of both mTORC1 and mTORC2 [116].

Rapamycin, discovered in 1975, is a macrocyclic lactone isolated from the soil bacterium *Streptomyces hygroscopicus*, and it has clinical applications including antifungal, immunosuppressant, and anticancer proprieties [117,118]. FDA approved this drug in 1997 for prevention of host-rejection during kidney transplants [119]. Preclinical studies have shown that rapamycin presents strong antiangiogenic and antiproliferative properties against a variety of human cancers such as the phase II study, which showed rapamycin potentiates the effect of paclitaxel in endometrial cancer cell lines [120].

Three different mechanisms of action have been proposed: first, the binding of the FKBP-12–rapamycin complex to mTOR that could lead dephosphorylation of downstream effector molecules such as S6K-1 and 4EBP1 [121]; second, the FKBP-12–rapamycin complex competes with phosphatidic acid to bind to the FRB domain of mTOR, blocking mTOR kinase function [122]; and third, the FKBP-12–rapamycin complex bounds to mTOR and destabilizes the mTOR–raptor–4EBP1/S6K-1 scaffold complex, leading to dephosphorylation of S6K-1 and 4EBP1 [123,124].

This inhibitor has limited bioavailability due to its poor aqueous solubility. In an effort to improve its pharmacokinetics, several rapamycin analogs, named rapalogs, have been developed, such as temsirolimus (CCI-779), everolimus (RAD001), and ridaforolimus (MK-8669/AP23573) [125-127].

Some studies have shown that these compounds are able to disrupt the mTORC2 complex in a dose-, time-, and cell type-dependent manner [24,128,129]. A possible mechanism by which rapamycin and rapalogs could inhibit mTORC2 relies on the interaction of newly synthesized mTOR molecules and rapamycin/rapalogs-FKBP12 complexes. In turn, this interaction would prevent mTOR from the interaction with RICTOR, thus inhibiting mTORC2. Indeed, it has been shown that prolonged exposure of cancer cells to rapamycin can promote its binding to mTOR before the assembly of the mTORC2 complex, with subsequent inhibition of the AKT-mediated signaling [24].

Rapamycin and its derivates exhibit a safe toxicity profile, being the side effects of skin rashes and mucositis dose dependent [130]. Other symptoms commonly described are fatigue, nausea, anemia, hypertriglyceridemia, hypercholesterolemia, and neutropenia [131]. Furthermore, temsirolimus and sirolimus are associated with significant rate of pulmonary toxicity [130,131]. Rare side effects of the aforesaid drugs include interstitial lung disease, risk of secondary lymphoma, and reactivation of latent infections [35].

Everolimus (Afinitor®), the oral mTOR inhibitor, has been approved by the FDA in 2009 for advanced renal cell cancer. Everolimus exhibit strong antiangiogenic and antiproliferative activity against various human cancer such as metastatic or unresectable pancreatic neuroendocrine tumors, subependymal giant cell astrocytoma [132], metastatic renal cell carcinoma, and advanced estrogen receptor (ER)-positive [133] and human epidermal growth factor receptor-2 (HER2)-negative breast cancer [134].

Several studies have been conducted to analyze the effectiveness of rapamycin and rapalogs alone and in combination with standard chemotherapy, hormonal therapy such as anti-VEGF inhibitors in the treatment of several types of cancers such breast, ovarian, cervical, and endometrial. Phase II studies are ongoing in order to test everolimus in combination with chemotherapy (cisplatin and gemcitabine) in patients with metastatic triple negative breast cancer (NCT01939418 and NCT01931163). In addition, a recent study of breast cancer (BOLERO-3) demonstrated that the combination of everolimus with trastuzumab and vinorelbine significantly prolonged progression-free survival (PFS) in patients with trastuzumab-refractory and taxane-pretreated, HER2-positive advanced breast cancer [135]. Moreover, another breast cancer study, BOLERO-1, evaluated patients treated with paclitaxel and trastuzumab with or without everolimus as first-line therapy [136]. Furthermore, clinical studies have evaluated the aromatase inhibitor letrozole in combination with everolimus in patients with metastatic endometrial carcinoma (NCT01068249) and breast cancer (NCT00107016).

Temsirolimus (Torisel®), the first rapamycin analog to be FDA approved as an anticancer drug, is an intravenous injection drug and gets converted into rapamycin *in vivo* [137]. This drug was valued with bevacizumab or in combination with chemotherapeutic agents in endometrial cancer cell lines, and results showed the increase progesterone mRNA expression and inhibition of ER mRNA expression [138,139]. Also, preliminary phase II study using temsirolimus in patients with metastatic cervical cancer showed positives results [140]. Another phase II clinical study (NCT01196429) evaluates additional effects of the temsirolimus combined with paclitaxel/carboplatin therapy have been conducted in patients with stages III/IV clear cell adenocarcinoma [141]. However, some studies failed to show the efficiency of temsirolimus in patients with persistent/recurrent epithelial ovarian cancer/primary peritoneal cancer showing a modest activity of this mTOR inhibitor, and the results were insufficient to justify further study in a phase III [142].

Ridaforolimus (MK-8669/AP23573), a non-rapamycin prodrug, is available in both oral and intravenous formulations. This mTOR inhibitor is actively being evaluated as either monotherapy or in combination with other therapies for treatment of various cancers, including sarcomas, endometrial, prostate, breast, and non-small cell lung cancer [143]. Studies had been conducted in patients with advanced endometrial cancer and clinical benefit response was reported in 33% of the patients [144]. Another phase II study using oral ridaforolimus in patients with advanced or recurrent endometrial cancer also showed partial response in 7.7% patients [145].

Although clinically promising, the efficacy of rapalogs is partially limited by the negative feedback loops in the mTOR pathway. With this regard, the exclusive inhibition of the mTORC1 complex by the rapalogs compromises the S6K-1-mediated feedback loop towards IRS-1, resulting in the activation of both the PI3K/AKT and the mitogen-activated protein kinase/extracellular signal-regulated kinases (MAPK/ERK) pathways, hence promoting compensatory cell survival, and the acquisition of chemoresistant phenotype [127,146,147]. Efforts have been made to overcome the previously mentioned clinical limitation by means of developing new generation mTOR inhibitors, which inhibit the catalytic activity of both mTORC1 and mTORC2 complexes.

7. ATP-competitive inhibitors

Although rapamycin is a potent allosteric mTORC1 inhibitor with clinical applications, a second-generation ATP-competitive inhibitor have been developed, including Torin1, Torin2, PP242, PP30, KU0063794, WAY-600, WYE-687, WYE-354, XL-388, INK-128, AZD-2014, AZD8055, and OSI-027 [148-153]. The ATP-competitive inhibitors of mTOR directly inhibit the mTOR kinase activity, affecting both mTORC1 and mTORC2 complexes simultaneously and suppress AKT activity.

http://dx.doi.org/10.5772/61676

ATP-competitive mTOR inhibitors represent a promising new approach to target the pathway with potentially grater tolerability and efficacy than rapamycin. It has been shown that ATP inhibitors displayed dramatic antiproliferative activity across a range of cancer cell lines [151,154,155].

Studies have been conducted with PP242 in colon cancer cells *in vitro* and *in vivo* showed decrease cell growth alone or in combination with MEK inhibitors [156]. Another ATP competitive inhibitor, Torin2, was developed to overcome the pharmacological limitations of Torin1 and it is a potent inhibitor of ATR, ATM, and DNA-PK [157,158]. Lung cancer cell treatment with Torin2 resulted in a prolonged block in negative feedback and consequent threonine-308 phosphorylation on AKT. These effects were associated with strong growth inhibition *in vitro* [159].

Studies conducted by Rodrik-Outmezguine and colleagues [160], comparing mTORC1 inhibition with rapamycin and AZD8055, revealed that rapamycin treatment led to an almost complete loss in the mTORC1 phosphorylation of S6K-1 (threonine-389) and increased phospho-AKT (serine-473). In contrast, AZD8055 treatment led to reductions in phospho-S6K-1 (threonine-389), phospho-4EBP1 (threonine-37/40, threonine-65, and threonine-70), and phospho-AKT (serine-473). Thereby, AZD8055 was a better inhibitor of mTORC1 in comparison to rapamycin. *In vivo* studies indicated that AZD8055 can inhibit tumor growth and AZD8055 showed promise as a therapeutic agent.

At present, there are several clinical trials focused on the examination of new agents, such as AZD-8055 (NCT00731263), OSI-027 (NCT00698243), and INK128 (NCT02142803), in a variety of human hematological malignancies and solid tumors, including breast cancer. Also some studies were conducted using GSK795 in patients with advanced platinum-resistant ovarian and showed interesting results as tumor regressions and CA125 decreases [161]. Phase I study are ongoing to evaluate the safety and toxicity profile of AZD2014 in combination with paclitaxel in patients with ovarian cancer (NCT02193633).

Despite the clinical improvements observed with the ATP-competitive inhibitor when compared to the rapalogs, the literature still acknowledges significant limitations that outcome from compensatory cellular events. With this regard, it has been found that loss of the feedback on PI3K results in compensatory activation of the MAPK/ERK cascade by mTOR downstream effectors, such as 4EBP1/eIF4E, maintaining cell proliferation [162]. Furthermore, it has been shown that chronic inhibition of mTORC2 induces the activation of AKT by its phosphorylation mediated by PDK-1, even in the absence of the priming serine-473 phosphorylation. Altogether, the referred mechanisms ultimately drive the acquisition of the resistant phenotype by the cancer cells [154,163].

8. Dual mTOR/PI3K inhibitors

Scientist have explored to shed light on strategies to overcome the limitations by concomitantly targeting two molecules in the PI3K/AKT/mTOR pathway, PI3K and mTOR, whereas the resistance mTOR inhibitors cloud arise via feedback PI3K activation. This molecular knowledge have stimulated the development of new inhibitors termed dual PI3K-mTOR inhibitors that include NVP-BEZ235, XL765, BGT226, PI-103, PF-04691502, PKI-587, and GDC-0980 [164-170]. Comparing with the other types of PI3K pathway inhibitors, dual PI3KmTOR inhibitors have the possible advantage of inhibiting all PI3K catalytic isoforms, mTORC1 and mTORC2 [171]. Therefore, these inhibitors may effectively turn off this pathway completely and display best efficacy in feedback inhibition normally observed with mTORC1 inhibitors [172]. However, it is not clear that dual PI3K-mTOR inhibitors will be tolerable at doses that effectively inhibit all p110 isoforms and mTOR [171].

The potential clinical value of the dual PI3K/mTOR inhibitors have been demonstrated by their significant inhibition of cell growth, the induction of apoptosis and/or autophagy [173] in a variety of tumor cancer cells [174-176]. In addition, these inhibitors have shown powerful effects in xenograft models of breast cancer [177], pancreatic cancer [178], melanoma [179], multiple myeloma [180], and RCC [181].

In agreement, dual PI3K/mTOR inhibitors have entered clinical trials either monotherapy or polytherapy. A single agent includes BEZ235/NVP-BEZ235 (NCT00620594) and BGT226 (NCT00600275 and NCT00742105) in advanced solid tumors and breast cancer, GDC-0980 (NCT00854126, NCT00854152, and NCT01455493) in non-Hodgkin lymphoma and endometrial carcinoma, and PF-04691502 (NCT00927823) and GSK2126458 (NCT00972686 and NCT01248858) in solid tumors. In combination with others agents, the treatment includes XL765 (Exelixis) with erlotinib (NCT00777699), letrozole (NCT01082068), and temozolomide (NCT00704080) in non–small cell lung cancer, breast cancer, and gliomas, respectively.

Both BEZ235 and XL765 have shown good tolerability, with adverse effects including diarrhea, anorexia, and nausea [49]. Furthermore, the combined therapy using rapamycin and dual PI3K/mTOR kinase inhibitor (PI-103) has been shown to be efficacious against human ovarian cells *in vivo* [183].

Inhibitor	**Trade name (company)**	**Drug target**	**Development stage**	**Tumor types**	**Reference**
LY294002	-	Pan-PI3K inhibitor	Preclinical	-	[57,58]
Wortmannin	-	Pan-PI3K inhibitor	Preclinical	-	[57,59,60]
PX-866	(Oncothyreon)	Pan-PI3K inhibitor	Phase II	Solid cancers, prostate, colorectal, glioblastoma, SCCHN, non-small cell lung cancer	[62,64]
NVP-BKM120	Buparlisib (Novartis)	Pan-PI3K inhibitor	Phase III	Non-small cell lung cancer, prostate, breast, GBM, colon	[65,66]

http://dx.doi.org/10.5772/61676

Inhibitor	Trade name (company)	Drug target	Development stage	Tumor types	Reference
XL147	Pilaralisib (Sanofi-Exelixis)	Pan-PI3K inhibitor	Phase II	Solid cancers, breast, breast, endometrial, ovarian, non-small cell lung cancer, glioblastoma, lymphoma	[69,72]
GDC-0941	Pictilisib (Genentech-Roche)	Pan-PI3K inhibitor	Phase II	Solid cancers, breast, non-small cell lung cancer, glioblastoma, non-Hodgkin's lymphoma	[75,81]
GSK-2636771	(GlaxoSmithKline)	PI3Kβ inhibitor	Phase I	Solid cancers (PTEN deficient), prostate	[84]
NVP-BYL719	Alpelisib (Novartis)	PI3Kα inhibitor	Phase II	Advanced solid tumors, SCCHN, breast, ovarian	[87,90]
GDC-0032	Taselisib (Genentech)	PI3Kα inhibitor	Phase III	Solid cancers, breast, non-small cell lung cancer	[91,93]
CAL-101	Idelalisib (Gilead Sciences)	PI3Kδ inhibitor	Phase III	Lymphomas, multiple myelomas, chronic lymphocytic leukemia, acute myeloid leukemia	[94,97,98]
KRX-0401	Perifosine (Pfizer)	AKT inhibitors	Phase II	Solid tumors, non-small cell lung cancer, colon, kidney, breast, gliomas, multiple myeloma, leukemia, lymphomas	[107,111,112,113]
GSK-690693	(GlaxoSmithKline)	ATP-competitive AKT inhibitor	Phase I	Hematologic malignancies	[114]
Rapamycin	Sirolimus (Wyeth)	Inhibits mTOR kinase by binding to FKBP12	Phase I	Glioblastoma, non-small cell lung cancer	[182]

Inhibitor	Trade name (company)	Drug target	Development stage	Tumor types	Reference
RAD001	Everolimus (Novartis)	Inhibits mTOR kinase by binding to FKBP12	Phase I/II/III (FDA has approved for RCC, 2009)	Metastatic renal cell carcinoma, breast cancer, melanoma, ovarian cancer, neuroendocrine tumors of the pancreatic origin (PNET), endometrial carcinoma	[56,133,134,135,136], NCT01939418, NCT01931163
CCI-779	Temsirolimus (Wyeth/Pfizer)	Inhibits mTOR kinase by binding to FKBP12	Phase I/II/III (FDA and European Medicine Agency have approved for RCC, 2007)	Non-small cell lung cancer; advanced solid tumors, metastatic renal cell carcinoma, hepatocellular carcinoma, cervical cancer, clear cell adenocarcinoma	[138,139,141]
MK-8669/AP23573	Ridaforolimus	Inhibits mTOR kinase by binding to FKBP12	Phase I/II/III	Sarcoma, bone, endometrial cancer	[144,145]
PP242		ATP competitive inhibitor of mTOR	Studies *in vitro* and *in vivo*	Colon cancer, acute myeloid leukemia	[156]
Torin2		ATP competitive inhibitor of mTOR	Studies *in vitro* and *in vivo*	Lung cancer	[159]
AZD8055		ATP competitive inhibitor of mTOR	Phase I	Advanced solid tumors, lymphoma	[183,184]
OSI-027		ATP competitive inhibitor of mTOR	Phase I	Advanced solid tumors, lymphoma	[185]
INK128		ATP competitive inhibitor of mTOR	Phase I	Glioblastoma, advanced solid tumors.	NCT02142803
GSK795		ATP competitive inhibitor of mTOR	Phase I	Advanced solid tumors	[134]
NVP-BEZ235	(Novartis)	Dual mTOR/PI3K	Phase I/II	Advanced solid tumors, breast cancer, prostate cancer	[94], NCT00620594

Inhibitor	Trade name (company)	Drug target	Development stage	Tumor types	Reference
BGT226	(Novartis)	Dual mTOR/PI3K	Phase I	Advanced solid tumors, breast cancer	[169], NCT00600275, NCT00742105
GDC-0980	(Genentech)	Dual mTOR/PI3K	Phase I/II	Non-Hodgkin lymphoma, endometriose	NCT00854126, NCT00854152, NCT01455493
PF-04691502	(Pfizer)	Dual mTOR/PI3K	Phase I	Advanced solid tumors	NCT00927823
GSK2126458	GlaxoSmithKline	Dual mTOR/PI3K	Phase I	Advanced solid tumors	NCT00972686, NCT01248858
XL765	(Exelixis)	Dual mTOR/PI3K	Phase I/II	Non-small cell lung cancer, breast cancer, gliomas	NCT00777699, NCT01082068, NCT00704080

Table 2. Overview of PI3K/AKT/mTOR pathway inhibitors.

9. Conclusions/future perspectives

Advances in molecular research have resulted in an improved understanding of cancer biology. There is strong preclinical rationale to support the continued development of PI3K/AKT/mTOR inhibitors, especially in some genetically defined cancer subtypes that may be the most sensitive to single-agent PI3K pathway inhibitors. These include cancers with PIK3CA activating mutations, mutations in PIK3R (p85 subunit), mutations or amplifications in one of the AKT isoforms or loss of PTEN. However, rational clinical trials design with a focus in identifying a patient population most likely to benefit from this strategy is imperative to the success of single-agent therapeutics.

The combination of PI3K/AKT/mTOR inhibitors with cytotoxic chemotherapy and other biological agents such as anti-HER2 compounds, EGFR inhibitors, and antiangiogenic agents may optimize the action of those agents in different pathways that control protein translation, cell growth, migration, metastasis, and angiogenesis. The successful development of the combinations will require determining the duration, doses, and schedules of targeted therapy and how to best incorporate it into standard treatment protocols. Several clinical trials are underway to prove the clinical use of the PI3K/AKT/mTOR inhibitors. The druggability of the components of the PI3K/AKT/mTOR signaling cascade, in addition to the enlightenment of the mutational landscape of human cancers, which points to the high frequency of genetic alterations and anomalous activation of the pathway, strongly suggests that targeting its elements might represent a useful treatment strategy in the fight against cancer.

Author details

Isabella S. Guimarães[1,2], Nayara G. Tessarollo[1,2], Paulo C.M. Lyra-Júnior[1,2], Diandra Z. dos Santos[1,3], Roger C. Zampier[1], Laura F.R.L. de Oliveira[1], Krislayne V. Siqueira[1], Ian V. Silva[2,4] and Leticia B.A. Rangel[1,2,3*]

*Address all correspondence to: lbarangel@yahoo.com

1 Laboratory of Cellular and Molecular Biology of Human Cancer, Department of Pharmaceutical Sciences, Federal University of Espirito Santo State, Brazil

2 Biotechnology Program, Federal University of Espirito Santo State, Brazil

3 Biochemistry and Pharmacology Program, Federal University of Espirito Santo State, Brazil

4 Department of Morphology, Health Sciences Center, Federal University of Espirito Santo State, Brazil

References

[1] Gomez-Pinillos A., Ferrari A.C. mTOR signaling pathway and mTOR inhibitors in cancer therapy. Hematology/Oncology Clinics of North America. 2012;26(3):483-505. DOI: 10.1016/j.hoc.2012.02.014

[2] Yuan T.L., Cantley L.C. PI3K pathway alterations in cancer: variations on a theme. Oncogene. 2008;27:5497–5510. DOI: 10.1038/onc.2008.245

[3] Li T., Wang G. Computer-aided targeting of the PI3K/Akt/mTOR pathway: toxicity reduction and therapeutic opportunities. International Journal of Molecular Sciences. 2014;15(10):18856-91. DOI: 10.3390/ijms151018856

[4] Bartholomeusz C., Gonzalez-Angulo, A.M. Targeting the PI3K signaling pathway in cancer therapy. Expert Opinion on Therapeutic Targets. 2012;16(1):121-30. DOI: 10.1517/14728222.2011.644788

[5] Kandoth C., McLellan M.D., Vandin F., Ye K., Niu B., Lu C., et al. Mutational landscape and significance across 12 major cancer types. Nature. 2013;502(7471):333-339. DOI: 10.1038/nature12634

[6] Vanhaesebroeck B., Guillermet-Guibert J., Graupera M., Bilanges B. The emerging mechanisms of isoform-specific PI3K signalling. Nature Reviews Molecular Cell Biology. 2010a;11 (5):329-341. DOI: 10.1038/nrm2882

[7] Vadas O., Burke J. E., Zhang X., Berndt A., Williams R. L. Structural basis for activation and inhibition of class I phosphoinositide 3-kinases. Science Signaling. 2011;4 (195):re2. DOI: 10.1126/scisignal.2002165

[8] Hawkins P.T., Anderson K.E, Davidson K., Stephens L.R. Signalling through class I PI3Ks in mammalian cells. Biochemical Society Transactions. 2006;34(5):647–662. DOI: 10.1042/BST0340647

[9] Patrucco E., Notte A., Barberis L., Selvetella G., Maffei A., Brancaccio M., et al. PI3Kgamma modulates the cardiac response to chronic pressure overload by distinct kinase-dependent and -independent effects. Cell. 2004;118(3): 375-387. DOI: 10.1016/j.cell.2004.07.017

[10] Hirsch E., Braccini L., Ciraolo E., Morello F., Perino A. Twice upon a time: PI3K's secret double life exposed. Trends in Biochemical Sciences. 2009;34(5): 244- 248. DOI: 10.1016/j.tibs.2009.02.003

[11] Dou Z., Chattopadhyay M., Pan J.A., Guerriero J.L., Jiang, Y. P., Ballou L.M., et al. The class IA phosphatidylinositol 3-kinase p110-beta subunit is a positive regulator of autophagy. Journal of Cell Biology. 2010;191 (4): 827-843. DOI: 10.1083/jcb.201006056

[12] Rauch J., Volinsky N., Romano D., Kolch W. The secret life of kinases: functions beyond catalysis. Cell Communication and Signaling. 2011;9(1):23. DOI: 10.1186/1478-811X-9-23

[13] Dou Z., Pan J.A., Dbouk H.A., Ballou L.M., DeLeon J.L., Fan Y., et al. Class IA PI3K p110b subunit promotes autophagy through Rab5 small GTPase in response to growth factor limitation. Molecular Cell. 2013;50 (1): 29-42. DOI: 10.1016/j.molcel.2013.01.022

[14] Vanhaesebroeck B., Vogt P.K., Rommel C. PI3K: from the bench to the clinic and back. Current Topics in Microbiology and Immunology. 2010b;347:1-19. DOI: 10.1007/82_2010_65

[15] Gaullier J.M., Simonsen A., D'Arrigo A., Bremnes B., Stenmark H, Aasland R. FYVE fingers bind PtdIns (3)P. Nature. 1998;394(6692):432-433.DOI: 10.1038/28767

[16] Mu F.T., Callaghan J.M., Steele-Mortimer O., Stenmark H., Parton R.G., Campbell P.L., et al. EEA1, an early endosome-associated protein. EEA1 is a conserved alpha-helical peripheral membrane protein flanked by cysteine "fingers" and contains a calmodulin-binding IQ motif. Journal of Biological Chemistry. 1995;270 (22):13503–13511.DOI: 10.1074/jbc.270.22.13503

[17] Stenmark H., Aasland R., Toh B.H., D'Arrigo A. Endosomal localization of the autoantigen EEA1 is mediated by a zinc-binding FYVE finger. Journal of Biological Chemistry. 1996;271 (39):24048–24054. DOI: 10.1074/jbc.271.39.24048

[18] Harlan J.E., Hajduk P.J., Yoon H.S., Fesik S.W. Pleckstrin homology domains bind to phosphatidylinositol-4,5-bisphosphate. Nature. 1994;371(6493):168–170. DOI: 10.1038/371168a0

[19] Cheever M.L., Sato T.K., de Beer T., Kutateladze T.G, Emr S.D., Overduin M. Phox domain interaction with PtdIns(3)P targets the Vam7 t-SNARE to vacuole membranes. Nature Cell Biology. 2001;3(7):613–8. DOI: 10.1038/35083000

[20] Ellson C.D., Gobert-Gosse S., Anderson K.E., Davidson K, Erdjument-Bromage H., Tempst P., et al. PtdIns(3)P regulates the neutrophil oxidase complex by binding to the PX domain of p40(phox). Nature Cell Biology. 2001;3(7):679-682. DOI: 10.1038/35083076

[21] Kanai F., Liu H., Field S.J., Akbary H., Matsuo T., Brown G.E., et al. The PX domains of p47phox and p40phox bind to lipid products of PI(3)K. Nature Cell Biology. 2001;3(7):675-678. DOI: 10.1038/35083070

[22] Song X., Xu W., Zhang A., Huang G., Liang X., Virbasius J.V., et al. Phox homology domains specifically bind phosphatidylinositol phosphates. Biochemistry. 2001;40(30):8940-8944. DOI: 10.1021/bi0155100

[23] Xu Y., Hortsman H., Seet L., Wong S.H., Hong W. SNX3 regulates endosomal function through its PXdomain-mediated interaction with PtdIns(3)P. Nature Cell Biology. 2001;3(7):658-666. DOI: 10.1038/35083051

[24] Sarbassov D.D., Ali S.M., Sengupta S., Sheen J.H., Hsu P.P., Bagley A.F., et al. Prolonged rapamycin treatment inhibits mTORC2 assembly and Akt/PKB. Molecular Cell. 2006;22(2):159-168. DOI: http://dx.doi.org/10.1016/j.molcel.2006.03.029

[25] Petrulea M.S., Plantinga T.S., Smit J.W., Georgescu C.E., Netea-Maier R.T. PI3K/Akt/mTOR: a promising therapeutic target for non-medullary thyroid carcinoma. Cancer Treatment Reviews. 2015;26. DOI: 10.1016/j.ctrv.2015.06.005

[26] Mukohara T. PI3K mutations in breast cancer: prognostic and therapeutic implications. Breast Cancer (Dove Medical Press). 2015;7:111-23. DOI: 10.2147/BCTT.S60696

[27] Hay N, Sonenberg N. Upstream and downstream of mTOR. Genes & Development. 2004;18(16):1926-45. DOI: 10.1101/gad.1212704

[28] Larue L., Bellacosa A. Epithelial–mesenchymal transition in development and cancer: role of phosphatidylinositol 3' kinase/AKT pathways. Oncogene. 2005;24(50): 7443-7454. DOI: 10.1038/sj.onc.1209091

[29] Manning B.D., Cantley L.C. Rheb fills a GAP between TSC and TOR. Trends of Biochemical Sciences. 2003;28(11):573-6. DOI: http://dx.doi.org/10.1016/j.tibs.2003.09.003

[30] Engelman J.A., Luo J., Cantley L.C. The evolution of phosphatidylinositol 3-kinases as regulators of growth and metabolism. Nature Reviews Genetics. 2006;7(8):606-19. DOI: 10.1038/nrg1879

[31] Jacinto E., Loewith R., Schmidt A., Lin S., Ruegg M.A., Hall A., et al. Mammalian TOR complex 2 controls the actin cytoskeleton and is rapamycin insensitive. Nature Cell Biology. 2004;6:1122–1128. DOI: 10.1038/ncb1183

[32] Vadlakonda L., Dash A., Pasupuleti M., Anil K. K., Reddanna P. The paradox of Akt-mTOR interactions. Frontiers in Oncology. 2013;3(165):1-9. DOI: 10.3389/fonc.2013.00165.

[33] Yin Y., Shen W.H. PTEN: a new guardian of the genome. Oncogene. 2008;27 (41): 5443-5453. DOI: 10.1038/onc.2008.241

[34] Chiang G.G., Abraham R.T. Targeting the mTOR signaling network in cancer. Trends in Molecular Medicine. 2007;13(10):433-42. DOI : http://dx.doi.org/10.1016/j.molmed.2007.08.001

[35] Leary A., Auclin E., Pautier P., Lhommé C. The PI3K/Akt/mTOR pathway in ovarian cancer: biological rationale and therapeutic opportunities. Ovarian Cancer—A Clinical and Translational Update. 2013;13:275-302. DOI: 10.5772/54170

[36] Stemke-Hale K., Gonzalez-Angulo A.M., Lluch A., Neve R.M., Kuo W.L., Davies M., et al. An integrative genomic and proteomic analysis of PIK3CA, PTEN, and AKT mutations in breast cancer. Cancer Research. 2008;68(15):6084-6091. DOI: 10.1158/0008-5472.CAN-07-6854

[37] Fresno V.J.A, Casado E., de Castro J., Cejas P., Belda-Iniesta C., González-Barón M.PI3K/Akt signalling pathway and cancer. Cancer Treatment Reviews. 2004;30(2): 193-204. DOI: 10.1016/j.ctrv.2003.07.007

[38] Tang J.M., He Q.Y., Guo R.X., Chang X.J. Phosphorylated Akt overexpression and loss of PTEN expression in non-small cell lung cancer confers poor prognosis. Lung Cancer. 2006;51(2):181-191. DOI: 10.1016/j.lungcan.2005.10.003

[39] Cheng H., Shcherba M., Pendurti G., Liang Y.,Piperdi B., Perez-Soler R. Targeting the PI3K/AKT/mTOR pathway: potential for lung cancer treatment. Lung Cancer Management. 2014;3(1):67-75. DOI: 10.2217/lmt.13.72

[40] Bellacosa A., de Feo D., Godwin A.K., Bell D.W., Cheng J.Q., Altomare D.A., et al. Molecular alterations of the AKT2 oncogene in ovarian and breast carcinomas. International Journal of Cancer. 1995;64(4):280-5. DOI: 10.1002/ijc.2910640412

[41] Shayesteh L., Lu Y., Kuo W.L., Baldocchi R., Godfrey T., Collins C., et al. PIK3CA is implicated as an oncogene in ovarian cancer. Nature Genetics. 1999;21:99-102. DOI: 10.1038/5042

[42] Campbell I.G., Russell S.E., Choong D.Y. Montgomery K.G., Ciavarella M.L., Hooi C.S. et al. Mutation of the PIK3CA gene in ovarian and breast cancer. Cancer Research. 2004;64:7678-81. DOI: 10.1158/0008-5472.CAN-04-2933

[43] Kuo K.T, Mao T. L., Jones S., Veras E., Ayhan A., Wang T.L., et al. Frequent activating mutations of PIK3CA in ovarian clear cell carcinoma. American Journal of Pathology. 2009;174(5): 1597–1601. DOI: 10.2353/ajpath.2009.081000

[44] Kinross K.M., Montgomery K.G., Kleinschmidt M., Waring P., Ivetac I., Tikoo A. et al. An activating Pik3ca mutation coupled with Pten loss is sufficient to initiate ovarian tumorigenesis in mice. Journal of Clinical Investigation. 2012;122(2):553-557. DOI: 10.1172/JCI59309

[45] Tanwar P.S., Zhang L., Kaneko-Tarui T., Curley M.D., Taketo M.M., Rani P. Mammalian target of rapamycin is a therapeutic target for murine ovarian endometrioid adenocarcinomas with dysregulated Wnt/β-catenin and PTEN. PLoS One. 2011;6(6):e20715. DOI: 10.1371/journal.pone.0020715

[46] Steuer-Vogt M.K., Bonkowsky V., Ambrosch P., Scholz M., Neiss A., Strutz J., et al. The effect of an adjuvant mistletoe treatment programme in resected head and neck cancer patients: a randomised controlled clinical trial. European Journal of Cancer. 2001;37(1):23-31. DOI: 10.1016/S0959-8049(00)00360-9

[47] Dancey J.E. Clinical development of mammalian target of rapamycin inhibitors. Hematology Oncology Clinics North of American. 2002;16(5):1101-14. PII: S0889-8588(02)00051-5

[48] Huang S., Houghton P.J. Inhibitors of mammalian target of rapamycin as novel antitumor agents: from bench to clinic. Current Opinion in Investigational Drugs. 2002;3(2):295-304. PMID: 12020063

[49] Wander S.A, Hennessy B.T, Slingerland J.M. Next-generation mTOR inhibitors in clinical oncology: how pathway complexity informs therapeutic strategy. Journal of Clinical Investigation. 2011;121(4):1231-1241. DOI: 10.1172/JCI44145

[50] Mabuchi S., Kawase C., Altomare D.A., Morishige K., Sawada K., Hayashi M., et al. mTOR is a promising therapeutic target both in cisplatin-sensitive and cisplatin-resistant clear cell carcinoma of the ovary. Clinical Cancer Research. 2009;15 (17): 5404-5413. DOI: 10.1158/1078-0432.CCR-09-0365

[51] Peng C.L., Lai P.S., Lin F.H., Yueh-Hsiu W.S., Shieh M.J. Dual chemotherapy and photodynamic therapy in an HT-29 human colon cancer xenograft model using SN-38-loaded chlorin-core star block copolymer micelles. Biomaterial. 2009;30:3614–3625. DOI: 10.1016/j.biomaterials.2009.03.048

[52] Zhang, P.; Hu, L.; Yin, Q.; Zhang, Z.; Feng, L.; Li, Y. Transferrin-conjugated polyphosphoester hybrid micelle loading paclitaxel for brain-targeting delivery: synthesis, preparation and in vivo evaluation. Journal of Controlled Release 2012;159:429–434. DOI: 10.1016/j.jconrel.2012.01.031

[53] Rodon J., Dienstmann R., Serra V., Tabemero J. Development of PI3K inhibitors: lessons learned from early clinical trials. Nature Reviews. Clinical Oncology. 2013;10(3): 143–153. DOI: 10.1038/nrclinonc.2013.10

[54] Yao J.C, Shah M.H., Ito T., Bohas C.L., Wolin E.M., Van Cutsem E., et al. RAD001 in Advanced Neuroendocrine Tumors, Third Trial (RADIANT-3) Study Group. Everolimus for advanced pancreatic neuroendocrine tumors. New England Journal of Medicine. 201;364(6):514-523. DOI: 10.1056/NEJMoa1009290.

[55] Hudes G., Carducci M., Tomczak P., Dutcher J., Figlin R., Kapoor A., et al. Temsirolimus, interferon alfa, or both for advanced renal-cell carcinoma. New England Journal of Medicine. 2007;356(22):2271–2281. DOI: 10.1056/NEJMoa066838

[56] Baselga J., CamponeM., Piccart M., Burris H.A., RugoH.S., Sahmoud T., et al. Everolimus in postmenopausal hormone-receptor-positive advanced breast cancer. New England Journal of Medicine. 2012;366(6):520–529. DOI: 10.1056/NEJMoa1109653

[57] Davies S.P., Reddy H., Caivano M., Cohen P. Specificity and mechanism of action of some commonly used protein kinase inhibitors. Biochemical Journal. 2000;351(1): 95-105.

[58] Vlahos C.J., Matter W.F., Hui K.Y., Brown R.F. A specific inhibitor of phosphatidylinositol 3-kinase, 2-(4-morpholinyl)-8-phenyl-4H-1-benzopyran-4-one (LY294002). Journal of Biological Chemistry.1994;269(7): 5241–5248.

[59] Knight Z.A., Shokat K.M. Chemically targeting the PI3K family. Biochemical Society Transactions. 2007;35(2):245–249. DOI: 10.1042/BST0350245

[60] Marone R., Cmiljanovic V., Giese B., Wymann M.P. Targeting phosphoinositide 3-kinase-moving towards therapy. Biochimica et Biophysica Acta. 2008;1784(1):159-185. DOI: 10.1016/j.bbapap.2007.10.003

[61] Garcia-Echeverria C., Sellers W.R. Drug discovery approaches targeting the PI3K/Akt pathway in cancer. Oncogene. 2008;27(41):5511–5526. DOI: 10.1038/onc.2008.246

[62] Ihle N.T, Williams R., Chow S., Chew W., Berggren M.I., Paine-Murrieta G., et al. Molecular pharmacology and antitumor activity of PX-866, a novel inhibitor of phosphoinositide-3-kinase signaling. Molecular Cancer Therapeutics. 2004;3(7):763-72.

[63] Ihle N.T., Paine-Murrieta G., Berggren M.I, Baker A., Tate W.R, Wipf P., et al. The phosphatidylinositol-3-kinase inhibitor PX-866 overcomes resistance to the epidermal growth factor receptor inhibitor gefitinib in A-549 human non-small cell lung cancer xenografts. Molecular Cancer Therapeutics. 2005;4(9):1349-1357. DOI: 10.1158/1535-7163.MCT-05-0149

[64] Hong D.S., Bowles D.W., Falchook G.S., Messersmith W.A., George G.C., O'Bryant C.L., et al. A multicenter phase I trial of PX-866, an oral irreversible phosphatidylinositol 3-kinase inhibitor, in patients with advanced solid tumors. Clinical Cancer Research. 2012;18(15):4173-82. DOI: 10.1158/1078-0432.CCR-12-0714

[65] Burger M., Pecchi S., Wagman A., Ni Z.J., Knapp M., Hendrickson T., et al. Identification of NVP-BKM120 as a potent, selective, orally bioavailable class I PI3 kinase inhibitor for treating cancer. ACS Medicinal Chemistry Letters. 2011;2(10):774-779. DOI: 10.1021/ml200156t

[66] Maira S.M., Pecchi S., Huang A., Burger M., Knapp M., Sterker D., et al. Identification and characterization of NVP-BKM120, an orally available pan-class I PI3-kinase inhibitor. Molecular Cancer Therapeutics. 2012;11(2):317-328. DOI: 10.1158/1535-7163.MCT-11-0474.

[67] Bendell J.C., Rodon J., Burris H.A., de Jonge M., Verweij J., Birle D., et al. Phase I, dose-escalation study of BKM120, an oral pan-Class I PI3K inhibitor, in patients with advanced solid tumors. Journal of Clinical Oncology. 2012;30(3):282-290. DOI: 10.1200/JCO.2011.36.1360

[68] Rodon J., Braña I., Siu L.L., De Jonge M.J., Homji N., Mills D., et al. Phase I dose-escalation and -expansion study of buparlisib (BKM120), an oral pan-Class I PI3K inhibitor, in patients with advanced solid tumors. Investigational New Drugs. 2014;32(4): 670-81. DOI: 10.1007/s10637-014-0082-9

[69] Edelman G., Bedell C., Shapiro G., Pandya S.S., Kwak E.L., Scheffold C., et al. A phase I dose-escalation study of XL147 (SAR245408), a PI3K inhibitor administered orally to patients (pts) with advanced malignancies. Journal of Clinical Oncology. 2010;28(15s):3004.

[70] Markman B., Dienstmann R., Tabernero J. Targeting the PI3K/Akt/mTOR pathway—beyond rapalogs. Oncotarget. 2010;1(7):530-543. PMC3248125

[71] Foster P., Yamaguchi K., Hsu PP., Qian F., Du X., Wu J., et al. The selective PI3K inhibitor XL147 (SAR245408) inhibits tumor growth and survival and potentiates the activity of chemotherapeutic agents in preclinical tumor models. Molecular Cancer Therapeutics. 2015;14(4):931-940. DOI: 10.1158/1535-7163.MCT-14-0833

[72] Shapiro G.I., Rodon J., Bedell C., Kwak EL., Baselga J., Braña I., et al. Phase I safety, pharmacokinetic, and pharmacodynamic study of SAR245408 (XL147), an oral pan-class I PI3K inhibitor, in patients with advanced solid tumors. Clinical Cancer Research. 2014;20(1):233-45. DOI: 10.1158/1078-0432.CCR-13-1777

[73] Soria J.C., LoRusso P., Bahleda R., Lager J., Liu L., Jiang J., et al. Phase I dose-escalation study of pilaralisib (SAR245408, XL147), a pan-Class I PI3K inhibitor, in combination with erlotinib in patients with solid tumors. Oncologist. 2015;20(3):245-6. DOI: 10.1634/theoncologist.2014-0449

[74] Tolaney S., Burris H., Gartner E., Mayer I.A., Saura C., Maurer M., et al. Phase I/II study of pilaralisib (SAR245408) in combination with trastuzumab or trastuzumab plus paclitaxel in trastuzumab-refractory HER2-positive metastatic breast cancer. Breast Cancer Research Treatment. 2015;149(1):151-161. DOI: 10.1007/s10549-014-3248-4

[75] Folkes A., Ahmadi K., Alderton W.K., Alix S., Baker S.J., Box G. et al. The identification of 2-(1H-indazol-4-yl)-6-(4-methanesulfonyl-piperazin-1-ylmethyl)-4-morpholin-4-yl-t hieno[3,2-d]pyrimidine (GDC-0941) as a potent, selective, orally bioavailable inhibitor of class I PI3 kinase for the treatment of cancer. Journal Medicinal Chemistry. 2008;51(18):5522-5532. DOI: 10.1021/jm800295d

[76] Sampath D., Belvin M., Guan J., Edgar K., Wallin J., Prior W.W., et al. Combination of class I PI3K inhibitor, GDC-0941, with standard of care therapeutics results in enhanced anti-tumor responses in human cancer models in vitro and in vivo. European Journal of Cancer Supplements. 2008;6(12):69-70. DOI: 10.1016/S1359-6349(08)72152-9

[77] Zou Z.Q., Zhang L.N., Wang F., Bellenger J, Shen Y.Z., Zhang X.H. The novel dual PI3K/mTOR inhibitor GDC-0941 synergizes with the MEK inhibitor U0126 in non-small cell lung cancer cells. Molecular Medicine Reports. 2012;5(2):503-8. DOI: 10.3892/mmr.2011.682

[78] Wallin J.J., Guan J., Prior W.W, Lee L.B, Berry L., Belmont L.D., Koeppen H., Belvin M., Friedman L.S., Sampath D. GDC-0941, a novel class I selective PI3K inhibitor, enhances the efficacy of docetaxel in human breast cancer models by increasing cell death in vitro and in vivo. Clinical Cancer Research. 2012;18(14):3901-11. DOI: 10.1158/1078-0432.CCR-11-2088

[79] Burrows N., Babur M., Resch J., Ridsdale S., Mejin M., Rowling E.J., et al. GDC-0941 inhibits metastatic characteristics of thyroid carcinomas by targeting both the phosphoinositide-3 kinase (PI3K) and hypoxia-inducible factor-1α (HIF-1α) pathways. Journal of Clinical Endocrinology and Metabolism. 2011;96(12):e1934-1943. DOI: 10.1210/jc.2011-1426

[80] Kwei K.A., Baker J.B., Pelham R.J. Modulators of sensitivity and resistance to inhibition of PI3K identified in a pharmacogenomic screen of the NCI-60 human tumor cell line collection. PLoS One. 2012;7(9):e46518. DOI: 10.1371/journal.pone.0046518

[81] Sarker D., Ang J.E., Baird R., Kristeleit R., Shah K., Moreno V., et al. First-in-human phase I study of pictilisib (GDC-0941), a potent pan-Class I phosphatidylinositol-3-kinase (PI3K) inhibitor, in patients with advanced solid tumors. Clinical Cancer Research. 2015;21(1):77-86. DOI: 10.1158/1078-0432.CCR-14-0947

[82] Jia S., Liu Z., Zhang S., Liu P., Zhang L., Lee S.H., et al. Essential roles of PI(3)K-p110[bgr] in cell growth, metabolism and tumorigenesis. Nature. 2008;454:776–779. DOI: 10.1038/nature07091

[83] Wee S., Wiederschain D., Maira S.M., Loo A., Miller C., deBeaumont R., et al. PTEN-deficient cancers depend on PIK3CB. Proceedings of the National Academy of Sciences. 2008;105:13057-13062. DOI: 10.1073/pnas.0802655105

[84] Ni J., Liu Q., Xie S., Carlson C., Von T., Vogel K., et al. Functional characterization of an isoform-selective inhibitor of PI3K-p110β as a potential anticancer agent. Cancer Discovery. 2012;2(5):425-433. DOI: 10.1158/2159-8290.CD-12-0003

[85] Rommel C., Camps M., Ji H. PI3K delta and PI3K gamma: partners in crime in inflammation in rheumatoid arthritis and beyond? Nature Reviews Immunology. 2007;7(3):191-201. DOI: 10.1038/nri2036

[86] U.S. Food and Drug Administration. U.S. Department of Health and Human Services. [Internet]. 2015. Available from: http://www.fda.gov/ICECI/Inspections/ucm250729.htm [Accessed: 2015-03-11]

[87] Fritsch C., Huang A., Chatenay-Rivauday C., Schnell C., Reddy A., Liu M., et al. Characterization of the novel and specific PI3Kα inhibitor NVP-BYL719 and development of the patient stratification strategy for clinical trials. Molecular Cancer Therapeutics. 2014;13(5):1117-29. DOI: 10.1158/1535-7163.MCT-13-0865

[88] Fritsch C.M., Schnell C., Chatenay-Rivauday C., Guthy D.A., de Pover A., Wartmann M., et al. NVP-BYL719, a novel PI3Kalpha selective inhibitor with all the characteristics required for clinical development as an anti-cancer agent. Cancer Research. 2012;3748. DOI: 10.1158/1538-7445.AM2012-3748

[89] Huang A., Fritsch C., Wilson C., et al. Single agent activity of PIK3CA inhibitor BYL719 in a broad cancer cell line panel. Cancer Research. 2012;3749. DOI: 10.1158/1538-7445.AM2012-3749

[90] Gonzalez-Angulo A.M., Juric D., Argiles G., Schellens J.H., Burris H.A, Berlin J., et al. Safety, pharmacokinetics, and preliminary activity of the {alpha}-specific PI3K inhibitor BYL719: results from the first-in-human study. Journal of Clinical Oncology. 2013;31:Abstract: 2531

[91] Ndubaku C.O., Heffron T.P., Staben S.T., Baumgardner M., Blaquiere N., Bradley E., et al. Discovery of 2-{3-[2-(1-isopropyl-3-methyl-1H-1,2-4-triazol-5-yl)-5,6 dihydrobenzo[f]imidazo[1,2-d][1,4]oxazepin-9-yl]-1H-pyrazol-1-yl}-2 methylpropanamide (GDC-0032): a β-sparing phosphoinositide 3-kinase inhibitor with high unbound exposure and robust in vivo antitumor activity. Journal of Medicinal Chemistry. 2013;56(11):4597-4610. DOI: 10.1021/jm4003632

[92] Wallin J.J., Edgar K.A., Guan J., Sampath D., Nannini M., Belvin M., et al. Abstract P2-17-01: the PI3K inhibitor GDC-0032 is selectively potent against PIK3CA mutant breast cancer cell lines and tumors. Cancer Research. 2013;73:P2-17-01. DOI: 10.1158/0008-5472.SABCS13-P2-17-01

[93] Juric D., Krop I., Ramanathan R.K., Xiao J., Sanabria S., Wilson T.R., et al. GDC-0032, a beta isoform-sparing PI3K inhibitor: results of a first-in-human phase Ia dose escalation study. In: AACR 104th Annual Meeting 2013; April 2013; Washington, DC; 73:LB–64.

[94] Yang Q., Modi P., Newcomb T., Qu C., Gandhi V. Idelalisib: first-in-class PI3K delta inhibitor for the treatment of chronic lymphocytic leukemia, small lymphocytic leukemia, and follicular lymphoma. Clinical Cancer Research. 2015;21(7):1537-1542. DOI: 10.1158/1078-0432.CCR-14-2034

[95] Herman S.E., Gordon A.L., Wagner A.J., Heerema N.A., Zhao W., Flynn J.M., et al. Phosphatidylinositol 3-kinase-δ inhibitor CAL-101 shows promising preclinical activity in chronic lymphocytic leukemia by antagonizing intrinsic and extrinsic cellular survival signals. Blood. 2010;116(12):2078-2088.

[96] Lannutti B.J., Meadows S.A., Herman S.E., Kashishian A., Steiner B., Johnson A.J., et al. CAL-101, a p110delta selective phosphatidylinositol-3-kinase inhibitor for the treatment of B-cell malignancies, inhibits PI3K signaling and cellular viability. Blood. 2011;117(2):591-594. DOI: 10.1182/blood-2010-03-275305

[97] Webb H.K., Chen H., Yu A.S., et al. Clinical pharmacokinetics of CAL-101, a p110{delta} isoform-selective PI3K inhibitor, following single- and multiple-dose administration in healthy volunteers and patients with hematological malignancies. ISRN Oncology. 2010;116(21):1774. DOI: 10.1155/2014/931858

[98] Kahl B.S., Spurgeon S.E., Furman R.R., Flinn I.W., Coutre S.E., Brown J.R., et al. A phase 1 study of the PI3Kδ inhibitor idelalisib in patients with relapsed/refractory mantle cell lymphoma (MCL). Blood. 2014;123(22):3398-3405. DOI: 10.1182/blood-2013-11-537555.

[99] Kondapaka S.B., Singh S.S., Dasmahapatra G.P., Sausville E.A., Roy K.K. Perifosine, a novel alkylphospholipid, inhibits protein kinase B activation. Molecular Cancer Therapeutics. 2003;2(11):1093-1103.

[100] Hilgard P., Klenner T., Stekar J., Nössner G., Kutscher B., Engel J. D-21266, a new heterocyclic alkylphospholipid with antitumour activity. European Journal of Cancer. 1997;33(3):442-446. DOI: 10.1016/S0959-8049(97)89020-X

[101] Yao C., Wei J.J., Wang Z.Y., Ding H.M., Li D., Yan S.C., et al. Perifosine induces cell apoptosis in human osteosarcoma cells: new implication for osteosarcoma therapy? Cell Biochemistry and Biophysics. 2013;65(2):217-227. DOI: 10.1007/s12013-012-9423-5

[102] Sun H., T. Yu, J. Li. Co-administration of perifosine with paclitaxel synergistically induces apoptosis in ovarian cancer cells: more than just AKT inhibition. Cancer Letters. 2011;310(1):118–128. DOI: 10.1016/j.canlet.2011.06.010

[103] Engel J.B., Schönhals T., Häusler S., Krockenberger M., Schmidt M., Horn E., et al. Induction of programmed cell death by inhibition of AKT with the alkylphosphocholine perifosine in in vitro models of platinum sensitive and resistant ovarian cancers. Archives of Gynecology and Obstetrics. 2011;283(3):603-10. DOI: 10.1007/s00404-010-1457-6

[104] Nyakern M., Cappellini A., Mantovani I, Martelli A.M. Synergistic induction of apoptosis in human leukemia T cells by the Akt inhibitor perifosine and etoposide through activation of intrinsic and Fas-mediated extrinsic cell death pathways. Molecular Cancer Therapeutics. 2006;5:1559-1570. DOI: 10.1158/1535-7163.MCT-06-0076

[105] Hideshima T., Catley L., Yasui H., Ishitsuka K., Raje N., Mitsiades C., et al. Perifosine, an oral bioactive novel alkylphospholipid, inhibits Akt and induces in vitro and

in vivo cytotoxicity in human multiple myeloma cells. Blood. 2006;107(10):4053-4062. DOI: http://dx.doi.org/10.1182/blood-2005-08-3434

[106] Xin Y., Shen X.D., Cheng L., Hong D.F., Chen B. Perifosine inhibits S6K1-Gli1 signaling and enhances gemcitabine-induced anti-pancreatic cancer efficiency. Cancer Chemotherapy and Pharmacology. 2014;73(4):711-719. DOI: 10.1007/s00280-014-2397-9

[107] Posadas E.M, Gulley J., Arlen P.M., Trout A., Parnes H.L., Wright J., et al. A phase II study of perifosine in androgen independent prostate cancer. Cancer Biology Therapy. 2005;4(10):1133-1137. DOI: 10.4161/cbt.4.10.2064

[108] Argiris A., Cohen E., Karrison T., Esparaz B., Mauer A., Ansari R., et al. Phase II trial of perifosine, an oral alkylphospholipid, in recurrent or metastatic head and neck cancer. Cancer Biology and Therapy. 2006;5(7):766-770. DOI: 10.4161/cbt.5.7.2874

[109] Knowling M., Blackstein M., Tozer R., Bramwell V., Dancey J., Dore N., et al. A phase II study of perifosine (D-21226) in patients with previously untreated metastatic or locally advanced soft tissue sarcoma: a National Cancer Institute of Canada Clinical Trials Group trial. Investigational New Drugs. 2006;24(5):435-439. DOI: 10.1007/s10637-006-6406-7

[110] Marsh Rde W., Rocha Lima C.M., Levy D.E., Mitchell E.P., Rowland Jr K.M., Benson A.B. A phase II trial of perifosine in locally advanced, unresectable, or metastatic pancreatic adenocarcinoma. American Journal of Clinical Oncology. 2007;30(1):26–31. DOI: 10.1097/01.coc.0000251235.46149.43

[111] Leighl N.B., Dent S., Clemons M., Vandenberg T.A., Tozer R., Warr D.G., et al. A phase 2 study of perifosine in advanced or metastatic breast cancer. Breast Cancer Research Treatment. 2008;108(1):87-92. DOI: 10.1007/s10549-007-9584-x

[112] Fu S., Hennessy B.T., Ng C.S., Ju Z., Coombes K.R., Wolf J.K., et al. Perifosine plus docetaxel in patients with platinum and taxane resistant or refractory high-grade epithelial ovarian cancer. Gynecologic Oncology. 2012;126(1):47-53. DOI: 10.1016/j.ygyno.2012.04.006

[113] Guidetti A., Carlo-Stella C., Locatelli SL., Malorni W., Mortarini R., Viviani S., et al. Phase II study of perifosine and sorafenib dual-targeted therapy in patients with relapsed or refractory lymphoproliferative diseases. Clinical Cancer Research. 2014;20(22):5641-5651. DOI: 10.1158/1078-0432.CCR-14-0770

[114] Rhodes N., Heerding D.A., Duckett D.R., Eberwein D.J., Knick V.B., Lansing T.J., et al. Characterization of an Akt kinase inhibitor with potent pharmacodynamic and antitumor activity. Cancer Research. 2008;68(7):2366-74. DOI: 10.1158/0008-5472.CAN-07-5783

[115] Feng Z., Zhang H., Levine A. J., Jin S. The coordinate regulation of the p53 and mTOR pathways in cells. PNAS, Proceedings of the National Academy of Sciences. 2005;102(23): 8204–8209. DOI: 10.1073/pnas.0502857102

[116] Guertin D.A., Sabatini D.M. The pharmacology of mTOR inhibition. Science Signalling. 2009;2(67):pe24. DOI: 10.1126/scisignal.267pe24

[117] Vezina C., Kudelski A., Sehgal S.N. Rapamycin (AY-22,989), a new antifungal antibiotic. I. Taxonomy of the producing streptomycete and isolation of the active principle. Journal of Antibiotics. 1975;28(10):721-726. DOI: http://doi.org/10.7164/antibiotics.28.721

[118] Singh K., Sun S., Vezina C. Rapamycin (AY-22,989), a new antifungal antibiotic. IV. Mechanism of action. Journal of Antibiotics. 1979;32(6):630-645. DOI: 10.7164/antibiotics.28.721

[119] Tsang C. K., Qi H., Liu L. F., Zheng, X.F.S. Targeting mammalian target of rapamycin (mTOR) for health and diseases. Drug Discovery Today. 2007;12(3–4): 112–24. DOI: 10.1016/j.drudis.2006.12.008

[120] Shafer A., Zhou C., Gehrig P.A., Boggess J.F., Bae-Jump VL. Rapamycin potentiates the effects of paclitaxel in endometrial cancer cells through inhibition of cell proliferation and induction of apoptosis. International Journal of Cancer. 2010;126(5): 1144-54. DOI: 10.1002/ijc.24837

[121] Oldham S., Hafen E. Insulin/IGF and target of rapamycin signaling: a TOR de force in growth control. Trends in Cell Biology. 2003;13(2):79-85. DOI: http://dx.doi.org/10.1016/S0962-8924(02)00042-9

[122] Fang Y., Vilella-Bach M., Bachmann R., Flanigan A., Chen J. Phosphatidic acid-mediated mitogenic activation of mTOR signaling. Science 2001;294(5548):1942-1945. DOI: 10.1126/science.1066015

[123] Hara K., Maruki Y., Long X., Yoshino K., Oshiro N., Hidayat S., et al. Raptor, a binding partner of target of rapamycin (TOR), mediates TOR action. Cancer Cell. 2002;110:177-189. DOI: http://dx.doi.org/10.1016/S0092-8674(02)00833-4

[124] Kim D.H., Sarbassov D.D., Ali S.M., King J.E., Latek R.R., Erdjument-Bromage H., et al. mTOR interacts with raptor to form a nutrient-sensitive complex that signals to the cell growth machinery. Cancer Cell. 2002;110:163-175. DOI: http://dx.doi.org/10.1016/S0092-8674(02)00808-5

[125] Liu Q., Chang J.W., Wang J., Kang S.A., Thoreen C.C., Markhard A., et al. Discovery of 1-(4-(4-propionylpiperazin-1-yl)-3-(trifluoromethyl)phenyl)-9-(quinolin-3-yl)benzo[h][1,6]naphthyridin-2(1H)-one as a highly potent, selective mammalian target of rapamycin (mTOR) inhibitor for the treatment of cancer. Journal of Medicinal Chemistry. 2010;53(19):7146-7155. DOI: 10.1021/jm101144f

[126] Alvarado Y., Mita M.M., Vemulapalli S., Mahalingam D., Mita A.C. Clinical activity of mammalian target of rapamycin inhibitors in solid tumors. Targeted Oncology. 2011;6(2):69-94. DOI: 10.1007/s11523-011-0178-5

[127] Zaytseva Y.Y., Valentino J.D., Gulhati P., Evers B.M. mTOR inhibitors in cancer therapy. Cancer Letters. 2012;319(1):1-7. DOI: 10.1016/j.canlet.2012.01.005

[128] Brown E.J., Albers M.W., Shin T.B., Ichikawa K., Keith C.T., Lane W.S., et al. A mammalian protein targeted by G1-arresting rapamycin-receptor complex. Nature. 1994;369(6483):756-758. DOI: 10.1038/369756a0

[129] Sabatini D.M., Erdjument-Bromage H., Lui M., Tempst P., Snyder S.H. RAFT1: a mammalian protein that binds to FKBP12 in a rapamycin-dependent fashion and is homologous to yeast TORs. Cell. 1994;78(1):35-43. DOI: http://dx.doi.org/10.1016/0092-8674(94)90570-3

[130] Vignot S., Faivre S., Aguirre D., Raymond E. mTOR-targeted therapy of cancer with rapamycin derivatives. Annals of Oncology. 2005;16(4):524-37. DOI: 10.1093/annonc/mdi113

[131] Duran I., Siu L.L., Oza A.M., Chung T.B., Sturgeon J., Townsley C.A., et al. Characterisation of the lung toxicity of the cell cycle inhibitor temsirolimus. European Journal of Cancer. 2006;42(12):1875-1880. DOI: http://dx.doi.org/10.1016/j.ejca.2006.03.015

[132] National Cancer Institute [Internet]. 2013. Available from: http://www.cancer.gov/about-cancer/treatment/drugs/fda-everolimus. [Accessed: 2015-05-20].

[133] Pavel M.E., Hainsworth J.D., Baudin E., Peeters M., Horsch D., Winkler R.E., et al. Everolimus plus octreotide long-acting repeatable for the treatment of advanced neuroendocrine tumours associated with carcinoid syndrome (RADIANT-2): a randomised, placebo-controlled, phase 3 study. Lancet. 2011;378(9808):2005-2012. DOI: 10.1016/S0140-6736(11)61742-X

[134] Burris H.A., Lebrun F., Rugo H.S., Beck J.T, Piccart M., Neven P., et al. Health-related quality of life of patients with advanced breast cancer treated with everolimus plus exmestane versus placebo plus exemestane in the phase 3, randomized, controlled, BOLERO-2 trial. Cancer. 2013;119(10):1908-1915. DOI: 10.1002/cncr.28010

[135] André F., O'Regan R., Ozguroglu M., Toi M., Xu B., Jerusalem G., et al. Everolimus for women with trastuzumab-resistant, HER2-positive, advanced breast cancer (BOLERO-3): a randomised, double-blind, placebo-controlled phase 3 trial. Lancet Oncology. 2014;15(6):580-91. DOI: 10.1016/S1470-2045(14)70138-X

[136] Hurvitz S.A., Dalenc F., Campone M., O'Regan R.M., Tjan-Heijnen V.C., Gligorov J., et al. A phase 2 study of everolimus combined with trastuzumab and paclitaxel in patients with HER2-overexpressing advanced breast cancer that progressed during prior trastuzumab and taxane therapy. Breast Cancer Research and Treatment. 2013;141(3): 437-446. DOI: 10.1007/s10549-013-2689-5

[137] Huang S., Houghton P.J. Targeting mTOR signaling for cancer therapy. Current Opinion of Pharmacology 2003;3:371–7. DOI: 10.1016/S1471-4892(03)00071-7

[138] Bae-Jump V.L., Zhou C., Boggess J.F., Gehring P.A. Synergistic effect of rapamycin and cisplatin in endometrial cancer cells. Cancer. 2009;115:3887:96. DOI: 10.1002/cncr.24431

[139] Temkin S.M., Fleming G. Current treatment of metastatic endometrial cancer. Cancer Control. 2009;16(1):38-45. PMID: 19078928

[140] Tinker A.V., Ellard S., Welch S., Moens F., Allo G., Tsao M.S., et al. Phase II study of temsirolimus (CCI-779) in women with recurrent, unresectable, locally advanced or metastatic carcinoma of the cervix. A trial of the NCIC Clinical Trials Group (NCIC CTG IND 199). Gynecologic Oncology 2013;130:269–74. DOI: 10.1016/j.ygyno.2013.05.008

[141] Takatori E., Shoji T., Miura Y., Takada A., Takeuchi S., Sugiyama T. Effective use of everolimus as salvage chemotherapy for ovarian clear cell carcinoma: a case report. Onco Targets and Therapy. 2014;7:165-169. DOI: 10.2147/OTT.S54745

[142] Behbakht K., Sill M.W., Darcy K.M., Rubin S.C., Mannel R.S., Waggoner S., et al. Phase II trial of the mTOR inhibitor, temsirolimus and evaluation of circulating tumor cells and tumor biomarkers in persistent and recurrent epithelial ovarian and primary peritoneal malignancies: a Gynecologic Oncology Group study. Gynecologic Oncology. 2011;123(1):19-26. DOI: 10.1016/j.ygyno.2011.06.022

[143] Zhang Y.J., Duan Y., Zheng X.F.S. Targeting the mTOR kinase domain: the second generation of mTOR inhibitors. Drug Discovery Today. 2011;16(7–8): 325–31. DOI: 10.1016/j.drudis.2011.02.008

[144] Colombo N., McMeekin S., Schwartz P., Kostka J., Sessa C., Gehrig P., et al. A phase II trial of the mTOR inhibitor AP23573 as a single agent in advanced endometrial cancer. Journal of Clinical Oncology. 2007;25(18):5516.

[145] Mackay H., Welch S., Tsao M.S., Biagi J.J., Elit L., Ghatge P., et al. Phase II study of oral ridaforolimus in patients with metastatic and/or locally advanced endometrial cancer; NCIC CTG IND 192. Journal of Clinical Oncology. 2011;29:s(5013).

[146] Guertin D.A, Sabatini D.M. Defining the role of mTOR in cancer. Cancer Cell. 2007;12(1):9-22. DOI: http://dx.doi.org/10.1016/j.ccr.2007.05.008

[147] Carracedo A., Pandolfi P.P. The PTEN-PI3K pathway: of feedbacks and cross-talks. Oncogene. 2008;27(41): 5527–5541. DOI: 10.1038/onc.2008.247

[148] García-Martínez J.M., Moran J., Clarke R.G., Gray A., Cosulich S.C., Chresta C.M., et al. Ku-0063794 is a specific inhibitor of the mammalian target of rapamycin (mTOR). Biochemical Journal. 2009;421(1):29-42. DOI: 10.1042/BJ20090489

[149] Feldman M.E., Apsel B., Uotila A., Loewith R., Knight Z.A., Ruggero D., et al. Active-site inhibitors of mTOR target rapamycin-resistant outputs of mTORC1 and mTORC2. PLoS Biology. 2009;7(2):e38. DOI: 10.1371/journal.pbio.1000038

[150] Yu K., Toral-Barza L., Shi C., Zhang W.G., Lucas J., Shor B., et al. Biochemical, cellular, and in vivo activity of novel ATP-competitive and selective inhibitors of the mammalian target of rapamycin. Cancer Research. 2009;69(15):6232-6240. DOI: 10.1158/0008-5472.CAN-09-0299

[151] Chresta C.M., Davies B.R., Hickson I., Harding T., Cosulich S., Critchlow S.E., et al. AZD8055 is a potent, selective, and orally bioavailable ATP-competitive mammalian target of rapamycin kinase inhibitor with in vitro and in vivo antitumor activity. Cancer Research. 2010;70(1):288-298. DOI: 10.1158/0008-5472.CAN-09-1751

[152] Yu K., Shi C., Toral-Barza L., Lucas J., Shor B., Kim J.E., et al. Beyond rapalog therapy. Preclinical pharmacology and antitumor activity of WYE-125132, an ATP-competitive and -specific inhibitor of mTORC1 and mTORC2. Cancer Research. 2010;70(2):621-631. DOI: 10.1158/0008-5472.CAN-09-2340

[153] Bhagwat V.S., Gokhale P.C., Crew A.P., Cooke A., Yao Y., Mantis C., et al. Preclinical characterization of OSI-027, a potent and selective inhibitor of mTORC1 and mTORC2: distinct from rapamycin. Molecular Cancer Therapeutics. 2011;10(8): 1394-1406. DOI: 10.1158/1535-7163.MCT-10-1099

[154] Thoreen C.C., Kang S.A, Chang J.W., Liu Q., Zhang J., Gao Y., et al. An ATP-competitive mammalian target of rapamycin inhibitor reveals rapamycin-insensitive functions of mTORC1. Journal of Biological Chemistry. 2009;284(12):8023-8032. DOI: 10.1074/jbc.M900301200

[155] Zhang H., Berel D., Wang Y., Li P., Bhowmick N.A., Figlin R.A., et al. A comparison of Ku0063794, a dual mTORC1 and mTORC2 inhibitor, and temsirolimus in preclinical renal cell carcinoma models. PLoS One. 2013;8(1):e54918. DOI: 10.1371/journal.pone.0054918

[156] Blaser B., Waselle L., Dormond-Meuwly A., Dufour M., Roulin D., Demartines N., et al. Antitumor activities of ATP-competitive inhibitors of mTOR in colon cancer cells.BMC Cancer. 2012;12:86. DOI: 10.1186/1471-2407-12-86

[157] Liu Q., Wang J., Kang S.A., Thoreen C.C., Hur W., Ahmed T., et al. Discovery of 9-(6-aminopyridin-3-yl)-1-(3-(trifluoromethyl)phenyl)benzo[h][1,6]naphthyridin-2(1H)-one (Torin2) as a potent, selective, and orally available mammalian target of rapamycin (mTOR) inhibitor for treatment of cancer. Journal of Medicinal Chemistry. 2011;54(5):1473-80. DOI: 10.1021/jm101520v

[158] Patricelli MP, Nomanbhoy TK, Wu J, Brown H, Zhou D, Zhang J, et al. In situ kinase profiling reveals functionally relevant properties of native kinases. Chemistry and Biology. 2011;18(6):699-710. DOI: 10.1016/j.chembiol.2011.04.011

[159] Liu Q., Xu C., Kirubakaran S., Zhang X., Hur W. Liu Y., et al. Characterization of Torin2, an ATP-competitive inhibitor of mTOR, ATM and ATR. Cancer Research. 2013; 73(8):2574-86. DOI: 10.1158/0008-5472

[160] Rodrik-Outmezguine V., Chandarlapaty S., Pagano N., Poulikakos P.I., Scaltriti M., Moskatel E., et al. mTOR kinase inhibition causes feedback-dependent biphasic regulation of AKT signaling. Cancer Discovery. 2011;3:248-259. DOI: doi: 10.1158/2159-8290.CD-11-0085

[161] Gungor H., Saleem A., Agarwal R., Blagden S.P, Michael A., Stronach M., et al. Pharmacokinetic (PK)/pharmacodynamic (PD) analysis of escalating repeat doses of the AKT inhibitor GSK2141795 (GSK795) in patients (pts) with ovarian cancer. Journal of Clinical Oncology. 2011;29(15):5064.

[162] Cope C.L., Gilley R., Balmanno K., Sale M.J., Howarth K.D., Hampson M., et al. Adaptation to mTOR kinase inhibitors by amplification of eIF4E to maintain cap-dependent translation. Journal of Cell Science. 2014;127(4):788-800. DOI: 10.1242/jcs.137588

[163] Ducker G.S., Atreya C.E., Simko J.P., Hom Y.K., Matli M.R., Benes CH., et al. Incomplete inhibition of phosphorylation of 4E-BP1 as a mechanism of primary resistance to ATP-competitive mTOR inhibitors. Oncogene. 2014;33(12):1590-1600. DOI: 10.1038/onc.2013.92

[164] Maira S.M., Stauffer F., Brueggen J., Furet P., Schnell C., Fritsch C., et al. Identification and characterization of NVP-BEZ235, a new orally available dual phosphatidylinositol 3-kinase/mammalian target of rapamycin inhibitor with potent in vivo antitumor activity. Molecular. Cancer Therapy. 2008;7(7):1851-1863. DOI: 10.1158/1535-7163.MCT-08-0017

[165] Park S., Chapuis N., Bardet V., Tamburini J., Gallay N., Willems L., et al. PI-103, a dual inhibitor of Class IA phosphatidylinositide 3-kinase and mTOR, has antileukemic activity in AML. Leukemia. 2008;22(9):1698–1706. DOI: 10.1038/leu.2008.144

[166] Mallon R., Hollander I., Feldberg L., Lucas J., Soloveva V., Venkatesan A., et al. Antitumor efficacy profile of PKI-402, a dual phosphatidylinositol 3-kinase/mammalian target of rapamycin inhibitor. Molecular Cancer Therapeutics. 2010;9(4):976–984. DOI: 10.1158/1535-7163.MCT-09-0954.

[167] Wallin J.J, Edgar K.A, Guan J., Berry M., Prior W.W, Lee L., et al. GDC-0980 is a novel class I PI3K/mTOR kinase inhibitor with robust activity in cancer models driven by the PI3K pathway. Molecular Cancer Therapeutics. 2011;10(12):2426-36. DOI: 10.1158/1535-7163.MCT-11-0446

[168] Cheng H., Li C., Bailey S., Baxi S.M., Goulet L., Guo L., et al. Discovery of the highly potent PI3K/mTOR dual inhibitor PF-04979064 through Structure-based drug design. ACS Medicinal Chemistry Letters. 2012;4(1):91-97. DOI: 10.1021/ml300309h

[169] Markman B., Tabernero J., Krop I., Shapiro G.I., Siu L., Chen L.C., et al. Phase I safety, pharmacokinetic, and pharmacodynamic study of the oral phosphatidylinositol-3-kinase and mTOR inhibitor BGT226 in patients with advanced solid tumors. Annals of Oncology. 2012;23(9):2399-408. DOI: 10.1093/annonc/mds011

[170] Papadopoulos K.P., Tabernero J., Markman B., Patnaik A., Tolcher A.W., Baselga J., et al. Phase I safety, pharmacokinetic, and pharmacodynamic study of SAR245409 (XL765), a novel, orally administered PI3K/mTOR inhibitor in patients with advanced solid tumors. Clinical Cancer Research. 2014;20(9):2445-56. DOI: 10.1158/1078-0432.CCR-13-2403

[171] Courtney K.D., Corcoran R.B., Engelman J.A. The PI3K pathway as drug target in human cancer. Journal of Clinical Oncology. 2010;28(6):1075-1083. DOI: 10.1200/JCO.2009.25.3641

[172] O'Reilly K.E., Rojo F., She Q.B., Solit D., Mills G.B., Smith D., et al. mTOR inhibition induces upstream receptor tyrosine kinase signaling and activates Akt. Cancer Research. 2006;66(3):1500- 1508. DOI: 10.1158/0008-5472.CAN-05-2925

[173] Liu T.J., Koul D., LaFortune T., Tiao N., Shen R.J., Maira S.M., et al. NVP-BEZ235, a novel dual phosphatidylinositol 3-kinase/mammalian target of rapamycin inhibitor, elicits multifaceted antitumor activities in human gliomas. Molecular Cancer Therapy. 2009;8(8):2204–2210. DOI: 10.1158/1535-7163

[174] Santiskulvong C., Konecny G.E., Fekete M., Chen K.Y., Karam A., Mulholland D., et al. Dual targeting of phosphoinositide 3-kinase and mammalian target of rapamycin using NVP-BEZ235 as a novel therapeutic approach in human ovarian carcinoma. Clinical Cancer Research. 2011;17(8):2373–2384. DOI: 10.1158/1078-0432.CCR-10-2289

[175] Sanchez C.G., Ma C.X., Crowder R.J., Guintoli T., Phommaly C., Gao F., et al. Preclinical modeling of combined phosphatidylinositol-3-kinase inhibition with endocrine therapy for estrogen receptor-positive breast cancer. Breast Cancer Research. 2011;13(2):1-17. DOI: 10.1186/bcr2833

[176] O'Brien N.A., McDonald K., Tong L., von Euw E., Kalous O., Conklin D., et al. Targeting PI3K/mTOR overcomes resistance to HER2-targeted therapy independent of feedback activation of AKT. Clinical Cancer Research. 2014;20(13):3507-3520. DOI: 10.1158/1078-0432.CCR-13-2769

[177] Schnell C.R., Stauffer F., Allegrini P.R., O'Reilly T., McSheehy P.M., Dartois C., et al. Effects of the dual phosphatidylinositol 3-kinase/mammalian target of rapamycin inhibitor NVP-BEZ235 on the tumor vasculature: implications for clinical imaging. Cancer Research. 2008;68(16):6598–6607. DOI: 10.1158/0008-5472.CAN-08-1044

[178] Cao P., Maira S.M., Garcia-Echeverria C., Hedley D.W. Activity of a novel, dual PI3 kinase/mTor inhibitor NVP-BEZ235 against primary human pancreatic cancers grown as orthotopic xenografts. British Journal of Cancer. 2009;100(8):1267–1276. DOI: 10.1038/sj.bjc.6604995

[179] Marone R., Erhart D., Mertz A.C., Bohnacker T., Schnell C., Cmiljanovic V., et al. Targeting melanoma with dual phosphoinositide 3-kinase/mammalian target of rapamycin inhibitors. Molecular Cancer Research. 2009;7(4):601–613. DOI: 10.1158/1541-7786.MCR-08-0366

[180] McMillin D.W., Ooi M., Delmore J., Negri J., Hayden P., Mitsiades N., et al. Antimyeloma activity of the orally bioavailable dual phosphatidylinositol 3- kinase/mammalian target of rapamycin inhibitor NVP-BEZ235. Cancer Research. 2009;69(14): 5835-5842. DOI: 10.1158/0008-5472.CAN-08-4285

[181] Cho D.C., Cohen M.B, Panka D.J, Collins M., Ghebremichael M., Atkins M.B., et al. The efficacy of the novel dual PI3- kinase/mTOR inhibitor NVP-BEZ235 compared with rapamycin in renal cell carcinoma. Clinical Cancer Research. 2010;16(14):3628–3638. DOI: 10.1158/1078-0432.CCR-09-3022

[182] Cloughesy T.F., Yoshimoto K., Nghiemphu P., Brown K., Dang J., Zhu S., et al. Antitumor activity of rapamycin in a Phase I trial for patients with recurrent PTEN-deficient glioblastoma. PLoS Medicine. 2008;5(1):e8. DOI: 10.1371/journal.pmed.0050008

[183] Naing A., Aghajanian C., Raymond E., Olmos D., Schwartz G., Oelmann E., et al. Safety, tolerability, pharmacokinetics and pharmacodynamics of AZD8055 in advanced solid tumours and lymphoma. British Journal of Cancer. 2012;107(7):1093-9. DOI: 10.1038/bjc.2012.368

[184] Asahina H., Nokihara H., Yamamoto N., Yamada Y., Tamura Y., Honda K., et al. Safety and tolerability of AZD8055 in Japanese patients with advanced solid tumors; a dose-finding phase I study. Investigational New Drugs. 2013;31(3):677-84. DOI: 10.1007/s10637-012-9860-4

[185] Tan D.S., Dumez H., Olmos D., Sandhu S.K., Hoeben A., Stephens A.W. First-in-human phase I study exploring three schedules of OSI-027, a novel small molecule TORC1/TORC2 inhibitor, in patients with advanced solid tumors and lymphoma. Journal of Clinical Oncology. 2010;28:(15s).Abstract: 3006

Chapter 8

Radiotherapy and Chemotherapy Treatments in Head and Neck Cancer Patients — Protocol for Management Before, During and After RTP

Paula Bonar Alvarez, Mario Perez-Sayans García,
Maria Elena Padín Iruegas and Abel García-García

Additional information is available at the end of the chapter

http://dx.doi.org/10.5772/60397

1. Introduction

The term oral cancer is used as a synonym for squamous cell carcinoma, which constitutes 90% of malignant neoplasms. Surgery, radiotherapy and chemotherapy are the election treatments. The selection of an only treatment or combination depends principally on the location of the tumour, its size, histological subtype, stage and the patient's general state of health. Surgery and RTP tend to be used alone to treat cases of non-metastatic disease (stages I and II), whereas more advanced cancers (III and IV) are treated by surgery in combination with radiotherapy and/or chemotherapy. It is important to bear in mind that the surgeries these patients undergo are aggressive. They provoke aesthetic and functional alterations that affect the patient's quality of life.

Prior to undergoing radiotherapy treatment, it is important that patients with head and neck cancer undergo a dental evaluation. This is because surgery provokes big aesthetic and functional alterations. Therefore, patients who already show deficient oral health before treatment are likely to leave their oral hygiene, increasing the gravity of complications.

There are a number of complications that appear in the head and neck region, not only during treatment but also, after. These include mucositis, dental caries and xerostomia. In this paper, we will describe the adverse, acute and late complications, as well as the treatment guidelines. Furthermore, we will develop a patient management protocol for before, during and after radiotherapy.

2. Head and neck cancer

The term oral cancer is used as a synonym for oral squamous cell carcinoma (OSCC), which accounts for 90% of all head and neck cancers and 3-4% of malignancies [1, 2]. The incidence of head and neck cancer has increased significantly over the past 20 years. Over 575,000 new oral cancer cases are annually diagnosed in the world [3]. According to data published in 1998 by Spanish National Epidemiology Centre, in our country, the number of deaths by oral, pharyngeal and labial cancer amounted to 1,891 of men and 374 of women. In Spain, incidence accounts for 12 to 15 cases per 100,000 men/year and two to four cases per 100,000 women/year [4]. However, the figures are now matching up. This is because some women are adopting harmful habits, which were traditionally attributable to men. The disease mainly affects men over 40 years of age, with a peak of maximum incidence in their 60s [5, 6].

The etiology of cancer has multiple factors. The main risk factors are smoking and alcohol. Despite showing synergistic effects, these are independent risk factors, as shown in a study by Castellsagué et al. [6, 7]. In some cases of solar ultraviolet radiation in lip cancer, infections, diets low in fruit and vegetables, immunodepression, bad oral hygiene and the presence of genetic factors can have a relevant effect.

Patients diagnosed with this cancer are treated by surgery, radiotherapy (RTP), chemotherapy (QTP) or a combined treatment. The choice of a unique or combined treatment depends on the location of the tumour, its extension, histological subtype, tumour stage and the patient's general condition. Surgery and RTP are used in isolation to treat cases of non-metastatic disease (stages I and II). However, advanced stages (III and IV) require concomitant RTP and QTP. In the early stages, the treatment of choice is surgery. With this, the tumour is eliminated with safety margins. This is achieved with or without cervical emptying, depending on the location, size or suspicion of regional metastasis. Once the cervical emptying is completed and analysed, if the structures are affected, subsequent treatment with RTP is evaluated. Advanced stages can be treated with surgery followed by RTP but this combination only cures a minority of patients and fewer than 30% will be alive at five years. With these treatments, tumour control and survival rates are unsatisfactory. Only 30% of patients will be alive after three years, while 60-70% of patients will have a loco-regional recurrence and/or will develop distant metastasis, which, ultimately, is the main cause of death in these patients [8].

QTP, in addition to RTP and surgery, is associated with a better general survival rate in patients with oral or oropharyngeal cancer. Induction QTP can extend survival from 8% to 20% and concomitant adjuvant chemo-radiotherapy can prolong survival up to 16%.

QTP consists of the administration of cytotoxic drugs that are capable of destroying and inhibiting the growth and reproduction of malignant cells [9]. In head and neck cancers, the most extensively used drugs are bleomycin, cisplatin, methotrexate, 5-fluorouracil, vinblastine and cyclophosphamide [10]. QTP can be developed by administering one or more chemotherapeutic drugs. The use of isolated drugs (mono-chemotherapy) has proven useless in the induction of significant complete or partial responses. Thus, the current trend is polychemotherapy, which affects the cellular populations in different cell-cycle phases. This is achieved by using the synergistic action of the drugs, decreasing the development of resistance to them and promoting a higher response per administered dose [10]. The most used combinations

http://dx.doi.org/10.5772/60397

include cisplatin and 5-fluorouracil; cisplatin, 5-fluorouracil and taxol or cisplatin, bleomycin and methotrexate. Cytostatic drugs offer better results in tumours with a significant growth fraction and/or early distant or frequent dissemination such as lymphomas (90% growth fraction). This is not the case for squamous cell carcinoma, which is the most common head and neck malignancy (25% growth fraction). Therefore, QTP is usually associated with another therapeutic modality [11].

RTP can be applied locally (brachytherapy) or externally (teletherapy). The external radiotherapy is the classic way to administer radiotherapy with a remote radiation source of the organism. Sources of external irradiation are low voltage (X-ray), supervoltage (cobalt 60), megavoltage (linear accelerator) and electron beam (power source). Of these, the most widely used treatments for head and neck therapy are cobalt-60 and the linear particle accelerator [12]. External radiotherapy requires a division of the dose and a longer period to carry it out, consisting of a weekly dose of 10 Gy, 2 Gy daily for five days and two days of rest, usually spread out over a period of 5-7 weeks. Fractioned RTP allows a full high dose in the tumour, respecting the normal adjacent tissue and decreasing toxicity. It also conditions the response in healthy and tumour tissues by repairing injuries. This is because, compared to tumour tissue, normal tissue repairs damaged DNA better, especially at low doses. It also promotes the reoxygenation of tumour cells, increasing their radiosensitivity and the repopulation of the tissue between fractions. This is particularly the case during weekends when the area is not irradiated, thereby reducing the early effects [13]. The radiation dose depends on the location and type of tumour and whether the RTP is used alone or combined with other treatment modalities. When the RTP is exclusive, the dose is usually between 60 Gy and 80 Gy, whereas the dose administered post-surgically is 50-60 Gy [1].

On the other hand, brachytherapy is a method that uses ionizing radiation. It places radioactive material in the proximity of or within the tumour. There are different modalities of brachytherapy, of which interstitial RTP is the most frequently used for head and neck tumours. In this modality, Iridium 192 (Ir192) and Iodine 125 (I125) are the most frequent radioactive sources.

RTP and QTP are combined to improve therapeutic results, increasing loco-regional tumour control and distant metastasis [14].

There are different ways to classify the effects produced by RTP on head and neck regions, as are shown in Table 1,2, 3 [10, 15-17].

EFFECTS	ACUTE	LATE
	Mucositis	Necrosis of soft tissue
	Radiodermatitis	Trismus
	Opportunist infections	Osteoradionecrosis (ORN)
	Xerostomia	Post-radiation caries
	Alteration in taste	

Table 1. Acute and late effects of RTP.

CHRONOLOGY	IMMEDIATE	MEDIUM TERM	LONG TERM
	Mucositis	Post-radiation caries	Osteoradionecrosis
	Alteration in taste	Opportunist infections	Tooth disorder
	Xerostomia	Necrosis of soft tissue	
	Radiodermatitis	Trismus	

Table 2. Chronology of RTP: immediate, medium term and long term effects.

EVOLUTION	REVERSIBLE	IRREVERSIBLE
	Mucositis	Xerostomia
	Radiodermatitis	Alteration in taste
	Xerostomia	Post-radiation caries
	Alteration in taste	Osteoradionecrosis
	Opportunist infections	Tooth disorder
	Necrosis of soft tissue	
	Trismus	

Table 3. Evolution of RTP: reversible and irreversible effects.

2.1. Acute complications of radiotherapy

a. Mucositis is the inflammation of the oral-oropharynx as a result of the cytotoxic effects of RTP. It is the most common complication that appears among patients who have been irradiated with neck and head cancer, with an incidence of 80 %. Mucositis is dose-dependent and therefore, it disappears with the end of the aggression [18]. The risk and its gravity depend on the characteristics of the treatment such as doses, size of the irradiated zone and its division.

The first sign is erythema, which appears when a dose of 10 Gy is accumulated (first week) and persists up to 15 days after the end of the RTP treatment. The point of maximum symptomatology is when there are accumulated doses of 60-70 Gy [19, 20]. Clinically, the mucosa is erythematous and edematous so it can become ulcerated and infected by fungi [19, 21]. The pain that accompanies mucositis can be so intense that it alters the patient's quality of life, limiting their basic oral functions such as speaking, swallowing saliva or eating [21].

Mucositis can be classified in four degrees, according to the intensity of the mucosa [16, 22]:

Grade 0: None (Figure 1).

Grade 1: Erythaema (Figure 2 and 3).

Grade 2: Erythaema, ulcers but capable of ingesting solids (Figure 4).

http://dx.doi.org/10.5772/60397

Grade 3: Ulcers, requiring liquid diet (Figure 5).

Grade 4: Oral feeding is impossible (Figure 6).

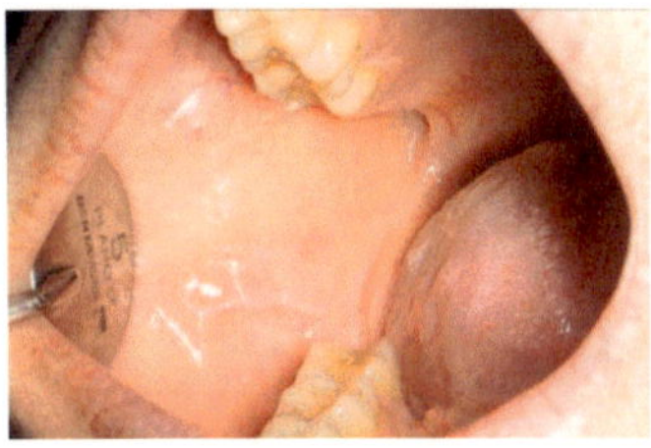

Figure 1. Grade 0.

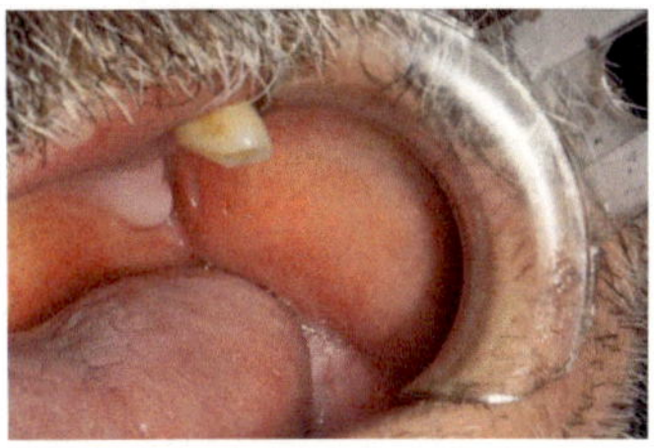

Figure 2. Grade 1.

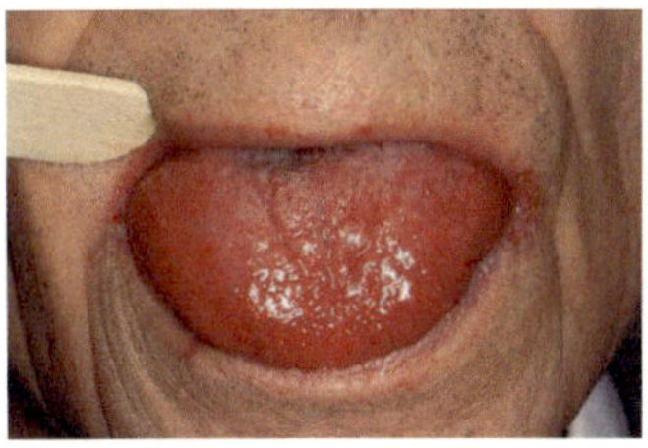

Figure 3. Grade 1.

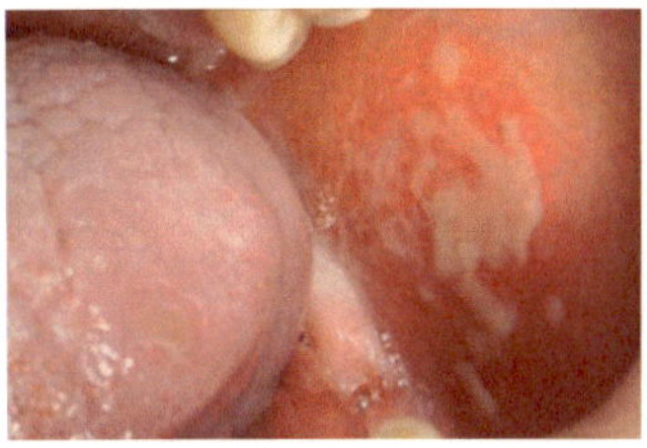

Figure 4. Grade 2.

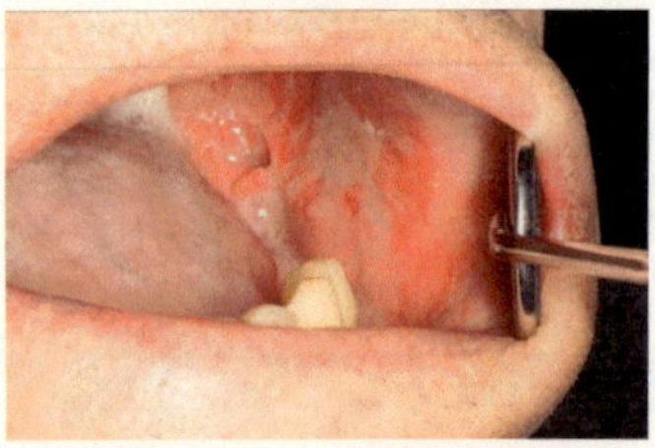

Figure 5. Grade 3.

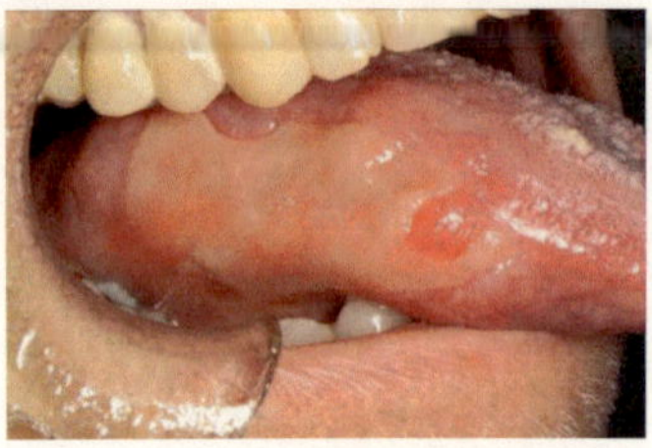

Figure 6. Grade 4.

b. RTP facilitates the surge of opportunist infections, mainly Candida (Figure 7 and 8) as a result of the reduction of saliva, the use of dentures, deficient oral hygiene and the persistence of habits such as smoking or drinking [23]. These types of infections tend to disappear with topical anti-fungal drugs. However, irradiated patients frequently have to use more effective systemic drugs [24].

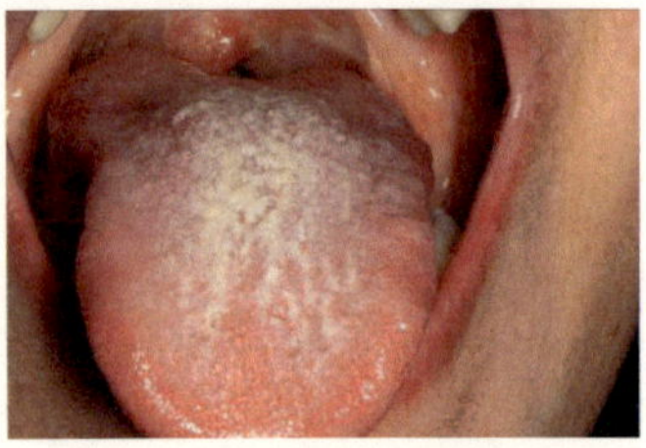

Figure 7. Candidiasis during RTP.

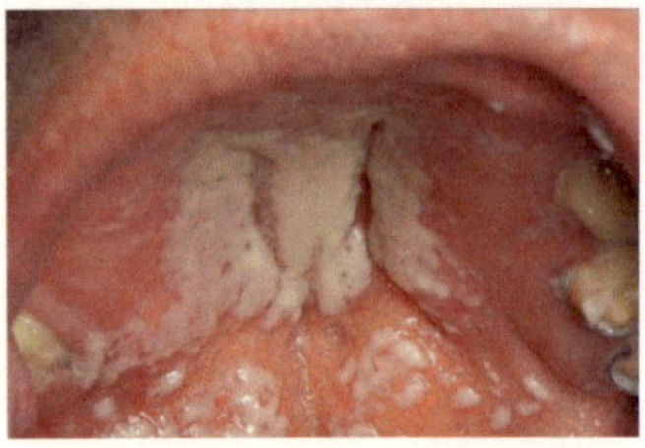

Figure 8. Candidiasis during RTP.

http://dx.doi.org/10.5772/60397

c. Radiodermatitis is considered as skin and subcutaneous tissue toxicity. Depending on its severity, it is classified in three different levels. Transitory erythaema is produced by the congestion of dermal papillae within the first 24 hours. A dose of 3 Gy is enough to trigger it (Figure 9 and 10). A dose of 25 Gy will produce an acceleration of the skin flaking process, which is manifested as a significant decrease of thickness. This will then become dark, atrophic and flaky, which is called dry radiodermatitis (Figure 11). A 50-70 Gy dose will cause a delayed erythaema, followed by a superficial necrobiosis and the formation of skin scabs. If these lesions progress, bleeding vesicula easily appears, which is called wet radiodermatitis (Figure 12). These lesions are cured when the RTP treatment has ended, leaving scars on the skin. These can be white and esclerotic telangiectastic. Follicles are destroyed and, on occasions, pigmentations can appear [10].

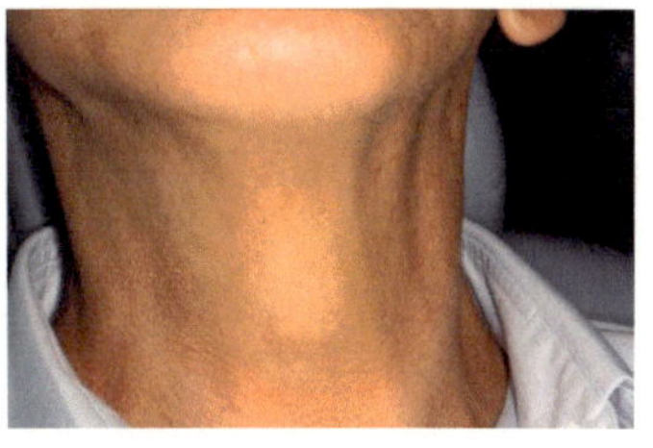

Figure 9. Radiodermatitis: Grade 0, 5 sessions of RTP.

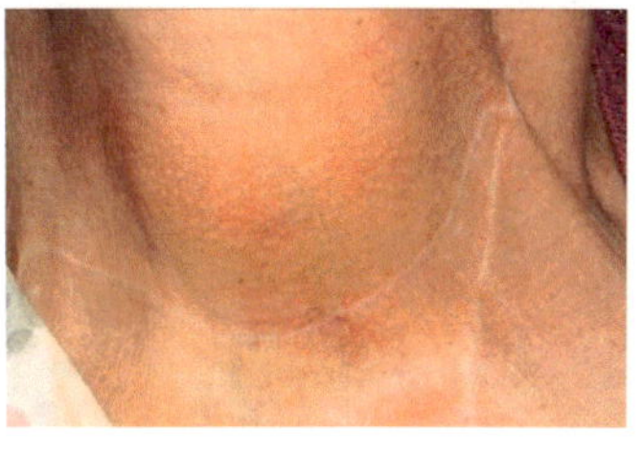

Figure 10. Radiodermatitis Grade I, 10 sessions of RTP.

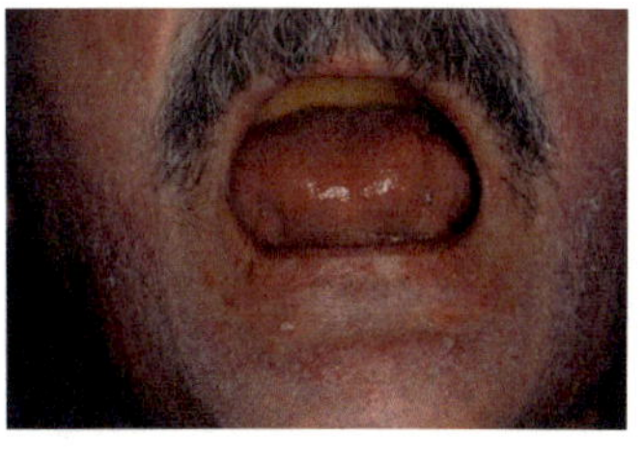

Figure 11. Radiodermatitis: Grade II, 17 sessions of RTP.

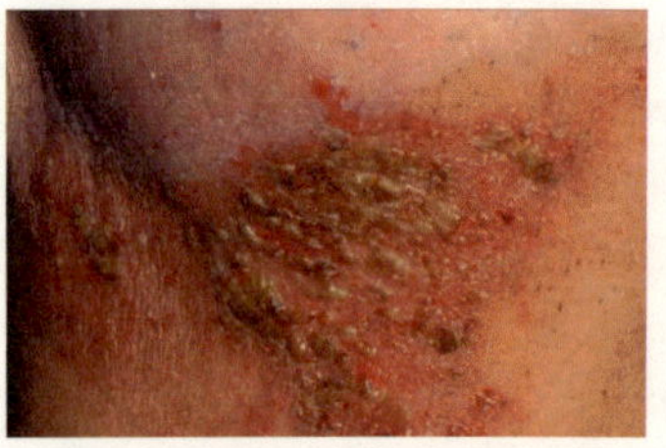

Figure 12. Radiodermatitis Grade III, 24 sessions of RTP.

d. Most patients suffer xerostomia or salivary hypofunction due to RTP in head and neck cancers. This usually appears within the first weeks of radiation. In low doses (under 30 Gy), it is believed that the damage can be reversible. However, higher doses (over 60-70 Gy) result in an irreversible and permanent xerostomia. With the latter, there is a significant degeneration of the acini, which is reflected by concomitant inflammation and fibrosis of the interstitium (Figure 13).

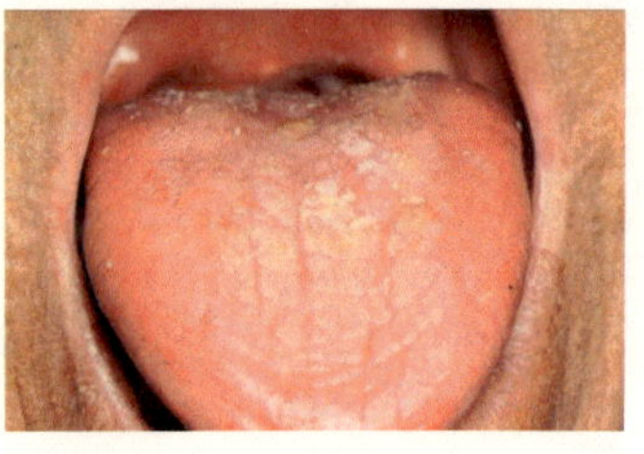

Figure 13. Rough tongue due to salivary hypofunction.

e. Salivary hypofunction (a resting saliva flow of less than 0.2 ml per minute or a stimulated flow of less than 0.7 ml per minute) is caused by the damage of direct ionizing radiation of the salivary glands' cells [25]. This is the most persistent effect in patients submitted to RTP for head and neck tumours. It is characterized by changes in the amount and quality of saliva (more viscous and scarce). It produces oral discomfort and pain, a higher risk of dental caries, oral infection, difficulty of speech and disfagia. This has a damaging effect on the patient's quality of life [26-28]. The reduction of salivary flow can also increase the susceptibility of the dental caries and takes into account the integrity of the mucosa [29].

f. The alteration in taste is a result of direct radiation of the taste buds and receptors of taste, as well as changes in the saliva [30-32]. It contributes to loss of appetite, which results in the patient's weight loss. It appears 15 days after the treatment starts from the 4 Gy and it reaches its maximum once the RTP is finished. In most cases, the sense of taste gradually returns to normal or almost normal levels one year after radiotherapy [33]. However, some

http://dx.doi.org/10.5772/60397

patients can experience a residual reduction of taste (hypogeusia), permanent damage to the sense (disgeusia) and the loss of taste (ageusia) [34, 35].

2.2. Late complications of radiotherapy

a. There is a necrosis of soft tissue characterized by an ulcer located in the irradiated tissue, without the presence of residual malignancy (Figure 14 and 15). It is usually a painful condition and the tissues present a pale colour and lack of flexibility [36].

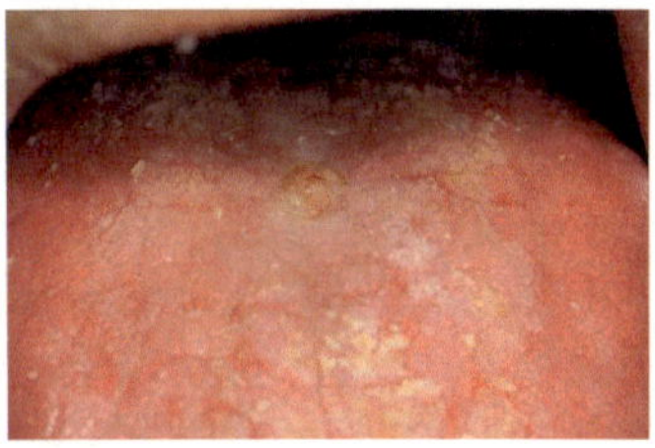

Figure 14. Necrosis of soft tissue two months after finishing RTP.

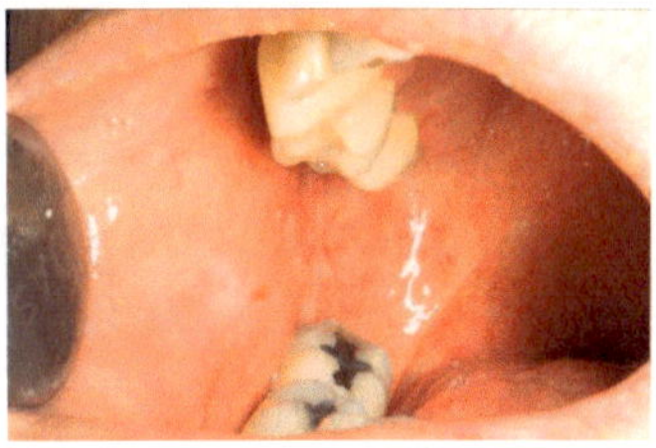

Figure 15. Necrosis of soft tissue two months after finishing RTP.

b. Trismus is characterized by a reduction in the opening due to the contraction and even fibrosis of the masticating muscles and the ATM (Figure 16). It appears between three and six months after radiation [23]. It can result in eating and communication problems. It also impacts oral hygiene and the use of prosthesis, as well as the development of dental treatments.

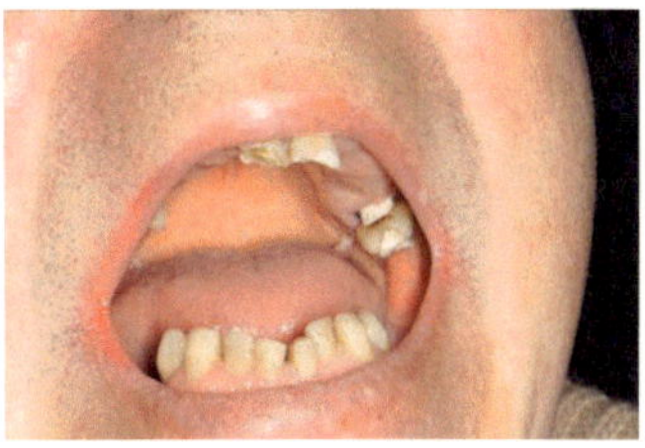

Figure 16. Still suffering from trismus one and a half years after finishing the RTP.

c. Osteoradionecrosis could be the most severe RTP complication [38]. It is defined as an area of bone exposure in a previously irradiated area, of at least six weeks of evolution and in absence of tumour recurrence [37]. ORN is the result of reduced vascularity of periodontal bone, the periosteum. It causes hypovascular, hypocellular and hypoxic tissue, where the capacity of bone repair and regeneration is severely compromised [38-40]. It can be asymptomatic or it can produce pain, dysaesthesia or anesthesia, depending on its relation with the dental nerve. Patients report halitosis, trismus and dysgeusia. Patients find that ORN impacts food in the lesion and they have difficulties in chewing and swallowing, as well as exhibiting phonation [36]. In most cases, the condition is chronic, developing gradually and becoming wider and painful [38, 41].

There are risk factors that can bring about ORN. These can be related to the tumour, with the patient and with the treatment. With regard to factors that depend on the patient, we fundamentally focus on the realization of post radiotherapy extractions. In fact, the development of ORN with no previous surgery has proved to be extremely strange (incidence of 2.7% after five years). Some other determinant factors are poor oral hygienic, previous irradiations of the zone and the presence of periodontitis. Further factors include bad habits such as tobacco and alcohol. Depending on the treatment, the risk factors are the administrated dose, its division, the RTP type and the irradiated zone. Ultimately, the risk factors, depending on the tumour, include the anatomical localization, the proximity of other bone structures and the size of the tumour. These factors must be taken into account because they increase the risk of ORN and if we are aware of them, we can prevent it.

Most ORN cases take place in the jaw. Here, vascularization is deficient and there is high bone density (Figure 17, 18 and 19). Clinical manifestations of ORN may include pain, orofacial fistulas, exposure of the necrotic bone, pathological fractures and suppuration [42].

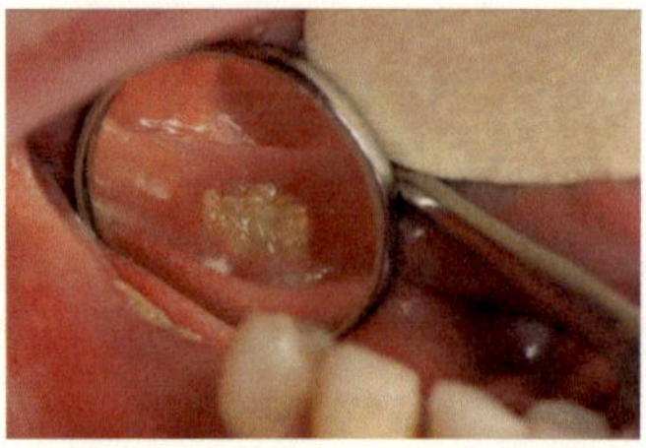

Figure 17. ORN in the jaw after extraction post-RTP.

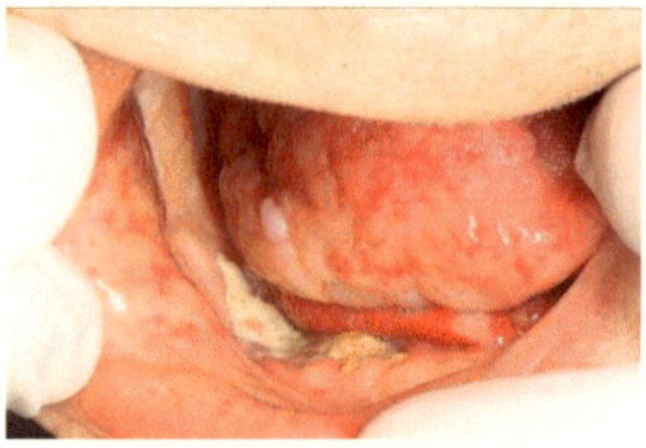

Figure 18. ORN in the jaw after extraction post-RTP.

http://dx.doi.org/10.5772/60397

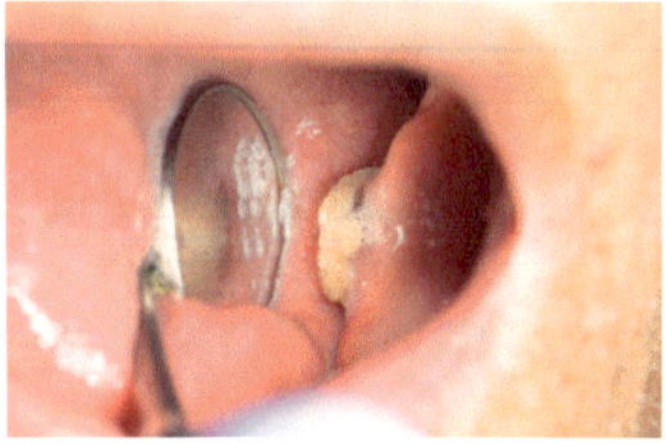

Figure 19. ORN after four months of finishing the RTP. Extraction had been carried out pre-RTP.

One third of ORN cases are spontaneous, although most cases occur due to teeth removal during radiotherapy or during an insufficient healing time after pre-RTP extractions. According to Starcke, Shannon, Murray and Makkonen, when the pre-RTP tooth removal is performed correctly and a certain period passes, a significant increase of osteorradionecrosis is not observed [43-45].

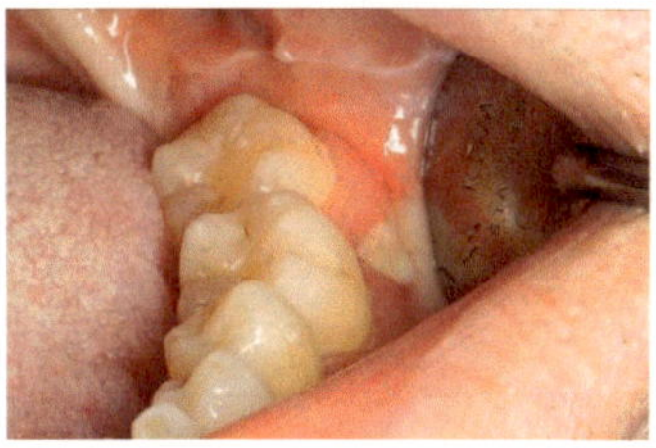

Figure 20. Spontaneous ORN in the jaw after RTP.

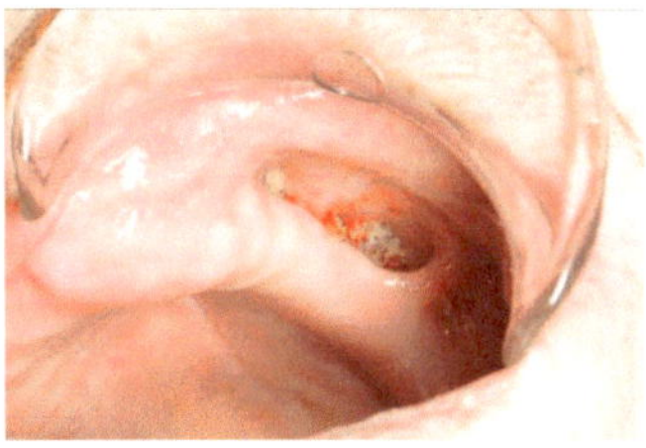

Figure 21. ORN after extraction post-RTP.

Incidence of ORN is two times higher in patients with teeth, although poor dental hygiene and continued drinking and smoking can also contribute to its quick appearance [46]. A higher incidence of osteoradionecrosis has been observed after receiving doses of over 65 Gy. This depends on the fractioning of radiation and the treatment with QTP or surgery in the irradiated area [47] (Figure 22 and 23 - case report of ORN that, after seven months of treatment, positively developed chlorhexidine.).

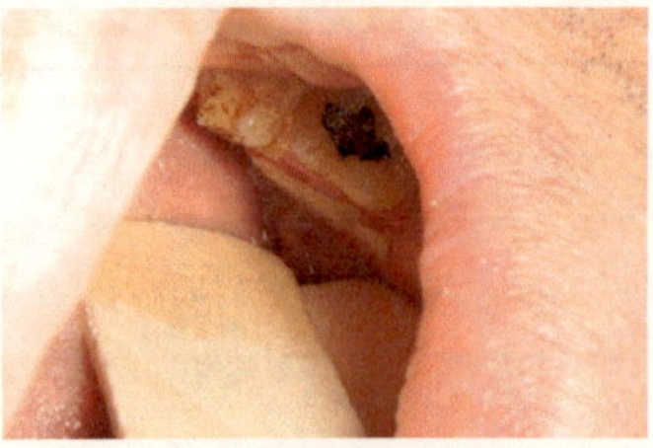

Figure 22. ORN two months after finishing the RTP, without previous extractions.

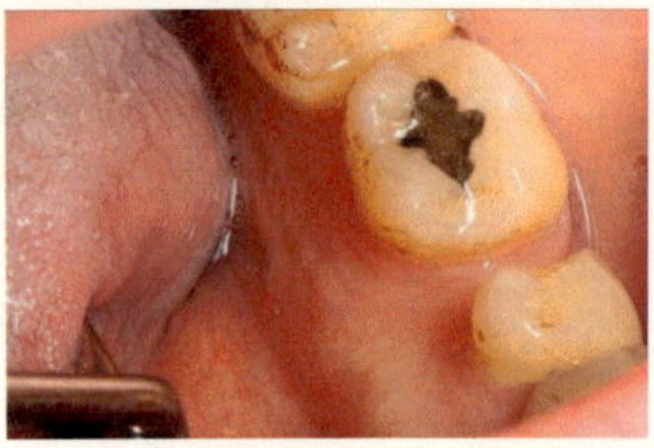

Figure 23. After seven months of good oral hygiene and rinses with chlorhexidine and chlorhexidine gel, it has progressed favourably.

d. Dental caries are very frequent in post-radiation starting three months after RTP has ended. There is a collapse and detachment of the enamel prisms that mainly affect the incisal edges, cuspids and cervical region of the teeth [10] (Figure 24). This is the result of a quantitative and qualitative alteration in the saliva, with a decrease of its stopping capacity. This favours the development of an acidogenic-cariogenic bacterial flora. A change towards a soft carbohydrate-rich diet, poor dental hygiene and the deterioration of motivation also influences this (Figure 25).

For irradiated patients, dietary changes - a softer or liquid diet with a higher concentration of carbohydrates - combined with a decrease in saliva, results in a change in the microbiota. This becomes increasingly cariogenic. This, in addition to poor dental hygiene, results in a demineralization of the enamel and the destruction of crowns and the cervical area. Here, the cement and dentin is exposed to the oral environment, producing increased dental sensitivity [48].

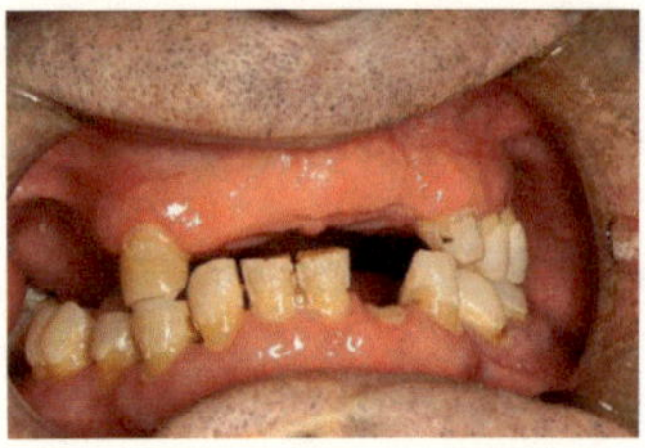

Figure 24. Dental wear during RTP.

http://dx.doi.org/10.5772/60397

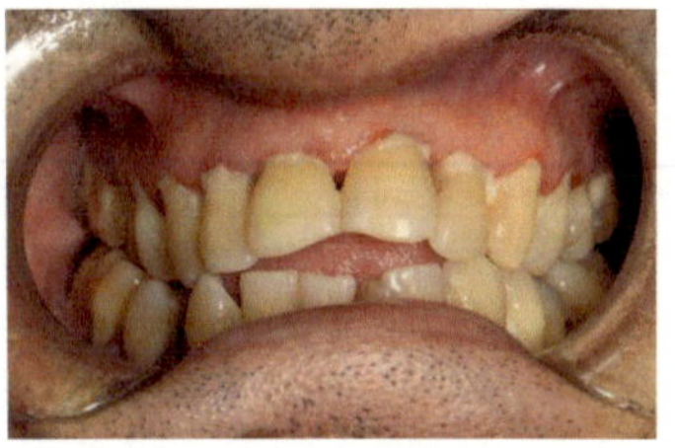

Figure 25. Accumulation of plaque due to poor hygiene during RTP.

3. Protocol for management before RTP

In literature of this subject area, there are articles published on the management of complications in patients with head and neck cancer. These mainly focus on mucositis, radiodermatitis and osterradionecrosis. However, in order for this to be prevented, we must monitor the patient before, during and after radiotherapy. In this chapter, therefore, we will focus on the management of the radiated patient, mainly before radiotherapy. This is because there are few protocols and we believe that these are necessary in order to minimize the risks during treatment.

Figure 26 and 27: Orthopantomography of a patient before beginning the RTP and two years after finishing the RTP.

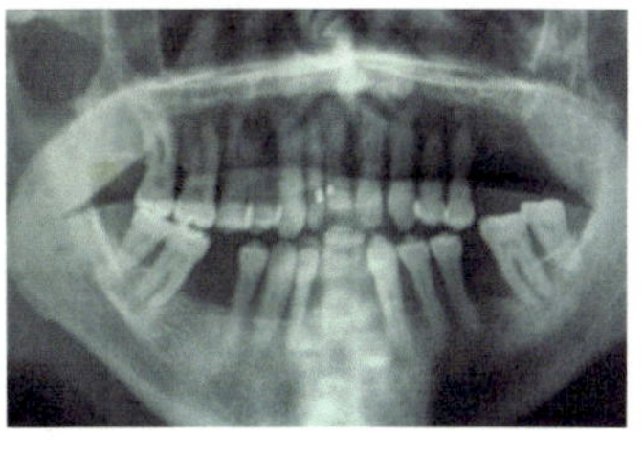

Figure 26. Before RTP.

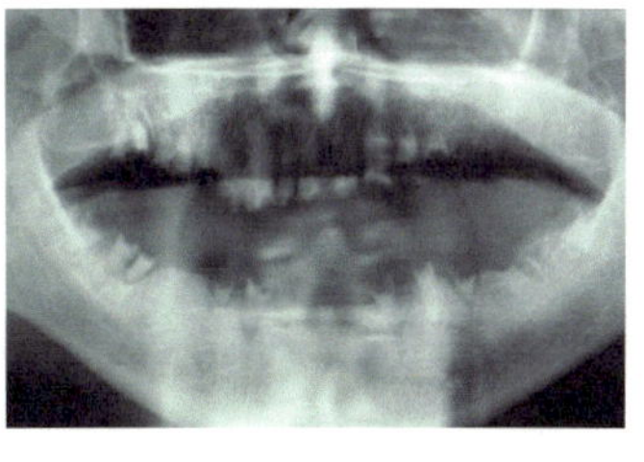

Figure 27. After RTP.

3.1. First visit

During the first visit, we collect the clinical history including the patients' personal data: age, gender, family medical history, personal medical history, current medical problems, medication, allergies and harmful habits. All patients are referred with an oncological report, including their medical history: tumour diagnosis, tumour stage and tumour treatment. A mouth X-ray is also included to evaluate the dental status. A bucodental exploration is developed to assess the oral situation of the patient and evaluate different therapeutic needs, covering the RTP protocol.

3.1.1. RTP protocol

1. All patients must bring orthopantomography and report your oncological data.

2. Medical history is covered.

3. On each visit, a radiographical series from the patient is necessary - extraoral (mouth closed, neck and maximum opening of the mouth) and intraoral (maxima intercuspidation, lateral intercuspidation, top and lower arcades, buccal mucosa and tongue), as is shown in Figures 28-38.

4. An exploration of the mucosa is developed (yugal mucosa, lips, tongue, gums, bottom of the vestibule, floor of the mouth, palate, etc.), in order to discard any pre-existing lesion.

5. A dental and periodontal exploration is developed with the assistance of a probe and mirror. The degree of dental hygiene is determined using the Silnesloe index [49].

Grade 0: Absence of dental plaque.

Grade 1: Plaque not visible but could be extracted from the gingival third of the tooth using the probe.

Grade 2: Moderate build-up of plaque in the gingival region that could easily be seen.

Grade 3: Abundance of plaque in the same region, possibly covering the neighbouring teeth.

6. The maximum interincisal distance is measured with callipers (a trismus is a bucal opening of less than 40 mm).

7. A culture is carried out. The sample is taken from the back of the tongue and the readings are at 24-48-72 hours. The sample is taken from the back of the tongue using a cotton swab, depositing it in an agar-sabourand plate and placing it in the furnace for 72 hours.

8. The status of the saliva function is assessed using a chart paper strip (1 cm thick by 17 cm length, with 1 cm not charted), introduced in a polyethylene bag. This is called a Global Saliva Test, in rest and stimulated [50]. The section of non-charted strip is extracted from the bag for testing. The end is then folded in a right angle and inserted in the oral cavity, below the tongue. When closing the lips, these will slightly touch the polyethylene bag. The saliva produced is accumulated in the lingual vallecule during the five minutes of the test's duration. During this time, the strip slowly soaks. Once this time has ended, it is

http://dx.doi.org/10.5772/60397

retrieved from the mouth and the wet charted strip is immediately read. Subsequently, the stimulation test is carried out by depositing some drops of citric acid at 4% in the oral cavity and repeating the same process.

Figures 28-39: Radiographical series from the patient going to treatment with RTP.

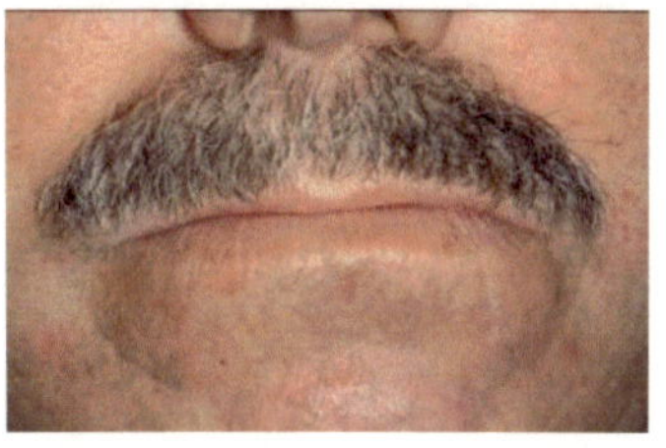

Figure 28. Mouth closed.

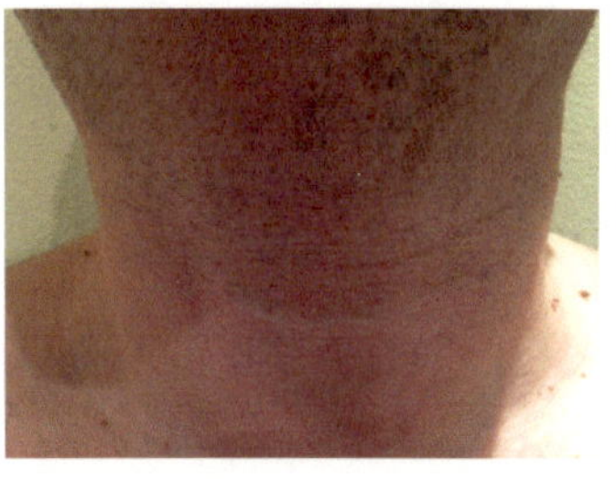

Figure 29. Neck.

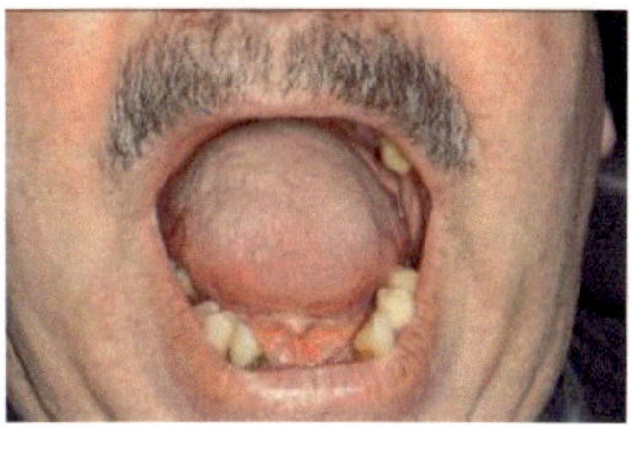

Figure 30. Maximum opening of the mouth.

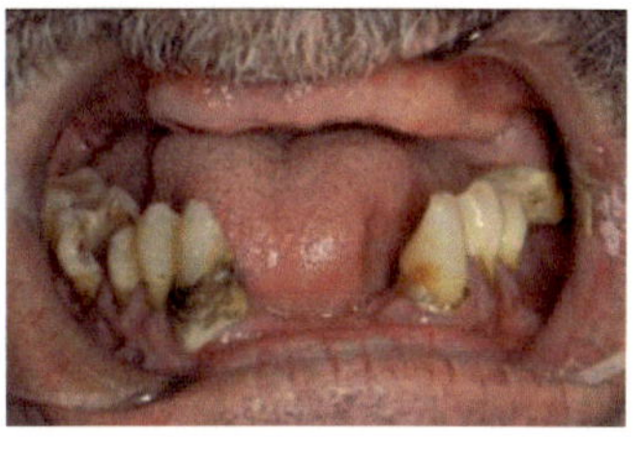

Figure 31. Maximum intercuspidation.

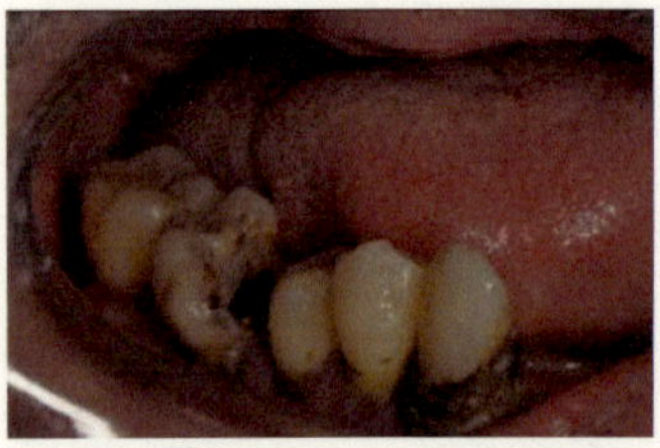

Figure 32. Right lateral intercuspidation.

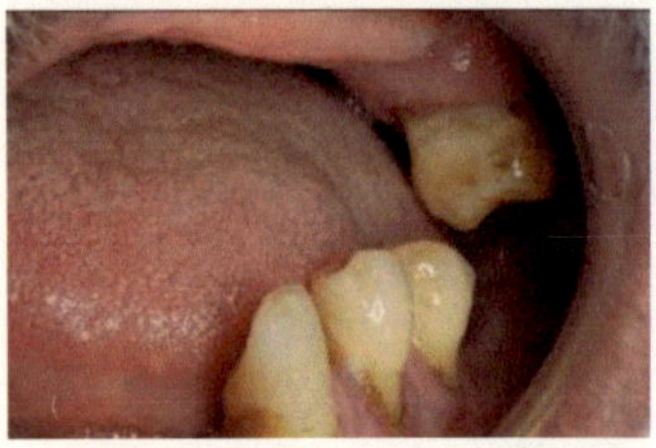

Figure 33. Left lateral intercuspidation.

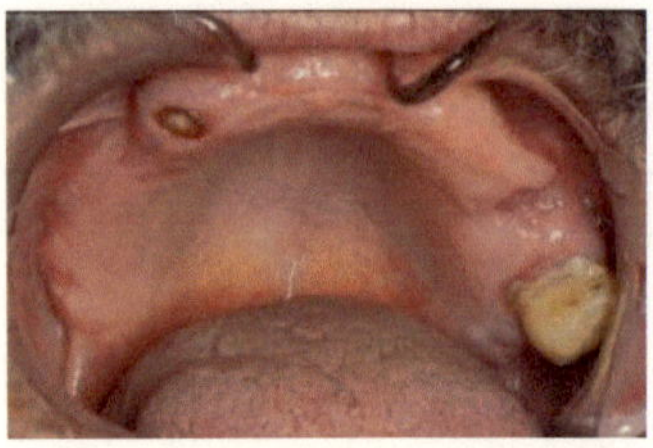

Figure 34. Top arcade.

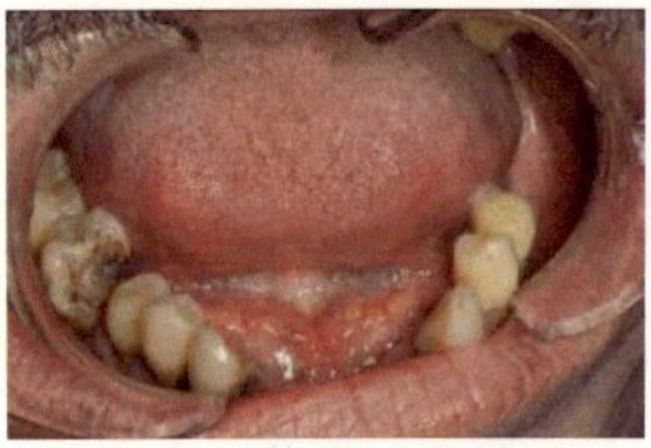

Figure 35. Lower arcade.

http://dx.doi.org/10.5772/60397

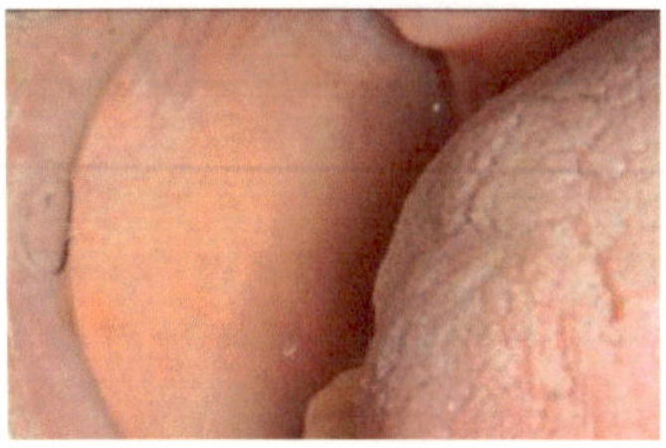

Figure 36. Right buccal mucosa.

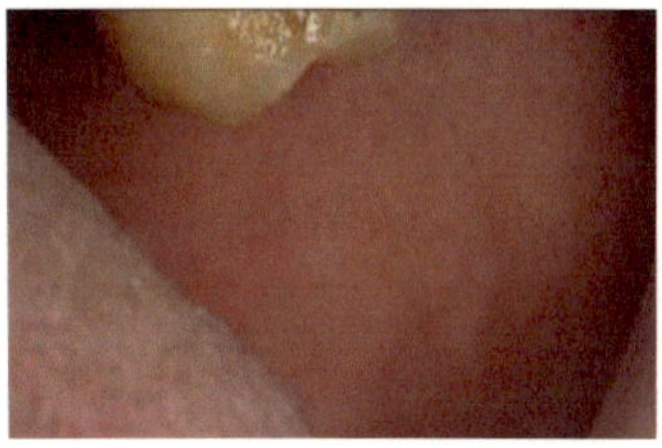

Figure 37. Left buccal mucosa.

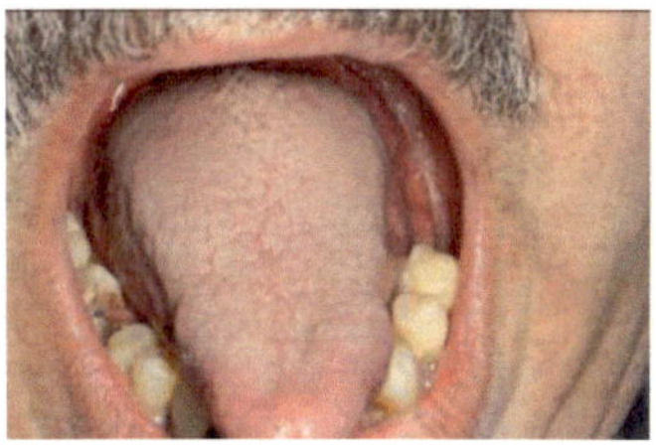

Figure 38. Tongue.

9. Once the odontogram is covered, with the assistance of an ortopantomography, the therapeutic needs will be defined:

    - Extraction (if this is necessary, all patients will sign an informed consent explaining all the possible complications).
    - Seals/endodontics.
    - Treatment for oral candidiasis (mycostatin - mouth wash three times a day for three minutes for four weeks).
    - Tartar removal, scaling and root planning.
    - Remove irritants that graze (traumatic prosthesis and sharp teeth).
    - Motivation in oral hygiene - strongly recommend a daily teeth brushing for at least three times a day with toothpaste with high fluoride content. Apart from Fluoridation

plan in patients with teeth - preparation of individual trays for the daily application of sodium fluoride gel at 1.24%, five minutes/day, indefinitely and mouth wash with chlorhexidine.

10. If extractions are recommended [51, 52], the prognosis of the tooth itself, the patient's motivation and their ability to follow oral hygiene instructions plays a role. All teeth with a questionable prognosis should be extracted before RTP:

- Caries (non-restorable).
- Active periodontal disease (symptomatic teeth).
- Moderate and severe periodontal disease (≥ 5 mm bags) especially with advanced bone loss, mobility and furcation involvement.
- Partial impaction or incomplete eruption, especially of third molars, which are not fully covered by the alveolar bone or in contact with the oral cavity.
- Extensive periapical lesions (if not chronic or well localized).
- Root fragments that are not completely covered by alveolar bone or show radiolucency.
- Teeth near the tumour or in the tumour.
- Lack of opposing teeth.
- Compromised hygiene.

When developing extractions, patients should be handled as follows [52-54].

- Antibiotic prophylaxis for patients who need it, as recommended by the ADA.
- Rinse with antiseptic mouthwash - chlorhexidine digluconate 0.12% for one minute.
- Anaesthetic technique:
- Anaesthesia with vasoconstrictor.
- Minimal trauma - regularization of the alveolar process by approximation of edges.
- Non-absorbable 4.0 silk suture.
- Antibiotics, Amoxicillin 750 mg 1/8 hours /7 days is prescribed.
- Post-operative treatment: analgesic-anti-inflammatory medication (ibuprofen 600 mg) and antiseptic mouthwash, chlorhexidine digluconate 0.12%.
- Minimum number of sessions, starting with mandibular extractions.

Most authors agree that the minimum delay time for RTP treatment is 15-20 days [39, 44, 52, 55]. While others indicate that, in the case of complex surgical procedures, patients must wait four to six weeks [10, 54].

http://dx.doi.org/10.5772/60397

Management before RTP
1. Report your oncological data.
2. Clinical history and bucodental exploration.
3. Orthopantomography.
4. Bucodental exploration.
5. The therapeutic needs will be defined: seals, endodontics and extractions.
6. Instructions and motivation in oral hygiene.
7. Global Saliva Test, in rest and stimulated.
8. Maximum interincisal distance.
9. Culture and identification of candidiasis.

4. Protocol for management during RTP

Patients who are to receive radiation therapy experience three main acute complications that cause functional disability and hinder the development of normal life. These are mucositis, radiodermitis and xerostomia. Weekly monitoring is required, i.e., we must see the patient once a week during the eight weeks that the treatment usually lasts. The main symptoms appear after the fifth dose of radiation. Thus, on each visit, we usually develop the following measurements covered in the protocol.

4.1. RTP protocol

a. Degree of mucositis.

b. Degree of radiodermatitis.

c. Degree of oral hygiene - Silnesloe index [49].

d. Presence of ORN.

e. Eliminate possible graze, if the patient has removable/complete prosthesis.

f. Dental state and instructions in oral hygiene.

g. Saliva amount by means of TSG I and TSG II [50].

h. Culture at mid-treatment and at the end.

i. Maximum interincisal distance at mid-treatment and at the end.

j. Radiographical series from the patient is necessary - extraoral (mouth closed, neck and maximum opening of the mouth) and intraoral (maxima intercuspidation, lateral intercuspidation, top and lower arcades, buccal mucosa and tongue).

k. Motivation in oral hygienic, strongly recommend a daily teeth brushing for at least three times a day with toothpaste with high fluoride content. Apart from Fluoridation plan in patients with teeth - preparation of individual trays for the daily application of sodium fluoride gel at 1.24%, five minutes/day, indefinitely and mouth wash with clorhexidine

During the radiotherapy treatment - and even 18 months later - no surgery technique should be used with these patients and if an endodontic treatment is necessary, dental apex cannot be surpassed. We advise exercises and jaw movements in order to prevent trismus and, in this way, the maximum opening can be kept.

We must insist on instructions on oral hygienic to prevent rampant caries. As these patients suffer from intense pain in the oral cavity, we can advise a soft brush so as not to irritate the mucosa, accompanied by a soft diet and anticariogenic

Fundamentally, these patients report dryness of the mouth and less saliva. The quality of saliva changes - it feels thicker which causes rampant caries. That, added to the functional disability produced by mucosistis, leads patients to abandon oral hygiene. As a result, their dental status worsens. Therefore, our treatment is based on prescribing oral rinses and insisting on the acquisition of oral hygiene habits. Basically, the purpose of it is to relieve symptoms using a formula. This includes using lidocaine hydrochloride 1% and chlorhexidine digluconate 0.12% before meals to help reduce swallowing pain [56-61].

Patients must drink at least half a litre of water a day to get a good hydration. There is a possibility of cryotherapy, above all in mucositis and occasioned by quimotherapics. Therefore, patients must thaw ice in their mouths every 30 minutes [62, 63].

Nowadays, there are saliva substitutes (sprays or gels that temporarily wet the oral mucosa - these are palliative) and stimulants (lemon drops, chewing gum with xylitol and sialogogues, among which the pilocarpine is the most important). Pilocarpine is an on-selective cholinergic agonist, which stimulates the salivary secretion. However, in our protocol, it is not recommended due to its various side effects [64, 65]. We recommend drinking water to hydrate, diet tips and good oral hygiene

As saliva decreases, the sense of taste disappears. Thus, a zinc element can be useful for the restoration of protein responsible for the regulation of pores in taste buds. It is also important to drink an abundance of liquids with meals and to slowly chew. This will liberate flavours and stimulate saliva [32, 66].

As for mucositis, large ulcerations appear in the mucosa of the oropharynx and oral cavity. Curing this disease usually takes three weeks. However, up to two months may pass before they start to subside [15, 56-58, 67]. In terms of management, we must differentiate pain control [68] and functional disability [60, 62, 69] by combining oral solutions (lidocaine hydrochloride 1% and chlorhexidine digluconate 0.12%) and a liquid or soft diet.

The election of treatment in the first phase of ulceration is to prevent infection. This can be achieved through good oral hygiene and antimicrobial agents, such as clorhexidine mouthwash, povidone iodine and hyaluronic acid gels, which form a film that restructures the epitelio. With these measures, the bacteria colonization in injuries with ulcerous mucositis is prevented but its apparition is not [70].

http://dx.doi.org/10.5772/60397

As previously stated, these patients experience a lot of pain and so it is necessary to use anti-inflammatories. These include Benzydamine, which is used as a mouthwash and reduces concentrations of tumour necrosis factors. This is efficient in the reduction of intensity and the lasting of injuries in the mucosa [71].

There are cytoprotective agents that eliminate free radicals acting as antioxidants. In this group, we have amifostine, prostaglandins and sucralfalte. The amifostine is a protector against the xerostomia during the radiotherapy treatment. It reduces its gravity and duration. However, it has multiple adverse effects and so its use is limited [72, 73]. Sucralfate adheres to the walls of the ulcer and constitutes a superficial barrier in the gastrointestinal tract. As a result, the oropharingeo pain is reduced but mucositis is not prevented. Sucralfate has some antibacterial activity so it aids the healing of injuries and stimulates the synthesis of the prostaglandins [74-77].

It is difficult to specify which treatment should be elected as each patient responds differently to radiotherapy. Our experience is that chlorexidine and hyaluronic acid [78] do no aid aggressive injuries. Thus, in different cases of mucositis III and IV, we recommend the use of, topic corticoids, mainly 0.5% Triamcinolone Acetonid, three times a day for three weeks. We also recommend oral rinses or creams, depending on whether the injuries are unique or multiple. The injuries develop favourably but as it is a corticoid, we have to suspend it gradually [79, 80]. Keefe et al. affirm that the high-level mucositis pain can be relieved with potent analgesic such as opiaceous [81].

Furthermore, we reviewed written studies on this subject and found that there are currently no published articles referring to the association between the administration of cortisone and the presence of recurrences in the head and neck. Moreover, if there are references in other locations, such as the prostate or the skin, it remains the treatment of choice [82-84].

Nowadays, there are new therapies (biological response modifiers) conducted in the investigation phase. These eliminate the mucositis, mainly reducing the minimum development of the mucositis and, specifically, various growth factors. They also contribute to the biological process of mucosity destruction [85]. In this group, we mention palifermine keratinocyte growth factor. In advanced degree cases, this sees reduced mucositis but has secondary effects and thus, its use is restricted [86-88].

Low-energy laser therapy is an effective method for the prevention and management of mucositis. It is used to accelerate the regeneration of tissues and stop swelling and pain [89-92].

It is also important to get a basic medium so that there is no mycosis. Thus, as a preventative measure, we recommend bicarbonate water rinses before meals (dilute a spoonful of bicarbonate in 200 ml of water). Additionally, in the case of candidiasis, the treatment of choice is Nystatin (topical antifungal). Here, we suggest rinsing three times a day, for three minutes over a period of four weeks. Optimal oral hygiene is crucial in order to reduce the risk of oral mucositis [89]. In cases that do not respond to the topical treatment or severe infections, we recommend systemic antifungal such as fluconazole, 150 mg. - daily doses for two weeks [93].

Little can be done to improve the toxicity of the skin, aside from moisturizing several times a day and not covering the area so it does not keep moisture. We also recommend leaving it to air dry.

Patients usually experience weight loss due to difficulties in swallowing caused by mucositis. Taste alterciones causes a loss of appetite and dietary recommendations are necessary.

Management During RTP
1. Revisions, once a week, during treatment with radiotherapy valued: a) Degree of mucositis. b) Degree of radiodermatitis. c) Degree of oral hygiene. d) Presence of ORN. e) Eliminate possible graze, if the patient has removable/complete prosthesis. f) Dental state and instructions in oral hygiene. g) Saliva amount by means of TSG I and TSG II. h) Culture at mid-treatment and at the end. i) Maximum interincisal distance at mid-treatment and at the end.
2. Treatment of complications.
3. Instructions of oral hygiene.
4. Liquid or soft diet.
5. Avoid extractions.
6. Remove toxic habits.
7. Remove any mechanical trauma to the oral mucosa.
8. Exercise to reduce trismus.

5. Protocol for management After RTP

Patients are monitored one month after finishing RTP treatment, as well as at three months, six months, nine months, 12 months and 18 months. From then onwards, patients are reviewed semi-annually. A new OPG requested 12 months after ending RTP.

In each of the reviews, the oral condition of the patient is assessed to establish treatment needs, developing the following examinations that are covered in the protocol.

5.1. RTP protocol

1. Odontogram with the current situation after undergoing RTP, dental and periodontal status.
2. Rating of oral hygiene: the Silnesloe index [49]

http://dx.doi.org/10.5772/60397

Grade 0: Absence of dental plaque.

Grade 1: Plaque not visible but can be extracted from the gingival third of the tooth using the probe.

Grade 2: Moderate build-up of plaque in the gingival region that can easily be seen.

Grade 3: Abundance of plaque in the same region, possibly covering the neighbouring teeth.

3. Maximum interincisal distance is measured with a calliper (trismus is a mouth opening of <40mm). Different exercises, which should be carried out in order to increase the oral opening, are explained to the patient.

4. The state of the salivary function is quantitatively assessed by a Global Saliva Test (TSG), both at rest (TSG I) and stimulated (TSG II), following the technique described by López-Jornet et al. [50].

5. A culture of the lingual dorsum is developed for isolation and identification of the candida species. The clinical form of candidiasis (subclinical, erythaematous, pseudomembranous) is assessed.

6. Mucositis and residual radiodermatitis are evaluated.

7. Avoid complete or removable prosthesis until six months post RTP. Weekly monitoring is essential to prevent damages in the mucosa and always add soft filler.

8. An exhaustive inspection of the oral cavity to early diagnose the recurrences.

9. Radiographical series from the patient is necessary - extraoral (mouth closed, neck and maximum opening of the mouth) and intraoral (maxima intercuspidation, lateral intercuspidation, top and lower arcades, buccal mucosa and tongue).

10. Motivation in oral hygienic - strongly recommend a daily teeth brushing for at least three times a day with toothpaste with high fluoride content. Apart from Fluoridation plan in patients with teeth - preparation of individual trays for the daily application of sodium fluoride gel at 1.24%, five minutes/day, indefinitely and wash mouth with clorhexidine.

Patient attending the annual review after finishing the RTP. We see good oral and dental hygiene and healthy appearance of mucous.

Follows the same pattern (mouth closed, neck, maximum opening of the mouth, maximum intercuspidation, right and left lateral intercuspidation, top and lower arcade, right and left buccaal mucosa and tongue).

Patient who comes to review after 14 months of finishing RTP. He has lost four lower incisive and the root-canal therapy we sent to keep them up to remove them.

The first Figure 39 shows the patient's condition before the RTP. Siguentes figures show the patient's current state (mouth closed, neck, maximum opening of the mouth, maximum intercuspidation, right and left lateral intercuspidation, top and lower arcade, right and left buccaal mucosa and tongue).

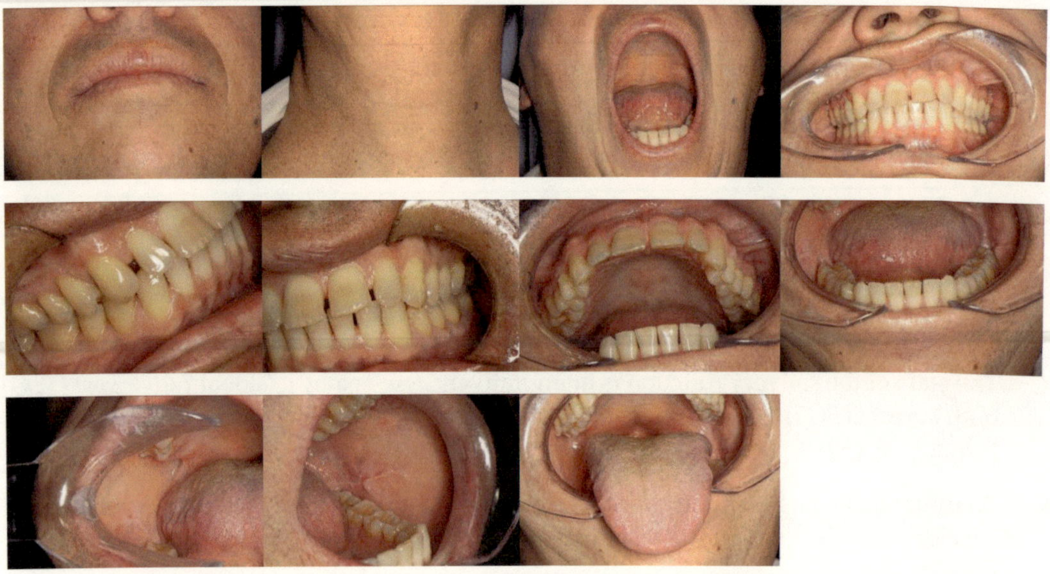

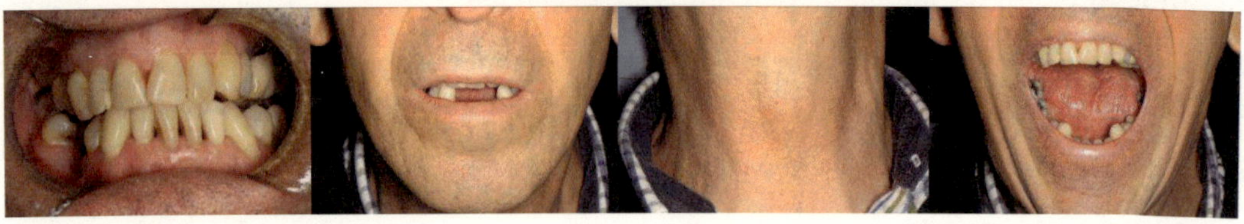

Figure 39. Before RTP

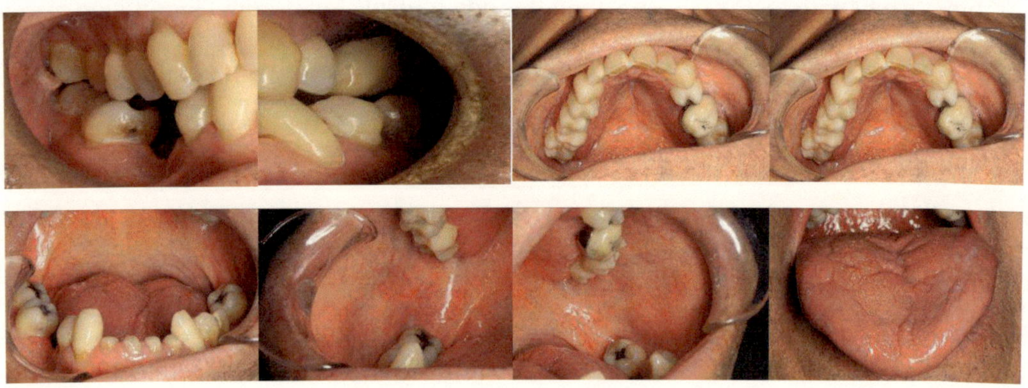

The figures below show the oral health status of different patients after one year of finishing the RTP. Here, you can see the various statuses of rampant caries and poor oral hygiene, except in a case where there is excellent oral hygiene

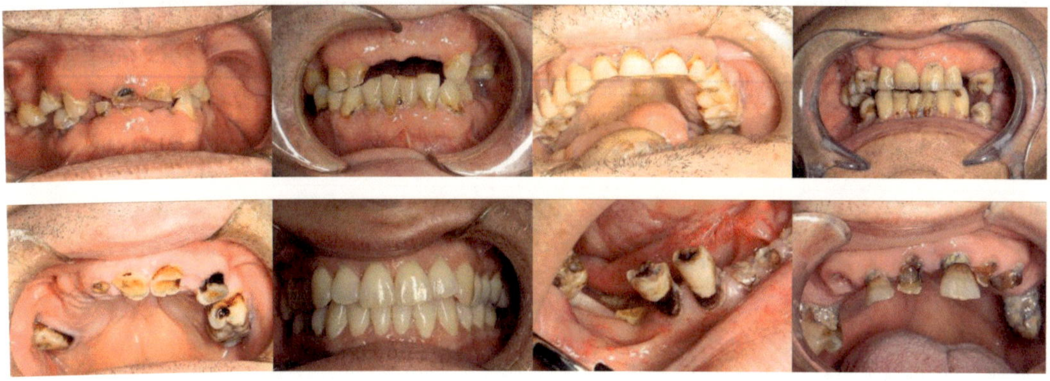

5.2. Assessment of osteoradionecrosis

1. It is classified according to the grade of bone affectation [94, 95]. The time of apparition after RTP and the association to exodoncias are valued either pre or post RTP.

Stage I: Osteoradionecrosis superficial - soft-tissue ulceration is minimal and only the exposed cortical bone is necrotic.

Stage II: Osteoradionecrosis localized - the exposed cortical bone and underlying medullary bone are necrotic.

IIA: Soft-tissue ulceration is minimal.

IIB: Soft-tissue necrosis (including orocutaneous fistulation).

Stage III: Osteoradionecrosis diffuse - bone necrosis full thickness of a segment (ability to pathological fracture).

IIIA: Soft-tissue ulceration is minimal.

IIIB: Soft-tissue necrosis (including orocutaneous fistulation).

2. Diagnosis

It is based on the clinical findings and medical history of the patient with the confirmation of a radiology study and biopsy - exposed area of bone necrosis due to tissue-irradiation, minimum cure of three to six months, without evidence of local healing and neoplastic absence enfermdad [38, 41, 96].

The symptoms can manifest months or years after the radiation of the patient. The injuries appear as ulcerations, with the exposure of rough and necrotic bone. In some cases, the injuries are discovered during a visual inspection of the cavity or due to the incommodity in a determined part of the mouth.

3. Treatment

In the first stage, a conservative treatment must be carried out. First, all irritants of the mouth are eliminated such as tobacco, alcohol and removable/complete prosthesis. Then, good oral hygiene and oral rinse with clorixidine 0,12 is carried out three times a day and a gel of clorhexidine is applied on the injuries three or four times a day.

In stage II, there is symptomatology and so the previous actions must be completed with an antibiotic treatment. In these cases, we can do a curettage of the exposed part until vital and vascular zone [97].

In stage III, pain can be intense and fistulization, suppuration and fractures can occur. Here, more radical surgery is needed to eliminate the osteolytic zone remaining vascularized [98].

5.3. Extraction post-RTP

The criteria established by Sulaiman et al. and Jansma et al. should be followed. After radiation therapy, it is necessary to delay any surgery for 18 months in order to reduce risks. The recommendations below should be followed [52, 53]:

- Rinse with antiseptic mouthwash - chlorhexidine digluconate 0.12%, one minute.
- Anaesthetic technique:
- -Anaesthesia without vasoconstrictor - truncal block, infiltrative anaesthesia, never intraligamental anaesthesia.
- Minimal trauma, alveolectomy, regularization of the alveolar process with no rotary instruments.
- Primary sealing with mucoperiosteal flaps.
- Non-absorbable 4.0 silk suture.
- Always prophylactic antibiotic (Amoxicillin 750mg 1/8 hours/10 days, if allergic to penicillin, a combination of spiramycin and metronidazole (Rhodogil®) is prescribed - two every eight hours, for 10 days).
- Post-operative treatment: analgesic-anti-inflammatory medication (Ibuprofen 600mg) and antiseptic mouthwash chlorhexidine digluconate 0.12%, plus antibiotics.
- Space the extractions in time.

Management After RTP
1. Patients are monitored one month after finishing RTP treatment, as well as at three months, six months, nine months, 12 months and 18 months. From then onwards, patients are reviewed semi-annually. A new OPG is requested 12 months after the end of the RTP.
a) Residual mucositis and radiodermatitis.
b) Grade of oral hygiene - oral hygiene motivation.
c) Presence of ORN.
d) Oral dental status.
e) Global Saliva Test (TSG), both at rest (TSG I) and stimulated (TSG II).

http://dx.doi.org/10.5772/60397

Management After RTP
f) Culture. g) Maximum interincisal distance.
2. Avoid extractions at least 18 months after finishing the RTP.
3. Avoid performing or complete/removable prosthesis for three to six months post-RTP.
4. Stimulate oral apertuta through exercises.
9. Treatment of Complications.
10. Diagnosis of recurrences.

6. Conclusions

Prior to initiating RTP treatment, all patients should be protocoled to ensure that they present optimal oral conditions. In this way, local and systemic complications can be minimized during and after treatment and measures that can be adopted to reduce adverse effects can be established. We consider it vital to quantify resting and stimulated saliva production prior to the commencement of RTP, as any previously existing xerostomia must be treated to prevent complications during RTP. The utility of an oral assessment should be explained and the importance of maintaining good oral health should be stressed.

Author details

Paula Bonar Alvarez[1], Mario Perez-Sayans García[1,2*], Maria Elena Padín Iruegas[3] and Abel García-García[4]

*Address all correspondence to: perezsayans@gmail.com

1 Oral Medicine, Oral Surgery and Implantology Unit. Faculty of Medicine and Dentistry. Santiago de Compostela, Spain

2 Instituto de Investigación Sanitaria de Santiago (IDIS), Santiago de Compostela, Spain

3 Human Anatomy and Embryology area. Faculty of Physiotherapy. Department of functional biology and health sciences, Pontevedra, Spain

4 Oral Medicine, Oral Surgery and Implantology Unit. Department of Maxillofacial Surgery, Complejo Hospitalario Universitario, Spain

References

[1] Barnes L, Eveson J, Reichart P, Sidransky D. *World Health Organization Classification of Tumours: Pathology and Genetics of Head and Neck Tumours.* 2005.

[2] Bagan J, Sarrion G, Jimenez Y. 'Oral cancer: Clinical Features'. *Oral Oncol* 2010;46(6): 414-417.

[3] Black R, Bray F, Ferlay J, Parkin D. 'Cancer Incidence and Mortality in the European Union: Cancer Registry Data and Estimates of National Incidence for 1990'. *Eur J Cancer* 1997;33(7):1075-1107.

[4] Moore SR, Johnson N, Pierce AM, Wilson DF. 'The Epidemiology of Mouth Cancer: A Review of Global Incidence'. *Oral Dis* 2000;6(2):65-74.

[5] Ord RA, Blanchaert RH. *Oral Cancer: The Dentist's Role in Diagnosis, Management, Rehabilitation, and Prevention.* Quintessence Pub.; 2000.

[6] Little JW. *Tratamiento Odontológico del Paciente Bajo Tratamiento Médico.* : Elsevier España; 1998.

[7] Castellsagué X, Quintana MJ, Martínez MC, Nieto A, Sanchez MJ, Juan A, et al. 'The Role of Type of Tobacco and Type of Alcoholic Beverage in Oral Carcinogenesis'. *International Journal of Cancer* 2004;108(5):741-749.

[8] Marcial VA, Pajak TF. 'Radiation Therapy Alone or in Combination with Surgery in Head and Neck Cancer'. *Cancer* 1985;55(S9):2259-2265.

[9] Caballero M, Grau JJ, Casellas S, Bernal-Sprekelsen M, Blanch JL. 'The Role of Chemotherapy in Advanced Oral Cavity Cancer'. *Acta Otorrinolaringologica* (English Edition) 2009;60(4):260-267.

[10] (10) Ceballos A, Bullón P, Gándara J, Chimenos E, Blanco A, Martínez-Sahuquillo A, et al. *Medicina Bucal Práctica.* Danú, SL 2000.

[11] Pignon J, Bourhis J, Domenge C, Designe L. 'Chemotherapy Added to Locoregional Treatment for Head and Neck Squamous-Cell Carcinoma: Three Meta-Analyses of Updated Individual Data'. *The Lancet* 2000;355(9208):949-955.

[12] Laramore GE. 'Role of Particle Radiotherapy in the Management of Head and Neck Cancer'. *Curr Opin Oncol* 2009;21(3):224-231.

[13] Steel GG. *Basic Clinical Radiobiology.*

[14] Cox JD, Stetz J, Pajak TF. 'Toxicity Criteria of The Radiation Therapy Oncology Group (RTOG) and the European Organization for Research and Treatment of Cancer (EORTC)'. *International Journal of Radiation Oncology* Biology* Physics* 1995;31(5): 1341-1346.

http://dx.doi.org/10.5772/60397

[15] Sciubba JJ, Goldenberg D. 'Oral Complications of Radiotherapy'. *The Lancet Oncology* 2006;7(2):175-183.

[16] Scully C, Sonis S, Diz P. 'Oral Mucositis'. *Oral Dis* 2006;12(3):229-241.

[17] World Health Organization. *WHO Handbook For Reporting Results of Cancer Treatment.* 1979.

[18] Raber-Durlacher JE, Elad S, Barasch A. 'Oral Mucositis'. *Oral Oncol* 2010;46(6): 452-456.

[19] Ray-Chaudhuri A, Shah K, Porter R. 'The Oral Management of Patients Who Have Received Radiotherapy to the Head and Neck Region'. *Br Dent J* 2013;214(8):387-393.

[20] Scully C, Epstein JB. 'Oral Health Care for the Cancer Patient'. *European Journal of Cancer. Part B: Oral Oncology* 1996;32(5):281-292.

[21] Epstein JB, Schubert M. 'Oropharyngeal Mucositis in Cancer Therapy'. *Oncology* 2003;17(12):1767-1776.

[22] Seto BG, Kim M, Wolinsky L, Mito RS, Champlin R. 'Oral Mucositis in Patients Undergoing Bone Marrow Transplantation'. *Oral Surgery, Oral Medicine, Oral Pathology* 1985;60(5):493-497.

[23] Singh N, Scully C, Joyston-Bechal S. 'Oral Complications of Cancer Therapies: Prevention and Management'. *Clin Oncol* 1996;8(1):15-24.

[24] Meurman JH, Grönroos L. 'Oral and Dental Health Care of Oral Cancer Patients: Hyposalivation, Caries and Infections'. *Oral Oncol* 2010;46(6):464-467.

[25] Dirix P, Nuyts S, Vander Poorten V, Delaere P, Van Den Bogaert W. 'The Influence of Xerostomia After Radiotherapy on Quality of Life'. *Supportive Care In Cancer* 2008;16(2):171-179.

[26] Cooper JS, Fu K, Marks J, Silverman S. 'Late Effects of Radiation Therapy in the Head and Neck Region'. *International Journal of Radiation Oncology* Biology* Physics* 1995;31(5):1141-1164.

[27] Schweiger JW. 'Oral Complications Following Radiation Therapy: A Five-Year Retrospective Report'. *J Prosthet Dent* 1987;58(1):78-82.

[28] Mandel ID. 'The Role of Saliva in Maintaining Oral Homeostasis'. *J Am Dent Assoc* 1989 Aug;119(2):298-304.

[29] Chambers MS, Toth BB, Martin JW, Fleming TJ, Lemon JC. 'Oral and Dental Management of the Cancer Patient: Prevention and Treatment of Complications'. *Supportive Care in Cancer* 1995;3(3):168-175.

[30] Mossman K. 'Gustatory Tissue Injury in Man: Radiation Dose Response Relationships and Mechanisms of Taste Loss'. *The British Journal of Cancer. Supplement* 1986;7:9.

[31] Spielman A. 'Chemosensory Function and Dysfunction'. *Critical Reviews in Oral Biology & Medicine* 1998;9(3):267-291.

[32] Cowart B. 'Taste Dysfunction: A Practical Guide for Oral Medicine'. *Oral Dis* 2011;17(1):2-6.

[33] Tomita Y, Osaki T. 'Gustatory Impairment and Salivary Gland Pathophysiology in Relation to Oral Cancer Treatment'. *Int J Oral Maxillofac Surg* 1990;19(5):299-304.

[34] Andrews N, Griffiths C. 'Dental Complications of Head and Neck Radiotherapy: Part 1'. *Aust Dent J* 2001;46(2):88-94.

[35] Conger AD. 'Loss and Recovery of Taste Acuity in Patients Irradiated to the Oral Cavity'. *Radiat Res* 1973;53(2):338-347.

[36] Jham BC, Freire, Addah Regina Da Silva. 'Oral Complications of Radiotherapy in the Head and Neck'. *Revista Brasileira de Otorrinolaringologia* 2006;72(5):704-708.

[37] Balogh JM, Sutherland SE. 'Osteoradionecrosis of the Mandible: A Review'. *J Otolaryngol* 1989 Aug;18(5):245-250.

[38] Marx RE. 'Osteoradionecrosis: A New Concept of its Pathophysiology'. *Journal Of Oral And Maxillofacial Surgery* 1983;41(5):283-288.

[39] Beumer J, Harrison R, Sanders B, Kurrasch M. 'Preradiation Dental Extractions and the Incidence of Bone Necrosis'. *Head Neck Surg* 1983;5(6):514-521.

[40] Epstein JB, Rea G, Wong FL, Spinelli J, Stevenson-Moore P. 'Osteonecrosis: Study of the Relationship of Dental Extractions in Patients Receiving Radiotherapy'. *Head Neck Surg* 1987;10(1):48-54.

[41] Mcleod NM, Bater MC, Brennan PA. 'Management of Patients at Risk of Osteoradionecrosis: Results of Survey of Dentists and Oral & Maxillofacial Surgery Units in the United Kingdom, and Suggestions for Best Practice'. *British Journal Of Oral And Maxillofacial Surgery* 2010;48(4):301-304.

[42] Brown D, Evans A, Sándor G. *Hyperbaric Oxygen Therapy in the Management of Osteoradionecrosis of the Mandible.* 2004.

[43] Starcke E, Shannon I. 'How Critical is the Interval Between Extractions and Irradiation in Patients With Head and Neck Malignancy?' *Oral Surgery, Oral Medicine, Oral Pathology* 1977;43(3):333-337.

[44] Murray CG, Herson J, Daly TE, Zimmerman S. 'Radiation Necrosis of the Mandible: A 10 Year Study. Part II. Dental Factors; Onset, Duration and Management of Necrosis'. *International Journal Of Radiation Oncology* Biology* Physics* 1980;6(5):549-553.

[45] Makkonen T, Kiminki A, Makkonen T, Nordman E. 'Dental Extractions in Relation to Radiation Therapy of 224 Patients'. *Int J Oral Maxillofac Surg* 1987;16(1):56-64.

http://dx.doi.org/10.5772/60397

[46] Curi MM, Lauria L. 'Osteoradionecrosis of the Jaws: A Retrospective Study of the Background Factors and Treatment in 104 Cases'. *Journal Of Oral And Maxillofacial Surgery* 1997;55(6):540-544.

[47] Granström G. 'Radiotherapy, Osseointegration and Hyperbaric Oxygen Therapy'. *Periodontol* 2000 2003;33(1):145-162.

[48] Kielbassa AM, Hinkelbein W, Hellwig E, Meyer-Lückel H. 'Radiation-Related Damage to Dentition'. *The Lancet Oncology* 2006;7(4):326-335.

[49] Silness J, Löe H. 'Periodontal Disease in Pregnancy II. Correlation Between Oral Hygiene and Periodontal Condition'. *Acta Odontologica* 1964;22(1):121-135.

[50] López-Jornet P, Camacho-Alonso F, Bermejo-Fenoll A. 'A Simple Test for Salivary Gland Hypofunction Using Oral Schirmer's Test'. *Journal Of Oral Pathology & Medicine* 2006;35(4):244-248.

[51] Epstein J, Stevenson-Moore P. 'Periodontal Disease and Periodontal Management in Patients with Cancer'. *Oral Oncol* 2001;37(8):613-619.

[52] Jansma J, Vissink A, Spijkervet FK, Roodenburg JL, Panders AK, Vermey A, et al. 'Protocol for the Prevention and Treatment of Oral Sequelae Resulting from Head and Neck Radiation Therapy'. *Cancer* 1992;70(8):2171-2180.

[53] Sulaiman F, Huryn JM, Zlotolow IM. 'Dental Extractions in the Irradiated Head and Neck Patient: A Retrospective Analysis of Memorial Sloan-Kettering Cancer Center Protocols, Criteria, and End Results'. *Journal Of Oral And Maxillofacial Surgery* 2003;61(10):1123-1131.

[54] Silvestre-Donat F, Plaza A, Serrano M. Revisiones. 'Prevención y Tratamiento de las Complicaciones Derivadas de la Radioterapia en Pacientes Con Tumores de Cabeza y Cuello'. *Medicina Oral* 1998;3(3):136-147.

[55] Bruins HH, Koole R, Jolly DE. 'Pretherapy Dental Decisions in Patients With Head and Neck Cancer: A Proposed Model for Dental Decision Support'. *Oral Surgery, Oral Medicine, Oral Pathology, Oral Radiology, And Endodontology* 1998;86(3):256-267.

[56] Cawley MM, Benson LM. 'Current Trends in Managing Oral Mucositis'. *Clin J Oncol Nurs* 2005;9(5):584-592.

[57] Biswal BM. 'Current Trends in the Management of Oral Mucositis Related to Cancer Treatment'. *Malays J Med Sci* 2008 Jul;15(3):4-13.

[58] Trucci VM, Veeck EB, Morosolli AR. 'Current Strategies for the Management of Oral Mucositis Induced by Radiotherapy or Chemotherapy'. *Revista Odonto Ciência (Journal Of Dental Science)* 2009;24(3):309-314.

[59] *Strategies for Managing Radiation-Induced Mucositis in Head and Neck Cancer. Seminars in Radiation Oncology*: Elsevier; 2009.

[60] Blanco Carrión A. 'Nueva Fórmula Magistral en Forma de Colutorio Para Lesiones Dolorosas de la Mucosa Oral'. *REVISTA EUROPEA DE ODONTOESTOMATOLOGIA* 1996;8:169-172.

[61] Stone R, Fliedner MC, Smiet A. 'Management of Oral Mucositis in Patients With Cancer'. *European Journal of Oncology Nursing* 2005;9:S24-S32.

[62] Lalla RV, Sonis ST, Peterson DE. 'Management of Oral Mucositis in Patients Who Have Cancer'. *Dent Clin North Am* 2008;52(1):61-77.

[63] Wong HM. 'Oral Complications and Management Strategies for Patients Undergoing Cancer Therapy'. *The Scientific World Journal* 2014;2014.

[64] Zimmerman RP, Mark RJ, Tran LM, Juillard GF. 'Concomitant Pilocarpine During Head and Neck Irradiation is Associated With Decreased Posttreatment Xerostomia'. *International Journal Of Radiation Oncology* Biology* Physics* 1997;37(3):571-575.

[65] Niedermeier W, Matthaeus C, Meyer C, Staar S, Müller R, Schulze H. 'Radiation-Induced Hyposalivation and its Treatment With Oral Pilocarpine'. *Oral Surgery, Oral Medicine, Oral Pathology, Oral Radiology, and Endodontology* 1998;86(5):541-549.

[66] Joshi VK. 'Dental Treatment Planning and Management for the Mouth Cancer Patient'. *Oral Oncol* 2010;46(6):475-479.

[67] Sonis ST. 'Oral Mucositis in Cancer Therapy'. *J Support Oncol* 2004;2(6 Suppl 3):3-8.

[68] Cheng KK. 'Oral Mucositis, Dysfunction, and Distress in Patients Undergoing Cancer Therapy'. *J Clin Nurs* 2007;16(11):2114-2121.

[69] Trucci VM, Veeck EB, Morosolli AR. 'Current Strategies for the Management of Oral Mucositis Induced by Radiotherapy or Chemotherapy'. *Revista Odonto Ciência (Journal Of Dental Science)* 2009;24(3):309-314.

[70] Keefe DM, Schubert MM, Elting LS, Sonis ST, Epstein JB, Raber-Durlacher JE, et al. 'Updated Clinical Practice Guidelines for the Prevention and Treatment of Mucositis'. *Cancer* 2007;109(5):820-831.

[71] Epstein JB, Silverman S, Paggiarino DA, Crockett S, Schubert MM, Senzer NN, et al. 'Benzydamine Hcl for Prophylaxis of Radiation-Induced Oral Mucositis'. *Cancer* 2001;92(4):875-885.

[72] Rades D, Fehlauer F, Bajrovic A, Mahlmann B, Richter E, Alberti W. 'Serious Adverse Effects of Amifostine During Radiotherapy in Head and Neck Cancer Patients'. *Radiotherapy and Oncology* 2004;70(3):261-264.

[73] Wasserman TH, Brizel DM, Henke M, Monnier A, Eschwege F, Sauer R, et al. 'Influence of Intravenous Amifostine on Xerostomia, Tumor Control, and Survival After Radiotherapy for Head-and-Neck Cancer: 2-Year Follow-Up of a Prospective, Randomized, Phase III Trial'. *International Journal of Radiation Oncology* Biology* Physics* 2005;63(4):985-990.

http://dx.doi.org/10.5772/60397

[74] Epstein JB, Wong FL. 'The Efficacy of Sucralfate Suspension in the Prevention of Oral Mucositis Due to Radiation Therapy'. *International Journal of Radiation Oncology* Biology* Physics* 1994;28(3):693-698.

[75] Brown DT, Miller CH, Maupin DE. 'The Effect of Sucralfate on the Growth of Cariogenic Streptococci'. J *Prosthet Dent* 1991;66(2):256-260.

[76] Etiz D, Erkal H, Serin M, Küçük B, Hepari A, Elhan A, et al. 'Clinical and Histopathological Evaluation of Sucralfate in Prevention of Oral Mucositis Induced by Radiation Therapy in Patients With Head and Neck Malignancies'. *Oral Oncol* 2000;36(1): 116-120.

[77] 'Sucralfate Stimulation of Gastric PGE2 Synthesis-Possible Mechanism to Explain its Effective Cytoprotective Properties'. *Gastroenterology: WB SAUNDERS CO INDEPENDENCE SQUARE WEST CURTIS CENTER, STE 300, PHILADELPHIA, PA* 19106-3399; 1984.

[78] Barber C, Powell R, Ellis A, Hewett J. 'Comparing Pain Control and Ability to Eat and Drink With Standard Therapy Vs Gelclair: A Preliminary, Double Centre, Randomised Controlled Trial on Patients With Radiotherapy-Induced Oral Mucositis'. *Supportive Care in Cancer* 2007;15(4):427-440.

[79] Llamas Martínez S, Esparza Gómez G, Moreno López L, Cerero Lapiedra R. 'Corticoides: Su Uso en Patología de la Mucosa Oral'. *Medicina Oral* 2003;8(4):248-259.

[80] González-Moles M. 'The Use of Topical Corticoids in Oral Pathology'. *Med Oral Patol Oral Cir Bucal* 2010;15:E827-E831.

[81] Keefe DM, Schubert MM, Elting LS, Sonis ST, Epstein JB, Raber-Durlacher JE, et al. 'Updated Clinical Practice Guidelines for the Prevention and Treatment of Mucositis'. *Cancer* 2007;109(5):820-831.

[82] Dietrich K, Schned A, Fortuny J, Heaney J, Marsit C, Kelsey K, et al. 'Glucocorticoid Therapy and Risk of Bladder Cancer'. *Br J Cancer* 2009;101(8):1316-1320.

[83] Severi G, Baglietto L, Muller DC, English DR, Jenkins MA, Abramson MJ, et al. 'Asthma, Asthma Medications, and Prostate Cancer Risk'. *Cancer Epidemiol Biomarkers Prev* 2010 Sep;19(9):2318-2324.

[84] Jensen AØ, Thomsen HF, Engebjerg M, Olesen AB, Friis S, Karagas M, et al. 'Use of Oral Glucocorticoids and Risk of Skin Cancer and Non-Hodgkin's Lymphoma: A Population-Based Case–Control Study'. *Br J Cancer* 2008;100(1):200-205.

[85] Von Bültzingslöwen I, Brennan MT, Spijkervet FK, Logan R, Stringer A, Raber-Durlacher JE, et al. 'Growth Factors and Cytokines in the Prevention and Treatment of Oral and Gastrointestinal Mucositis'. *Supportive Care in Cancer* 2006;14(6):519-527.

[86] Spielberger R, Stiff P, Bensinger W, Gentile T, Weisdorf D, Kewalramani T, et al. 'Palifermin for Oral Mucositis After Intensive Therapy for Hematologic Cancers'. *N Engl J Med* 2004;351(25):2590-2598.

[87] Schmidt E, Thoennissen NH, Rudat A, Bieker R, Schliemann C, Mesters RM, et al. 'Use of Palifermin for the Prevention of High-Dose Methotrexate-Induced Oral Mucositis'. *Ann Oncol* 2008 Sep;19(9):1644-1649.

[88] Vadhan-Raj S, Trent J, Patel S, Zhou X, Johnson MM, Araujo D, et al. 'Single-Dose Palifermin Prevents Severe Oral Mucositis During Multicycle Chemotherapy in Patients With Cancera Randomized Trial'. *Ann Intern Med* 2010;153(6):358-367.

[89] Lalla RV, Latortue MC, Hong CH, Ariyawardana A, D'Amato-Palumbo S, Fischer DJ, et al. 'A Systematic Review of Oral Fungal Infections in Patients Receiving Cancer Therapy'. *Supportive Care in Cancer* 2010;18(8):985-992.

[90] Silva GBL, Mendonça EF, Bariani C, Antunes HS, Silva MAG. 'The Prevention of Induced Oral Mucositis With Low-Level Laser Therapy in Bone Marrow Transplantation Patients: A Randomized Clinical Trial'. *Photomedicine and Laser Surgery* 2011;29(1):27-31.

[91] Migliorati C, Hewson I, Lalla RV, Antunes HS, Estilo CL, Hodgson B, et al. 'Systematic Review of Laser and Other Light Therapy for the Management of Oral Mucositis in Cancer Patients'. *Supportive Care in Cancer* 2013;21(1):333-341.

[92] Posten W, Wrone DA, Dover JS, Arndt KA, Silapunt S, Alam M. 'Low-Level Laser Therapy for Wound Healing: Mechanism and Efficacy'. *Dermatologic Surgery* 2005;31(3):334-340.

[93] Pappas PG, Kauffman CA, Andes D, Benjamin DK,Jr, Calandra TF, Edwards JE,Jr, et al. 'Clinical Practice Guidelines for the Management of Candidiasis: 2009 Update by the Infectious Diseases Society of America'. *Clin Infect Dis* 2009 Mar 1;48(5):503-535.

[94] Schwartz HC, Kagan AR. 'Osteoradionecrosis of the Mandible: Scientific Basis for Clinical Staging'. *American Journal Of Clinical Oncology* 2002;25(2):168-171.

[95] Epstein JB, Wong FL, Stevenson-Moore P. 'Osteoradionecrosis: Clinical Experience and a Proposal for Classification'. *Journal of Oral and Maxillofacial Surgery* 1987;45(2):104-110.

[96] Peterson DE, Doerr W, Hovan A, Pinto A, Saunders D, Elting LS, et al. 'Osteoradionecrosis in Cancer Patients: The Evidence Base for Treatment-Dependent Frequency, Current Management Strategies, and Future Studies'. *Supportive Care in Cancer* 2010;18(8):1089-1098.

[97] Madrid C, Abarca M, Bouferrache K. 'Osteoradionecrosis: An Update'. *Oral Oncol* 2010;46(6):471-474.

http://dx.doi.org/10.5772/60397

[98] Pitak-Arnnop P, Sader R, Dhanuthai K, Masaratana P, Bertolus C, Chaine A, et al. 'Management of Osteoradionecrosis of the Jaws: An Analysis of Evidence'. European Journal of Surgical Oncology (EJSO) 2008;34(10):1123-1134.

Chapter 9

A Close Look at Neutropenia among Cancer Patients — Risk Factor and Management

Bassam Abdul Rasool Hassan,
Zuraidah Binti Mohd Yusoff and Saad Bin Othman

Additional information is available at the end of the chapter

http://dx.doi.org/10.5772/60794

1. Introduction

Neutrophil cells: were discovered by Elie Metchnikoff as an inflammatory immune response to rose thorns inserted in starfish larvae [1].

Neutrophils are a major type of white blood cell (WBC), and they represent about 45%-70% of all WBC. Neutrophils can also be referred to as poly-morphonucleat leucocytes or granulocytes, as their cytoplasm contains granules, which contains glycogen and antibacterial substances [2]. Neutrophils are synthesized and produced by hematopoietic stem cells in bone marrow. It takes 10 – 14 days to produce mature neutrophils. Neutrophils were first thought to have a short viability period of only 6-10 hours [2, 3], but in the late 1990s, it was that neutrophils may survive much longer. In addition, recent evidence has suggested that neutrophils may produce anti-inflammatory molecules and may promote the resolution of inflammation [4]. Moreover, it has been found that during inflammation or infection, neutrophils will migrate to the inflamed tissues, phagocytosis and remain active at site for about 2-6 days [2, 4, 5].

2. Synthesis and production of neutrophils cells

Neutrophil production and synthesis is a major activity of the bone marrow. In fact, two-thirds of blood cell synthesis in bone marrow is dedicated to the production of monocytes and granulocytes. Hematopoietic stem cells are characterized by little blood flow and low oxygen tension, while the more mature and actively dividing stem cells reside closer to the abluminal side of the sinusoids, the special vascular structure of the bone marrow. The chemokine receptor CXCR4 is essential for the homing of stem cells and more mature neutrophils to the bone marrow [6].

Deletion of CXCR4 causes mature neutrophils to be released from the bone marrow into circulation without affecting the life-span of circulating neutrophils [6, 7].

The production of neutrophils is extensive, with $1 - 2 \times 10^{11}$ cells being generated per day in a normal adult human. Granulocyte colony stimulating factor (G-CSF) is essential for tuning the production of neutrophils to meet the increased needs that occur during infections, but G-CSF is not absolutely required for granulocytopoiesis. Indeed, G-CSF null mice have approximately 25% residual granulocytopoiesis and still generate fully mature neutrophils [6]. The production of neutrophils is largely regulated by the rate of apoptosis of neutrophils in tissues. When macrophages and dendritic cells phagocytose apoptotic neutrophils in tissues, the production of interleukin 23 (IL-23) is reduced [6].

3. The role of neutrophils

Neutrophils are the body's first line of innate defense from micro-organismsand and inflammation. Neutrophils are able to bind to and ingest invading microorganisms such as bacteria, fungi, germs, or any foreign body in the blood by a process known as phagocytosis, most likely due to their defensive and/or phagocytic process is by their ability to release lytic enzymes from their granules and to produce reactive oxygen intermediates (ROI) [2, 3, 4, 8].

Neutrophils cells directly recognize surface-bound or freely secreted molecules produced by bacteria (i.e., pathogen-derived molecules), including peptidoglycan, lipoproteins, lipoteichoic acid, lipopolysaccharide (LPS), CpG-containing DNA, and flagellin. These pathogen-derived molecules, known as pathogen-associated molecular patterns, interact directly with a number of pattern-recognition receptors expressed on the cell surface of neutrophil cell. Pattern-recognition receptors play a role in the recognition of microbes by neutrophils, and the efficiency of phagocytosis by neutrophils is markedly enhanced if microbes are opsonized with serum host proteins, such as complement and/or antibody [9].

Neutrophils have receptors on their surface that help them to contact and bind to tissues and to the vascular endothelium near sites of infection or inflammation [2] and they are the first cells that migrate to the site of invasion or inflammation to start the clearance of infectious particles. In the events of invading foreign threat, they also send warning signals to other innate immune cells [1].

Thus the migration of neutrophils from the blood circulation to surroundings tissues is considered key in triggering host defense.

During the process of migration to site of invasive, neutrophils need to cross the vessel wall (transmigration). This takes place largely at postcapillary venules, where the vessel wall is rather thin, and the diameter of the vessel is sufficiently small that the neutrophils can make

http://dx.doi.org/10.5772/60794

contact with the vessel wall, and is yet not occluded by neutrophils when they arrest and make firm contact with the endothelium [6, 9, 10]. Neutrophil transmigration is a highly regulated process that requires the up-regulation of neutrophils and endothelial cell adhesion molecules. During neutrophil adhesion to endothelial cell, binding of neutrophils or endothelial cell adhesion molecules to their ligands may induce intracellular signaling pathways and downstream events, which may in turn modulate neutrophil transmigration. Indeed, the ligation of various adhesion molecules can initiate signal transduction pathways and induce subsequent cellular changes [11, 12].

Moreover, it has been found that neutrophils that migrate through tissues are more effective phagocytic cells than blood neutrophils that is non-migrating neutrophils [6]. Therefore, neutrophils have emerged as key components of the effector and regulatory circuits of the innate and adaptive immune systems, and this has led to a renewed interest in their biology [4]. Recent studies have shown that human neutrophils are a major source of cytokines, which are crucial for the survival, maturation, and differentiation of B cells, and are also involved in bone resorption [4].

4. Process of neutrophil cells penetration to the tissues

Migration of neutrophil cells from blood circulation into the surrounding tissues, this process consider as the key role that trigger host defense. Neutrophil transmigration across the vascular endothelium is a highly regulated process that requires the up-regulation of neutrophil and endothelial cell (EC) adhesion molecules. During neutrophil adhesion to ECs, binding of the neutrophil or EC adhesion molecules to their ligands may induce intracellular signaling pathways and downstream events, which may in turn modulate neutrophil transmigration. Indeed, the ligation of various adhesion molecules can initiate signal transduction pathways and induce subsequent cellular changes [11].

5. Neutropenia

Neutropenia is defined as a decrease in the absolute number of neutrophils in the blood. Clinically, neutropenia is defined as a decrease in the absolute neutrophil count (ANC) of more than two standard deviations below the normal range. Therefore, the patient is considered neutropenic when the ANC is lower than 1500 cells/μl (the normal level) [2, 3, 5, 13, 14]. An ANC above 1000 cells/μl will still confer normal protection against infection; therefore mild neutropenia is defined as an ANC 500 - 1000 cells/μl. There is a significant increase in the incidence of serious infection once ANC falls below 500 cells/μl, and moderate neutropenia is defined as an ANC of 200 - 500 cells/μl [2, 3, 13]. When ANC falls below 200 cells/μl it is defined as severe neutropenia. This condition is very serious and requires the patient to be admitted to the hospital and treated with antibiotics [3, 13], and patients with an ANC below 100 cells/μl are at the highest risk of infection. Hundred percent of the patients with ANC < 100 cells/μl lasting 3 weeks or more develop documented infection.

Neutropenia is usually diagnosed by a complete blood count (CBC) or full blood count (FBC). If the results show a low ANC then these tests are repeated [15]. If the repeated test shows the same results, a bone marrow biopsy is carried out to confirm the diagnosis. Bone marrow aspirate is taken from two sites, one from the middle of the bone and one from the solid, bonier part of the bone, usually from the large pelvic bone, the ilium, or the sternum [15].

Febrile neutropenia (i.e., neutropenia with fever) is mostly associated with chemotherapy, but it may also occur after irradiation of the bone marrow. In this chapter, the term febrile neutropenia is usually used to describe the occurrence of neutropenia (body temperature ≥38.3°C or oral temperature ≥38°C for more than hour) and an ANC of ≤ 500 cells/μl at the time of fever, or in the following 48 hours [2, 14, 15, 16, 17, 18].

6. Adverse effects

Neutropenia has many negative effects. One of these side effects is dose reduction of chemotherapy. Fifty percent (50%) of cancer patients received less than 85% of the prescribed doses because of neutropenia.

Neutropenia can also cause delays in chemotherapy treatment, which can lead to increase in cancer cell growth and tumor size. Both dose reduction and delay of chemotherapy can have serious effects on patients' lives, and may even lead to death [19, 20].

Neutropenia also has a dramatic and detrimental effect on the patients' quality of life. Fatigue is the predominant characteristic, which leads to a decrease in the ability to perform daily life activities. Patients describe fatigue as feeling weak and exhausted. Psychological problems were also reported by the patients, such as sadness, anxiety, reduced self-worth, and inability to fulfill normal roles [19, 20].

7. Neutropenia diagnosis

The diagnosis of neutropenia is usually made by performing the following tests:

7.1. Complete blood count

The first test to investigate the suspicion of neutropenia presence is to perform complete blood count (CBC) or full blood count (FBC) whereby the neutrophil numbers will be measured. If the results showed a low neutrophil count then these tests will be repeated in order to be certain that neutropenia is actually present [21].

7.2. Bone marrow aspirate/trephine biopsy

After performing a blood test, a bone examination could be carried out to confirm the results. Bone marrow biopsy is done by obtaining bone marrow aspirates from two sites that are from the middle of the bone and also from solid bonier part of the bone. This bone biopsy is performed with the patient under general anesthesia or local anesthesia with sedation. These bone marrow samples are usually taken from the large bones such as large pelvic bone, the ilium, or sometimes from the flat breastbone (i.e., the sternum) [21].

8. Causes of neutropenia

Demographic factors, hematological disorders, autoimmune diseases, infections, drugs reactions, and chemotherapy or radiotherapy play a major role in the etiology of neutropenia [2, 13, 17]. Neutrophil production is lower among older people; they are not as able to produce mature neutrophil as younger people, and ANC in White men is higher than that in Black men. Also neutropenia incidence seems to be higher in women than men [2, 13, 14]. Hematological diseases like leukemia, myelodysplastic syndrome, Hodgkin's and non-Hodgkin's diseases, and multiple myeloma have also been shown to cause neutropenia [2]. In these hematological diseases, severe destruction of bone marrow leads to the destruction of stem cells. This will result in the prevention of or decrease in neutrophil production, thus causing neutropenia [2]. Moreover, these hematological diseases can have an effect on the red blood cells (RBC) and platelet production which can lead to severe anemia and thrombocytopenia. Usually the patient will suffer from fever ≥ 38.5°C as well as gingivitis, bleeding, stomatitis, bone chills, and the patient might also collapse [22]. Neutropenia has also been associated with autoimmune diseases like systemic lupus erythromatosis (SLE). Neutropenia following SLE is usually mild and the patient may not suffer from serious bacterial infection. However patients with Sjören syndrome and rheumatoid arthritis may have severe neutropenia, leaving them at higher risk of bacterial or fungal infection [2]. Many drugs such as diuretics, chlorpromazine, and allopurinol have been shown to cause neutropenia, and two mechanisms for this have been suggested. The first postulates that the drug produces dose-dependent toxicity on cell production, protein synthesis, bone marrow, and cell survival. The second suggests a mechanism of drug-inducing immunological reactions, for example, the binding of drugs with the surface of the neutrophil cell, leading to cell destruction and neutropenia. These two mechanisms are not always seen; they happen in only a small percentage of patients. These two mechanisms also require a long duration of drug use [2].

9. Chemotherapy

Neutropenia is mostly associated with chemotherapy and radiotherapy. Chemotherapeutic drugs affect the production of folic acid as well as the synthesis of DNA, RNA and protein by acting as anti-metabolites, which lead to bone marrow destruction [2, 13, 14, 22]. Bone marrow destruction in turn leads to a decrease in neutrophil production. Therefore, chemotherapy and radiotherapy are considered to be the main causes of neutropenia and febrile neutropenia. Besides that, chemotherapeutic drugs kill and suppress all the cells that have a high rate of division or affect blood cells, bone cells, and neutrophil cells (Fortner *et al.*, 2005). The chemotherapeutic drugs actinomycin, asparaginase, cytarabine, busulfan, cisplatin, daunorubicin, etoposide, fluorouracil, ifosfamide, and methotrexate are highly associated with neutropenia development [2, 14, 23].

The link between chemotherapy and neutropenia was emphasized by Buffoni *et al.* (2006) who looked at the effect and toxicity of chemotherapeutic drugs on 30 non-small lung cancer patients treated with a combination of cisplatin and vinorelbine on day 1 and day 8 and repeated every 21 days. The major toxic effect associated with these chemotherapies was neutropenia 3 and 4 (63%). The treatment also caused three deaths, two of which were due to febrile neutropenia. Hence it can be concluded that even though the combination of cisplatin and vinorelbine was very effective in the treatment of lung cancer, it was also associated with neutropenia, some of which was fatal [24].

Yamanaka *et al.* (2007) conducted a study 1055 patients in Japan with advanced gastric cancer on oral fluoropyrimidine derivatives (S-1). The main important result of the study was that neutropenia incidence was an inadequate predictor of increased survival in these patients. Also the another important point of their study was that the absence of neutropenia indicated that the doses of the chemotherapeutics drugs were not intensive enough to cause neutropenia [25]. This point was also indicated in the observational retrospective study carried out in Penang Hospital on 117 solid tumor patients who were admitted between January 2003 and December 2006, and treated with various types of chemotherapy regimens. The highest chemotherapeutic regimen received in this study was (5-FU + epirubicin + cyclophosphamide) (47, 40.2%), followed by (gemcitabine + cisplatin) (6, 5.1%), and others. The majority of the patients in the study were on a 1-day chemotherapy administration schedule of (90, 76.9%), followed a schedule of more than one day (27, 23.1%). The statistical analysis of Chi-square test results showed insignificant associations between chemotherapy type and neutropenia incidence (P=0.798) and neutropenia severity (P=0.199). The same results were found between neutropenia incidence and chemotherapy administration schedule and duration (P=0.689) and neutropenia severity (P=0.434).

The main explanation for these results was that the doses of these drugs were not high enough to cause bone marrow suppression and lead to neutropenia. Moreover, the administration schedule for each drug was long enough to overcome neutropenia, and the high use of G-CSF likely played a major role in reducing the time and neutropenia severity. All these factors likely contributed to the non-significant association observed between neutropenia incidence and severity, and chemotherapeutics drugs and administration schedule [26]. The correct doses of chemotherapeutic drugs must be used in order to prevent the incidence of lethal neutropenia [27].

Another study looking at the association between neutropenia and chemotherapy drugs was conducted by Banerji *et al.* (2006) in the United Kingdom. The study involved 173 patients treated with etoposide and carboplatin. The results obtained from the study showed a significant association between neutropenia and the chemotherapy drugs (P <0.0001) [28].

However, different chemotherapy regimens are not associated with the same neutropenia severity. This difference is due to substantial variations in the resiliency of hematopoietic

http://dx.doi.org/10.5772/60794

tissues among cancer patients and chemotherapy tolerance. Moreover, severe neutropenia has been reported in patients with solid cancers, especially breast cancer patients, when treated with cyclophosphamide, methotrexate and 5-fluorouracil (CMF), suggesting that neutropenia is associated with the intensity of the chemotherapy regimens [8], for example, the doses of cytotoxic drugs such as epirubicin, cisplatin, doxorubicin, vincristine, capecitabine, carboplatin, and bleomycin were not high or intensive and they do not seem to cause severe neutropenia (i.e., neutropenia is considered a minor side-effect for these chemotherapies). But these low chemotherapy doses can cause other major adverse effects like nausea, vomiting, thrombocytopenia, alopecia, and anemia [29, 30, 31].

9.1. Role of route of chemotherapy administration

The route of chemotherapy administration could be either systematic which includes: intravenous (I.V), oral, and intramuscular (I.M) or local intrathecal, intraperitoneal, intra-arterial, and intrapleural. The most commonly used administration routes are the intravenous and the oral route. The advantage of administering chemotherapy by these two routes is that tumor cells throughout the body would be exposed to the chemotherapy. However, the disadvantage is that sensitive tissues such as in the bone marrow and mucosa will also be equally exposed to these chemotherapeutic drugs. So the main goal of I.V administration of chemotherapy is to achieve a systematic chemotherapy concentration that is effective for the cancer treatment of the cancer concerned [32]. When the chemotherapy is administered by the I.V. route, the entire dose of the chemotherapy drug will be in the blood circulation and produce its effect on the cancer cells. This will also lead to an increase in its adverse effect as compared to the oral route whereby the drugs will be slowly absorbed and the concentration will increase gradually thus not producing major side effects. But there will be no difference between the oral and the I.V. route in the part concerned with neutropenia incidence, onset, or severity, since neutropenia is related to chemotherapeutics intensity and effects but not with the route of administration [32, 33].

Jassem *et al*. (2003) focused on the effect of oral and I.V. administration of chemotherapeutic drugs on neutropenia incidence. In their study, 56 patients were treated with vinorelbine and cisplatin for their non-small cell lung cancer (NSCLC). On day 1 both drugs were given via I.V. route, and this was followed by cisplatin I.V. and vinorelbine oral on days 8, 15, and 22. The cycle was repeated every 28 days. The great and the predominant side effect observed was neutropenia, that is, 73% of the patients had grade 3 (severe) and 4 (life threatening) neutropenia and anemia had a lower percentage of incidences. Thus, Jassem and his colleagues' study demonstrated that the route of chemotherapy administration has no significant effect on their pharmacological action, since both routes produced similar efficacy and safety as well as similar side effects. However, the important point of their study was the new approach of I.V. administration on day 1, and oral administration on days 8, 15, and 22 which is more suitable and comfortable to the patients. However, the route of administration had no effect on the chemotherapy toxicity since neutropenia and anemia were still the major side effects produced by these chemotherapeutics drugs [34].

9.2. Impact of chemotherapy cycles and schedule on neutropenia

It is preferred to administer on a continuous basis for maximal cancer cell killing and to decrease the development of cancer cells resistance. However, chemotherapy toxicity results in the destruction of normal cells, and thus should be stopped for sufficient intervals so as to allow normal cells to recover. The duration of chemotherapy administration is known as chemotherapy cycle. Neutropenia incidence is mainly and highly associated with the first cycle of the chemotherapy more than the other or subsequent cycles. Indeed, the depletion of the bone marrow will lead to decreased production of the neutrophils and neutropenia which mainly occur with the first cycle of chemotherapy.

The association was determined by a study conducted in the United States of America by Crawford *et al.* (2005) The study included more than 4,000 cancer patients age ranged from 18 to 97 years. More than 100 different chemotherapeutic regimens were reported and the most frequently used chemotherapeutics were anthracyclines (35%), platinum compounds (33%) and fluorouracil (20%). Neutropenia occurrence after the first cycle of the chemotherapy was documented in 2,160 patients. Neutropenia with ANC nadir of $< 1 \times 109$ cell/ L was observed in 43% of the patients, while severe neutropenia (ANC nadir $< 0.5 \times 10^9$ cell/ L) was seen in 24% of the studied population. Fourteen percent of the patients had febrile neutropenia, while severe febrile neutropenia was found in 9% [35].

Another study in the United States conducted by Wolf *et al.* (2005) on 2,222 cancer patients showed that one-third of them were treated with fewer than four cycles of the chemotherapy due to complications. The most important result obtained was that half of the cases of neutropenia occurred during the first cycle of chemotherapy, especially among breast cancer patients [36].

The relationship between chemotherapy and neutropenia was also reported by Schallier *et al.* (2007). He conducted a study in Belgium on 48 non-small lung cancer patients treated with three cycles of paclitaxel, carboplatin, and gemcitabine. Schallier and his colleagues aimed to detect the toxicity of these chemotherapies after each cycle. The results of their study showed that the chemotherapy-induced neutropenia happened on days 8 and 15 of the first cycle. During the second cycle, 34 out of 42 patients developed neutropenia on day 15. Neutropenia was also prominent on day 15 of the third cycle, during which 24 out of 42 patients developed it. Therefore, the study showed that there was a strong relationship between chemotherapy cycle and neutropenia incidence. However, there was no significant relationship between chemotherapy cycle and neutropenia severity, which remained the same across the three cycles [37].

Neutropenia severity mainly increases due to chemotherapeutic drugs schedules [38]. Chemotherapeutic drugs are usually administered in a manner that will enhance their main benefits and reduce or prevent their toxic effects [32, 33, 39], but the duration of administration is also controlled by the pharmacokinetic and pharmacodynamic characteristics of the drug used, as some chemotherapeutic drugs can cause severe bone marrow suppression, such as the alkylating agent cyclophosphamide. These drugs are usually administered by pulse method, that is, for a short period (usually 1 day) followed by a long interval before the next dose is given. This will give time for both the bone marrow and neutrophils to recover [40]. When given on a longer administration schedule, drugs such as 5-flurouracil will lead to the inhibition of RNA synthesis of the cancer cells, thus killing them. However, when given as a single bolus dose they will lead to the inhibition of thymidylate synthesis, which will result in severe side-effects. On the other hand, paclitaxel, when given for more than 1 day, will mainly lead to severe toxicity and cause more destruction of the bone marrow. However, when given for 1 day, paclitaxel will render the desired anticancer effect, with fewer effects on bone marrow. The standard interval between each cycle, whether the cycle lasts 1 day or more, ranges from 21 to 28 days [32, 33, 39].

10. Prevalence and incidence of neutropenia

Neutropenia generally occurs in one out of three patients treated with chemotherapy. Once neutropenia happens, it may threaten the patient's life, and chemotherapy schedule or dose should be delayed in order to give the body a chance to produce new neutrophils [41, 42, 43, 44]. Although neutropenia is common during chemotherapy, severe neutropenia is not and can cause serious morbidity and mortality due to resulting infections. Epidemiological studies have shown a wide variation in neutropenia incidence according to geographic regions. The average incidence of neutropenia in the United States is 56.4 per million people. There are no, or very few studies that give an exact number of neutropenia prevalence [45].

11. Risk factors for neutropenia

11.1. Gender

The female gender is a risk factor for neutropenia and febrile neutropenia. The possible reason for the higher number of females than males with neutropenia is that the incidence of cancer in females is generally higher than that in males by a ratio of 1:1.3 [46]. Moreover, it has also been reported that 49% of the solid cancer patients who developed neutropenia during chemotherapy were diagnosed with breast cancer. Since breast cancer occurs mostly in females, this could also explain the higher number of females with neutropenia [17, 47]. A study by Wolf *et al.* (2005) in the United States looked at the risk factors associated with neutropenia among 2,222 patients. The main results showed that there were significant associations of neutropenia severity and gender (P= 0.001) and between complication and gender (P= 0.004) [47]. An observational retrospective study was conducted by Bassam *et al.* (2009) on solid cancer patients admitted to Penang Hospital in 2003 - 2006 who became neutropenic during chemotherapy. The results show an insignificant association between incidence and neutropenia severity with patients' demographic data, leading to the conclusion that the demographic data is not a risk factor for neutropenia incidence or severity. However, the main reason for this insignificance was the small sample size [18].

11.2. Age

Neutropenia is more common among the elderly (i.e., 50 years of age or older). Indeed these individual are already less able to produce mature neutrophil cells [2, 8, 13, 17]. According to the National Cancer Registry of Malaysia (2003), cancer incidence, especially breast cancer incidence, is more predominant at the age of 50 years or more. Yip and Omar Hasan Kasule (2005) reported that neutropenia occurred mostly in people aged 50 - 59 years and 75% of the neutropenic patients in their study were diagnosed with breast cancer [48, 49]. In his study, Crawford (2007) investigated 282 lymphoma cancer patients treated with cyclophosphamide, doxorubicin, vincristine and prednisolone (CHOP), and said that the incidence of neutropenia was predominant among individuals aged 65 years or more compared to younger than 65 years of age [50]. Moreover, in the United States, Voelker *et al.* (2004) carried out a retrospective study from 1991 to 1999 on 7,238 patients with non-Hodgkin lymphoma (NHL). The main objective was to find the major risk factors associated with initiation and duration of hospitalization among neutropenic patients after chemotherapy. The median age was 75 years (range: 66 to 100 years). About 22% of patients needed hospitalization and half were first admitted within the first 42 days of treatment. The mean duration of hospitalization was 55.7 ± 1.43 days and the median was 34 days. The risk factors found to be associated with hospital admission were patients' age, gender, chemotherapy type, history, and disease stage. The risk of hospitalization due to neutropenia increased with age until the age of 80 years [51]. So the study by Voelker *et al.* (2004) demonstrated a significant association between neutropenia and patients' age and gender. At these advanced ages, chemotherapy doses usually reduced and the administration of G-CSF (Filgrastim) is increased [17, 36].

11.3. Ethnic group

The ethnic group has been suggested to have a significant effect on ANC and therefore there is a relationship between these variables and neutropenia [13]. However, some specific types of cancers are highly associated with specific races. According to Kaur *et al.* (2007), breast cancer incidence in Penang mostly occurs among the Chinese (62.5%), followed by the Malays (26.7%), and the Indians (10.2%), and breast cancer is most highly associated with neutropenia (Wolf *et al.*, 2005), which could indicate that the ethnic group does play a role in the incidence of neutropenia [32, 52].

Moreover, in the United States, another study by Hershman *et al.* (2003) also showed that there is an association between ethnicity and neutropenia (WBC level) in breast cancer survivors. Their study was performed on African American and White American women with breast cancer (stage I and II) treated with chemotherapy. It showed that the WBC level in African American women was significantly lower than that of White American women. There was also a significant difference between the period of chemotherapy treatment of African American (19 women) versus White American women due to neutropenia. The explanation for the difference in period of treatment was said to be due to lower ANC. Besides that, neutropenia occurrence led to a delay in chemotherapy administration. Therefore, their study demonstrated a significant association between neutropenia occurrence and ethnicity [53].

12. Neutropenia and cancer type

12.1. Solid cancer

Neutropenia has been shown to be associated with solid tumors especially breast cancer, as about 25% of breast cancer patients develop neutropenia. Lyman and Wilmot (2006) and Wolf *et al.* (2005) found that among patients with solid cancer, breast cancer patients had the highest risk for developing severe neutropenia and febrile neutropenia during the first cycle of chemotherapy. Due to the neutropenia, 40% of the breast cancer patients had the chemotherapy delayed and about 25% had their chemotherapy treatment doses reduced. The possibility of breast cancer patients to develop neutropenia at point during chemotherapy was 78% [17, 32]. Patients with solid tumors usually have normal neutrophil cell function as compared to patients with hematological malignancies, whose neutrophil function is completely abnormal and thus would suffer from neutropenia. Patients with solid tumors are also not immunocompromised as are those with hematological malignancies, and many centers now consider solid tumor patients to have a low risk of neutropenia [54, 55]. A significant association was also found between cancer type and neutropenia duration, but not between cancer type and neutropenia severity [56]. The study by AL-Ahwal (2005) also showed that the association between neutropenia severity and solid cancer was not significant, but that co-morbidity of chemotherapy with solid cancer was significant. Among breast cancer with neutropenia, more than 75% of cases seemed to be associated with the type of chemotherapy employed, which was CMF [17]. In a retrospective study on 117 solid cancer patients with neutropenia conducted by Bassam and colleagues in Penang, the type of solid cancer played an insignificant role in the incidence and/or neutropenia severity. The main explanation for this result was that patients with a solid tumor are different from those with hematological malignancy, in the sense that solid tumor patients usually have normal neutrophil cell function. While, in case of hematological malignant patients where by their neutrophil cells function is completely abnormal and thus they suffer from neutropenia. In contrast, neutropenia occurrence among solid cancer patients usually starts after chemotherapy, and severe neutropenia may last for 7 - 10 days. Thus the main cause of neutropenia is not the presence of cancer itself, but the chemotherapeutic agents or drugs used. For this reason solid tumor patients who developed neutropenia are considered to be at low risk for neutropenia [26].

12.2. Hematological cancer

Patients with hematological malignancies are necessarily immunocompromised, either as a result of the malignancy or due to the therapeutic interventions used to manage it. Some hematological malignancies are associated with specific immune defects that predispose to infections with particular pathogens. For example, patients with acute leukemia have an increased risk of severe gram-negative bacterial infections as a result of quantitative or functional neutropenia. Patients with chronic lymphocytic leukemia and multiple myeloma are susceptible to invasive bacterial infections from staphylococci, streptococci, and especially pneumococcus. Patients with lymphoma have abnormalities of the cellular immune system that result in an increased risk of viral (e.g., herpes simplex) and fungal infections (e.g., cryptococcus). Moreover, therapeutic interventions such as corticosteroids, chemotherapy, stem cell transplant, and radiation also produce deficiencies in the host immune defense [57].

Neutropenia due to chemotherapy is the most common risk factor for severe bacterial infections in hematological malignancies. Impaired T-cell function in patients undergoing allogenic stem cell transplant is associated with an increased susceptibility to invasive viral infections. It can also induce alterations in host colonization, such as disruption of natural skin and mucosal barriers, and can interfere with nutrition, which can cause an increase in the risk of infection. Therefore, the degree of neutropenia either as a consequence of the disease or the therapy, is directly related to the incidence of serious bacterial and fungal infection in patients with hematological malignancies. There is a significant increase in the incidence of serious infection once ANC falls below 500 cells/μl. Patients with ANC below 100 cells/μl are at the highest risk of infection. The duration of neutropenia also contributes significantly to the risk of serious infections. Qualitative defects in neutrophil function have been described in hematological malignancies. These include defects in chemotaxis, phagocytosis, bactericidal capacity, and the absence of respiratory burst that accompanies phagocytosis. Additionally, chemotherapeutic regimens used in association with corticosteroids can decrease phagocytosis and neutrophil migration [57].

13. Management of neutropenia

13.1. Granulocyte colony stimulating factors

Granulocyte colony stimulating factors are glycoproteins that regulate the proliferation, differentiation, functional activity and survival of myeloid cells, which help in reducing the duration and neutropenia severity as a result of chemotherapy [8]. Moreover, G-CSF treatment can significantly reduce hospitalization period and frequency neutropenic patients, and reduce the amount of antibiotics used [8]. G-CSF such as Filgrastim (Neupogen®) can be used to prevent, reduce, or palliate neutropenia in patients treated with chemotherapy. Filgrastim has also been shown to decrease the incidence of febrile neutropenia and to improve survival. Moreover, G-CSF have also been shown to decrease neutropenia severity. Both G-CSF and granulocyte-macrophage colony stimulation factors (GM-CSF) (Sargramostim®) have been approved by the United States Food and Drug Administration for the treatment of neutropenia [2, 8]. But G-CSF use is preferred as it is more effective and has a lower side-effect [8]. A study on the efficacy of the G-CSF in reducing neutropenia among solid tumor and lymphoma patients receiving chemotherapy was carried out by Lyman *et al.* (2002). In their study, G-CSF was administered before the occurrence of fever and neutropenia. There were 1144 patients with eight trials, five with filgrastim and three with lenograstim. The results showed that G-CSF reduced the risk of febrile neutropenia (odd ratio [OR] 0.38, 95% [CI]: 0.29 - 0.49). However, the reduction of infection-related mortality was insignificant (OR= 0.6, 95% CI 0.3 - 1.22). There were no differences in treatment effect by cancer type. The study demonstrated that there was a significant association between the G-CSF and the reduction of neutropenia risk [58].

Juan *et al.* (2001) carried out a prospective study in Spain on 44 solid cancer patients between 1997 and 1999. The aim of the study was to compare the effectiveness of different doses of G-CSF (lenograstim) on neutropenia. The doses used were 263 micrograms/day (full dose) and 131.5 micro grams/ day (half dose). Of the 44 patients, 39 (88.6%) developed neutropenia after chemotherapy. A total of 120 courses of chemotherapy were given to the patients, full doses were given in 61 courses and half a dose of lenograstim was given in 59 courses. The results of the study showed that severe neutropenia was more common among patients who received low doses of lenograstim (20%) as compared to the full dose of lenograstim (12%), but the difference was not significant (P= 0.1). The frequency of fever and hospital admission was not affected. The mean ANC with full doses of lenograstim was higher than with half doses, but was again not significant (P= 0.324). Juan concluded that both doses of lenograstim had a similar efficacy in reducing neutropenia severity [59].

All the above studies showed that G-CSF should be the primary treatment for severe and febrile neutropenia. This is also in accordance with Malaysian treatment guidelines for febrile neutropenia (i.e., severe neutropenia) treatment [60], which indicate that G-CSF should be considered in patients with febrile neutropenia with high risk features. In the case of severe febrile neutropenia (ANC less than 0.1× 109 cells/L), or in the presence of signs and symptoms of infection, antibiotics, must, be used with G-CSF [8].

13.2. Antimicrobial therapy

Empirical antibiotic therapy is required in neutropenia especially, when it is combined with gram-negative bacterial infection, as this combination is associated with high mortality. This point is supported by Schimpff (2001), who mentioned that if fever is not taken seriously and the neutropenic patient is suffering from a bacterial infection, 40% will die within the first 48 hours [61]. This is because there are no reliable methods to determine whether neutropenic fever is due to bacterial infection or not. Thus, antimicrobial therapy must be started either as mono antibiotic therapy or a combination antibiotic therapy. This reduces the mortality of gram-negative infection by 10% [62]. Any empirical antibiotic used must have a wide range of activity, enough to cover the majority of potential pathogens. There are three different universal strategies for using antibiotics in the treatment of febrile neutropenia: (i) a combination of either beta-lactam with aminoglycoside, (ii) monotherapy with wide range beta-lactam, and (iii) both of the above strategies combined [62]. Most neutropenic patients are treated with a beta-lactam antibiotic such as ceftazidime which is widely used as a single empirical antibiotic for neutropenic fever because its effectiveness is very similar to combination therapy. Other beta-lactam antibiotics such as imipenem, ticarcillin and cefepime may also be used as monotherapy or in combination with metronidazole or aminoglycoside (amikacin and gentamicin) to overcome bacterial infection, especially gram-negative bacteria. Penicillin derivatives such as piperacillin and tazobactam can also be used alone or in combination with beta-lactam derivatives such as imipenem to overcome anaerobe bacterial infection. The new generations of beta-lactam antibiotics have shown wide protection against both gram-positive and gram-negative bacteria such as cefepime [63]. Therefore, ceftazidime or imipenem could be used as first-line treatment while awaiting the results of a culture and sensitivity test [2]. This is also in accordance with Malaysian antibiotic guidelines for febrile neutropenia (i.e., severe neutropenia) treatment [61, 64]. According to the United States Food and Drug Administration, there are many types of antibiotics that could be used to treat neutropenic patients. However, there are only a limited number of antibiotics that are effective for the treatment of febrile neutropenia (i.e., severe neutropenia). Ceftazidime is considered one of the most effective antibiotics and has been approved for the treatment of febrile neutropenic patients at different ages [65].

Combination therapy is also used when there is a need, when there is resistant bacteria in neutropenic patients, or even because of neutropenia severity [62]. In the United States, cephalosporin (mainly ceftazidime) is frequently used as an initial single empirical antibiotic for the treatment of febrile neutropenia. The combinations of cephalosporin plus vancomycin, third generation cephalosporin plus penicillin, or carbapenem plus aminoglycoside are also used. These combinations have been recommended for patients who were suspected to be or are suffering from resistance gram-negative bacterial infection [8]. The same result was found by De Pauw *et al.* (1994) who conducted a study on 692 cancer patients suffering from febrile neutropenia. In their study the patients either received 2g ceftazidime every 8 hours, or 14 - 16 g/ day of piperacillin, in 4 - 6 divided doses plus tobramycin 1.7 - 2 mg/kg of body weight every 8 hours. Their results showed that mortality due to infections was 6% with ceftazidime and 8% with piperacillin plus tobramycin. Adverse effects of ceftazidime occurred in 8% of patients, compared to 20% who received combination antibiotics. The main conclusion made by De Pauw and his colleagues was that ceftazidime as monotherapy was as effective as piperacillin plus tobramycin, and that ceftazidime was much safer in the treatment of febrile/ severe neutropenic patients [65].

Another study in Japan by Yano and Nakano (1996) looked at the use of antibiotic monotherapy in 43 patients suffering from hematological toxicity. Eighteen of these patients suffered from severe neutropenia (ANC < 500 cells/μl). The patients were treated with cefpirome or a combination of two beta-lactam antibiotics. The results showed that 89.5% of patients on cefpirome had a better quality of life, a decreased number of infusions, and a decrease in the frequency of antibiotic administration. Cefpirome use also led to a reduction in night urination, a low cost/benefit ratio and a reduction in nursing responsibilities. Due to this high efficacy rate, cefpirome monotherapy is therefore considered a first line treatment for patients with hematological diseases, and especially those with severe neutropenia, suffering from infection [66].

The effectiveness of antibiotic monotherapy was again supported by Tamura *et al.* (2001), who compared the effectiveness of antibiotic monotherapy and combination antibiotics in neutropenic patients. One hundred sixty five patients were enrolled in the study, with an average age of 52 years. Severe febrile neutropenia was found in the 60% of patients (ANC < 100 cells/ μl). The patients were divided into two groups. One group was treated with antibiotic monotherapy (either cefepime or carbapenem) and the other was treated with a combination of cefepime and aminoglycoside. Two- thirds of the patients from both groups showed that infection was overcome with antibiotic treatment. The conclusion was that the use of antibiotic monotherapy is as good and effective as combination antibiotics in the treatment of febrile neutropenic patients. As mentioned the use of antibiotic monotherapy (ceftazidime or cefepime) was also emphasized by the Malaysian Ministry of Health. Indeed, while the uses of dual therapy may be preferred in cases with severe neutropenia, a prolonged duration should be expected, as should complications, such as sepsis, hypotension, mucositis and recurrent episodes [67].

13.3. Antibiotics schedule

According to the guidelines from the Infectious Society of America, neutropenic patients who remained febrile but showed recovery in ANC on the third day of antibiotic therapy can either continue with antibiotic treatment for 7 days, or antibiotic treatment can be stopped on the fourth or fifth day. For those febrile neutropenic patients with no recovery in ANC, antibiotics should be continued, and can be discontinued after 2 weeks if examinations and cultures show no bacterial growth [68]. Hughes *et al.* (2002) reported that antibiotic schedule for neutropenic patients is mainly determined and controlled by ANC (i.e., neutropenia severity). Antibiotic treatment can be stopped after 3 days if there is no infection. Indeed, continuing antibiotic treatment until the neutropenia is resolved is not preferred as it could lead to increased drug toxicity and bacterial resistance. Thus, Hughes and his colleagues suggested a preferred treatment of antibiotics for 5 - 7 days; antibiotics could be stopped before 5 days if there is evidence of hematological recovery [69].

In Canada, a study by Tomiak *et al.* (1994) looked at the antibiotic schedule used in 134 febrile neutropenic patients and its effect on duration of hospital stay. The study showed that antibiotics can be stopped within 4 - 5 days especially for patients whose culture shows no bacterial infection. The association between neutropenia and antibiotic reduction was significant ($P<0.001$) [70].

14. Types of route antibiotics administration according to risk of infection

14.1. Low risk neutropenic patients (Oral therapy)

A recent review has reported that inpatient oral antibacterial therapy can be safely replaced with conventional intravenous treatment among low-risk patients with febrile neutropenia, namely, those who are clinically stable, who do not suffer from acute leukemia, pneumonia, severe soft tissue infection, and who do not have any evidence of organ failure. Among these patients single-agent quinolone was not inferior to combinations of quinolone with amoxicillin plus clavulanic acid, but the latter is preferred when laboratory test show gram-positive infections. Moreover, oral quinolone therapy should not be administered to patients who have already received quinolone as a prophylaxis [71].

14.2. High risk neutropenic patients

The majority of the treatment guidelines indicate that high-risk neutropenic patients need to be treated with using parenteral broad spectrum antibiotic therapy, that is using standard, hospital-based guidelines. For a long time, the most common approach was the selection and use of combination antimicrobial therapy (beta-lactam plus aminoglycoside antibiotics) [72].

14.3. Duration of therapy

According to the guidelines from the Infectious Society of America, neutropenic patients who remain febrile but show recovery in neutrophil cell count on the third day of antibiotic therapy could either continue with antibiotics treatment for 7 days or antibiotic treatments can be stopped on the fourth or fifth day.

For those neutropenic febrile patients with no recovery in the ANC it is preferred to continue antibiotics which could only be discontinued after 2 weeks when the examination and cultures show no bacterial growth [69].

14.4. Antifungal drugs

Fungal treatment is one of the most important steps for neutropenic patients. Even one positive blood culture for candida should be considered significant. Patients with disseminated candidiasis should be treated with fluconazole, which is as effective as amphotericin B and less toxic. If the patient is not stable and has already received fluconazole, amphotericin B is recommended. The treatment should continue until all signs of infections are resolved for a minimum of 2 weeks. Patients with invasive fungal infection are at risk of recurrent infection due to chemotherapy-induced neutropenia [73].

14.5. Antiviral drugs

The main characteristic of viruses is their simple structure, which helps them multiply. Viruses use the biochemical mechanisms of the host cell to produce new protein and genes. This makes the virus and the host cell identical and makes it difficult for the antiviral drug to distinguish the viral cell from the host cell. In the last couple of years, further information on the mechanism of viral multiplication has helped in the development of antiviral drugs such as acyclovir, which is effective against some herpes viruses. On the other hand, the increase in the use of immunosuppressive drugs had led to an increase in both bacterial and viral infections [74].

15. Conclusion

Neutropenia is a critical condition occurring among patients undergoing chemotherapy. It is strongly associated with a number of negative experiences that have an adverse effect on patients' quality of life. Neutropenia can lead to and is associated with critical infection of bacterial, fungal, or viral origin which may cause death if not treated. But survival in neutropenic patients can improve overtime with the uses of empirical antibiotic treatment (monotherapy or combination therapy). G-CSF is also a very effective treatment for neutropenia and febrile neutropenia.

http://dx.doi.org/10.5772/60794

Author details

Bassam Abdul Rasool Hassan[1*], Zuraidah Binti Mohd Yusoff[2] and Saad Bin Othman[2]

*Address all correspondence to: bassamsunny@yahoo.com

1 Department of Pharmacy, Faculty of Medicine, University of Malaya, Kuala Lumpur, Malaysia

2 Clinical Pharmacy Discipline, School of Pharmaceutical Sciences, Universiti Sains Malaysia (USM), Malaysia

References

[1] Kumar V., Sharma A. Neutrophils: Cinderella of innate immune system. International Immunopharmacology, 2010; 10, 1325 – 1334.

[2] Dale DC. Neutropenia. In: Herman NW. (ed.) Encyclopedia of Life Sciences. Chichester John Wiley & Son's, Ltd; 2005. p10 - 32.

[3] Frey RJ. Neutropenia. In: Donna O., Christine J., Karen B. (eds.) The Gale Encyclopedia of Medicine. Farmington Hills, Gale Research, An International Thomson Company; 1999. p77-89.

[4] Mantovani A., Cassatella MA., Costantini C., Jaillon S. Neutrophils in the activation and regulation of innate and adaptive immunity. Immunology, 2011; 11, 519-531.

[5] Walker R, Edwards C. Laboratory Data. In: Wynne HA., Edward C. (eds.) Clinical Pharmacy & Therapeutics. New York, Churchill Livingstone; 2003. p 111-124.

[6] Borregaard N. Neutrophils, from marrow to microbes. Immunity, 2010; 33, 657-670.

[7] Eash KJ., Means JM., White, DW., Link DC. CXCR4 is a key regulator of neutrophil release from the bone marrow under basal and stress granulopoiesis conditions. Blood, 2009; 113, 4711–4719.

[8] Dale DC. Neutropenia and the Problem of Fever and Infection in Patients with Cancer. In: Morstyn G, Lieschke GJ. (eds.) Hematopoietic growth factors in oncology: New Jersey, Human Press; 2004. p65-87.

[9] Kobayashi S., Voyich JM., Burlak C., Deleo FR. Neutrophils in the innate immune response. Archivum Immunologiae et Therapiae Experimentalis, 2005; 53, 505–517.

[10] Alcaide P, Auerbach S, Luscinskas FW. Neutrophil recruitment under shear flow: It's all about endothelial cell rings and gaps. Microcirculation, 2009; 16, 43-57.

[11] Woodfin A., Voisin MB., Nourshargh S. Recent developments and complexities in neutrophil transmigration. Current Opinion in Hematology, 2010; 17, 9-17.

[12] Qin W., Eddie T., Chiang ML., Jean L., Rick R., Paul A. Janmey DS., Claire MD. Changes in the biomechanical properties of neutrophils and endothelial cells during adhesion. Blood, 2001; 97, 660-668.

[13] Frey R, Granger J. Neutropenia. In: Thackery E. (ed) The gale encyclopedia of cancer, Detroit: Gale Group; 2002. p. 770-773.

[14] Linker CA. Blood. In: Tiernery LM., McPhee SJ. Papadakis MA. (eds.) Current medical diagnosis and treatment. New York, Appleton & Lange; 2000. p 222-238.

[15] Bolyard AA., Edwards C., Kinsey S., Schwinzer B., Zeidler C. Understanding severe chronic neutropenia, Oaks, CA, USA, Scnir; 1994.

[16] Bledsoe BE., Kufs D., Soltis CA. Hematology. In: Bledsoe BE., Porter RS., Cherry RA. (eds.) Paramedic Care / Principles and Practice. New Jersey: Pearson Prentice Hall; 2005. p100-122.

[17] AL-Ahwal MS. Pattern of febrile neutropenia in solid tumors - A hospital based study. Pakistan Journal of Medical Sciences, 2005; 21, 249-252.

[18] Lyman GH., Wilmot JP. Risks and consequences of chemotherapy-induced neutropenia. Clinical Cornerstone, 2006; 8, 12-18.

[19] Bassam H., Zuraidah MY., Saad BO., Neutropenia onset, severity and their association with demographic data. Asian Journal of Pharmaceutical and Clinical Research, 2009; 2, 51-53.

[20] Ashley J., Taylor D., Houts A. The experience of chemotherapy- induced neutropenia: quality-of-life interviews with adult cancer patients. Journal of Supportive Oncology 2004; 2, 66-67.

[21] Ropka ME., Faan RN., Padilla G. Assessment of neutropenia related quality of life in a clinical setting Oncology Nursing Society 2007; 34, 403-409.

[22] Verstraete M., Vrhaeghe R., Peerlinck K., Boogaerts M.A. Haematological Disorders. In: Speight TM., Holford NH. (eds.) A very's Drug Treatment. Auckland, Adis Press; 1997. p56-68.

[23] Kimble-Koda MA., Young LY., Kardjan WA., Guglielmo BJ. Infections in Neutropenic Patients. In: Troy D. (eds.) Hand Book of Applied Therapeutics, Philadelphia, Lippincott Williams & Wilkins; 2002. p203-241.

[24] Buffoni L., Dongiovanni D., Barone C., Fissore C., Ottaviani D., Dongiovanni V., Grillo R., Salvadori A., Birocco N., Schena M., Bertetto O. Fractionated dose of cisplatin (CDDP) and vinorelbine (VNB) chemotherapy for elderly patients with advanced non-small cell lung cancer: phase II trial. Lung Cancer 2006; 54, 353-357.

[25] Yamanaka T., Matsumoto S., Teramukai S., Ishiwata R., Nagai Y., Fukushima M. Predictive value of chemotherapy-induced neutropenia for the efficacy of oral fluoropyrimidine S-1 in advanced gastric carcinoma. British Journal of Cancer 2007; 97, 37-42.

[26] Hassan BAR, Zuraidah MY., Saad O., Association of neutropenia onset and severity with chemotherapy regimens and schedules. Asian Pacific Journal of Cancer Prevention, 2011; 12, 1425-1428.

[27] Di maio M., Gridelli C., Gallo C., Shepherd F., Piantedosi FV., Cigolari S., Manzione L., Illiano A., Barbera S., Robbiati SF., Frontini L., Piazza E., Ianniello GP., Veltri E., Castiglione F., Rosetti F., Gebbia V., Seymour L., Chiodini P., Perrone F. Chemotherapy-induced neutropenia and treatment efficacy in advanced non-small-cell lung cancer: a pooled analysis of three randomized trials. Lancet Oncology 2005; 6, 669-677.

[28] Banerji U., Ashley S., Coward J., Hughes S., Zee Y., Benepal T., Norton A., Eisen T., O'Brien M. The association of chemotherapy induced neutropenia on treatment outcomes in small cell lung cancer. Lung Cancer 2006; 54, 371-377.

[29] Kern WV. Current Epidemiology of Infections in Neutropenic Cancer Patients. In: Rolston KVI., Rubenstein EB., (eds.) Text book of febrile neutropenia. London: Martin Dunitz, Ltd; 2001. p.57-90.

[30] Bow EJ. Infection risk and cancer chemotherapy: the impact of the chemotherapeutic regimen in patients with lymphoma and solid tissue Malignancies. Journal of Antimicrobial Chemotherapy, 1998; 41, 1-5.

[31] Howland RD. Mycek MJ. (2006) Anticancer Drugs. In: Pharmacology 3rd edition. Philadelphia: Lippincott Williams & Wilkins; 2006. p. 435-484.

[32] Larsson PA., Carlsson G., Gustavsson B., Graf W., Glimelius B. Different intravenous administration techniques for 5-Fluorouracil pharmacokinetics and pharmacodynamic effects Acta Oncologica, 1996; 35(2): 207-212.

[33] Jassem J., Kosmidis P., Ramlau R., Zarogoulidis K., Novakova L., Breton J., Etienne PL., Seebacher C., Grivaux M., Ojala A., Aubert D., Lefresne F. Oral vinorelbine in combination with cisplatin: a novel active regimen in advanced non-small-cell lung cancer Annals of Oncology, 2003; 14, 1634-1639.

[34] Lyman G., Kuderer N., Djulbegovic B. Recombinant colony-stimulating factors reduce febrile neutropenia and infection in people receiving dose-intensive chemotherapy, but increase bone pain. American Journal of Medicine, 2002; 112, 406-411.

[35] Crawford J., Wolff D., Culakova E., Poniewierski M.S., Selby C., Dale D., Lyman G.H. First-cycle risk of severe and febrile neutropenia in cancer patients receiving systemic chemotherapy: results from a prospective nationwide study. Journal of Supportive Oncology, 2005; 3, 52-53.

[36] Wolff D., Culakova E., Poniewierski MS., Lyman GH., Dale DC. & Crawford, J. Predictors of chemotherapy-induced neutropenia and Its complications: results from a prospective nationwide registry. Journal of Supportive Oncology, 2005; 3, 24-25.

[37] Schallier D., Neynsa B., Fontainea C., Vande Steeneb J., De Meyc J., Meysmand M., De Grevea J. A novel triplet regimen with paclitaxel, carboplatin and gemcitabine (PACCAGE) as induction chemotherapy for locally advanced unresectable non small cell lung cancer (NSCLC). Lung Cancer, 2007; 56, 247-254.

[38] Rugo HS. Cancer. In: Tiernery, L. M., McPhee, S.J. & Papadakis, M.A. (ed.) Current Medical Diagnosis and Treatment. New York, Appleton & Lange; 2000. p.105-141.

[39] Glimelius B., Jakobsen A., Graf W., Berglund A., Gadeberg C., Hansen P., Kjaer M. Brunsgaard N., Sandberg E., Lindberg B., Sellstrom H., Lorentz T. Pahlman L. Bolus injection (2±4 min) versus short-term (10±20 min) infusion of 5-Fluorouracil in patients with advanced colorectal cancer: a prospective randomised trial. European Journal Of Cancer 1998; 34(5): 674-678.

[40] Scurr M., Judson I., Root T. Combination Chemotherapy and Chemotherapy Principles. In: Brighton D., Wood M. (eds.) Cancer Chemotherapy London, Churchill Livingstone; 2005. p 33-51.

[41] Neutropenia Association Inc. Neutropenia, causes, consequences and care. What is Neutropenia. Canada: Neutropenia Association Inc; 1993.

[42] Di Maio M., Gridelli C., Gallo C., Shepherd F., Piantedosi FV., Cigolari S., Manzione L., Illiano A., Barbera S., Robbiati SF., Frontini L., Piazza E., Ianniello GP., Veltri E., Castiglione F., Rosetti F., Gebbia V., Seymour L., Chiodini P., Perrone F. Chemotherapy-induced neutropenia and treatment efficacy in advanced non-small-cell lung cancer: a pooled analysis of three randomized trials. Lancet Oncology, 2005; 6, 669-677.

[43] Fortner BV., Schwartzberg L., Tauer K., Houts AC., Hackett, J., Stolshek BS. Impact of chemotherapy-induced neutropenia on quality of life: a prospective pilot investigation. Support Care Cancer 2005; 13, 522-528.

[44] Timmer-bonte JN., De Boo TM., Smit HJ., Biesma B., Wilschut FA., Cheragwandi SA., Termeer A., Hensing CA., Akkermans J., Adang EM., Bootsma GP. Tjan-Heijnen VC. Prevention of chemotherapy-induced febrile neutropenia by prophylactic antibiotics plus or minus granulocyte colony-stimulating factor in small-cell lung cancer: a Dutch randomized phase III study. Journal of Clinical Oncology, 2005; 23, 7974-7984.

[45] Munshi HG. Severe neutropenia: a diagnostic approach. Western Journal of Medicine, 2000; 172, 248-252.

[46] National Cancer Registry of Malaysia. Second Report of the National Cancer Registry Cancer Incidence in Malaysia. In: Malaysia MOH (ed.) National Cancer Registry; 2003. p. 1-141.

http://dx.doi.org/10.5772/60794

[47] Wolff D., Crawford J., Dale CD., Poniewierski MS., Lyman G.H. Risk of neutropenic complications based on a prospective nationwide registry of cancer patients initiating systemic chemotherapy. Journal of Support Oncology, 2005; 3, 56-57.

[48] National Cancer Registry of Malaysia. Second Report of the National Cancer Registry Cancer Incidence in Malaysia. In: Malaysia MOH (ed.): National Cancer Registry; 2003. p. 1-141.

[49] Yip C., Kasule OH. Epidemiology of breast cancer in Malaysia. International Medical Journal 2005; 4, 1.

[50] Crawford J. Update on neutropenia and myeloid growth factors. Supportive Oncology 2007; 5(4): 27-29.

[51] Voelker MD., Rubenstein LM., Chrischilles EA., Chen-Hardee SS., Link BK., Wright KB., Brooks JM. Delgado DJ. Time to first neutropenia hospitalization during first-course chemotherapy among newly diagnosed non-Hodgkin's lymphoma patients: national SEER-medicare study. Journal of Supportive Oncology 2004; 2: 40-41.

[52] Kaur G., Ismail R., Lee SK., Sabaratnam S., Ahmad N. Assessment of correlation between clinicopathological features and Lymph node metastases in breast cancer. The Internet Journal of Pathology, 2007; 5(2): 1528-8307.

[53] Hershman D., Weinberg M., Rosner Z., Alexis K., Tiersten A., Grann VR., Troxel A. Neugut AI. Ethnic neutropenia and treatment delay in African American women undergoing chemotherapy for early-stage breast cancer. Journal of the National Cancer Institute, 2003; 95: 1545-1548.

[54] Zia Rahman GE., Hwee-Yong Y., Fraschini G., Bodey G., Hortobagvi G. Chemotherapy-induced neutropenia and fever in patients with metastatic breast carcinoma receiving salvage chemotherapy. Cancer, 1997; 79: 1150-1157.

[55] Rolston KVI. Infections in Patients with Solid Tumors. In: Rolston KVI., Rubenstein EB. (eds.) Text Book of Febrile Neutropenia. London: Martin Dunitz Ltd; 2001. p. 91-109.

[56] Koasak Ü, Rolston KVI., Mullen CA. Fever and neutropenia in children with solid tumors is similar in severity and outcome to that in children with leukemia. Support Care Cancer, 2002; 10: 58-64.

[57] Sharma A., Lokeshwar N. Febrile neutropenia in haematological malignancies. Journal of Postgraduate Medicine, 2005; 51, 42-48.

[58] Lyman G., Kuderer N., Djulbegovic B. Recombinant colony-stimulating factors reduce febrile neutropenia and infection in people receiving dose-intensive chemotherapy, but increase bone pain. American Journal of Medicine 2002; 112, 406-411.

[59] Juan O., Campos JM., Caranana V., Sanchez JJ., Casan R., Alberola, V. A randomized, crossover comparison of standard-dose versus low-dose lenograstim in the prophylaxis of post-chemotherapy neutropenia. Support Care Cancer 2001; 9, 241-246.

[60] Clinical practice guidelines. Rational Antibiotic Utilisation in Selected Paerdiatric Conditions. In: Health Technology Assessment Unit, M. D. D. Putrajaya, Ministry of Health Malaysia, Academy of Medicine Malaysia; 2007.

[61] Schimpff CA. Fever and Neutropenia: an Historical Perspective. In: Rolston KVI., Rubenstein EB., (edS.) Text Book of Febrile Neutropenia. London: Martin Duntiz Ltd; 2001. p. 1-26.

[62] Rolston KVI. Infections in Patients with Solid Tumors. In: Rolston KVI., Rubenstein EB. (eds.) Text Book of Febrile Neutropenia. London: Martin Dunitz Ltd; 2001. p. 91-109.

[63] Clinical practice guidelines. Rational Antibiotic Utilisation in Selected Paediatric Conditions. In: Health Technology Assessment Unit, M. D. D. Putrajaya, Ministry of Health Malaysia, Academy of Medicine Malaysia. 2004.

[64] Alexander SW., Pizzo PA. Special considerations in children with fever and neutropenia. In: Rolston KVI., Rubenstein EB. (eds.) Text book of febrile neutropenia. London: Martin Dunitz Ltd; 2001. p. 65-78.

[65] De Pauw BE., Deresinski SC., Feld R., Lane-Allman EF., Donnelly JP. Ceftazidime compared with piperacillin and tobramycin for the empiric treatment of fever in neutropenic patients with cancer: A multi center randomized trial. Annals of Internal Medicine, 1994; 120, 834- 844.

[66] Yano K., Nakano Y. Clinical evaluation of monotherapy with cefpirome for infections complicating hematological disorders. Journal of Infect Chemother, 1996; 2, 75-78.

[67] Tamura K., Matsuoka H., Ikeda S., Masuda M., Tsukada j., Matsuishi H., Izumi Y., Saburi Y., Uike N., Okamura S., Kawano F., Utsunomiya A., Shibuya T., Imamura Y., Uozumi K., Hayashi M., Gondoh H. A Randomized trial of single versus combination antibiotic therapy for febrile neutropenic patients by Kyushu Hematology Organization For Treatment (K-HOT) Study Group. Clinical Oncology, 2001; 20, Abstract 1549.

[68] Leighl N., Feld R. Clinical Practical Guidlines in Patients With Fever and Neutropenia. In: Rolston KVI., Rubenstein EB. (eds.) Text Book of Febrile Neutropenia. London: Martin Dunitz Ltd; 2001. p. 560-583.

[69] Hughes WT., Armstrong D., Bodey GP., Bow EJ., Brown AE., Calandra T., Feld R., Pizzo PA., Rolston KVI., Shenep JL., Young L.S. Guidelines for the use of antimicrobial agents in neutropenic patients with cancer, Clinical Infectious Diseases; 2002 34, 730-751.

http://dx.doi.org/10.5772/60794

[70] Tomiak AT., Yau JC., Huan SD., Cripps MC., Goel R., Perrault DJ., Bourcier JD., Prosser IA., Soltys KM., Evans WK., Stewart DJ. Duration of intravenous antibiotics for patients with neutropenic fever. Annals of Oncology, 1994; 5, 441-445.

[71] Schimpff CA. Fever and Neutropenia: an Historical Perspective In: Rolston KVI., Rubenstein E.B., (eds.). Text Book of Febrile Neutropenia. London: Martin Duntiz Ltd; 2005. p. 1-26.

[72] Flaherty J. (1999) Infectious Complications of Oncology Therapy. In: Vokes EE., Golomb HM., (eds.). Oncologic Therapies. Berlin; Springer 1999.p. 228-244.

[73] Wiltink EHH., Janknegt R. Antiviral drugs. Pharmaceutisch Weekblad. 1991; 13 (2): 58-69.

Chapter 10

Current Concepts in Pancreatic Cancer

Zeeshan Ramzan, Phat Le, Payal Kapur and
Sergio Huerta

Additional information is available at the end of the chapter

http://dx.doi.org/10.5772/60451

1. Introduction

Pancreatic cancer is one of the most lethal malignancies, ranking as the fourth leading cause of death from cancer in the United States. Despite a variety of improved diagnostic and therapeutic approaches over the past several decades the mortality rate has not significantly improved. There is wide variation in the therapeutic approach to pancreatic cancer based upon multiple factors such as the stage at presentation, patient's coexisting medical comorbidities, etc. and at times the optimal treatment strategy is still controversial.

2. Epidemiology

Cancer of the exocrine pancreas was diagnosed in 45,220 patients in the United States in 2013. Underscoring its fatal nature, during the same year, 85% of patients (38,460) died from this disease [2]. Thus, despite only comprising 3% of all new cancer diagnoses, pancreatic cancer accounted for 6-7% of all deaths related to cancer [2]. Over the past 10 years, the similar incidence and the death rates emphasize that most pancreatic cancers are fatal as a result of late stage at diagnosis (Figure 1) [2-12]. Although, the gap between the yearly incidence and mortality of pancreatic cancer has slightly widened over the past ten years, most patients diagnosed with cancer will succumb to this deadly disease (Figure 2).

The average age at diagnosis is 60 to 65 years. The etiology of pancreatic cancer is not known, but several risk factors have been identified. For instance, men have a slightly higher incidence compared to women (Relative Risk [RR] 1.35) and Black men have a 30-40% higher rate in incidence compared to White men [13]. Cigarette smoking is the best well-recognized environmental risk factor for the development of pancreatic cancer. Current smokers have a RR of

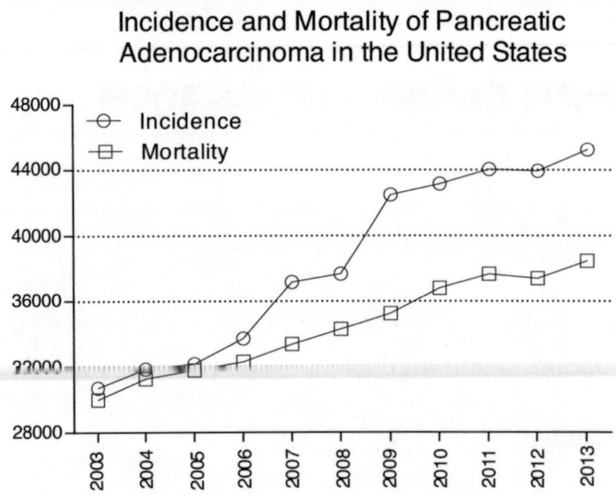

Figure 1. Incidence of Adenocarcinoma of the pancreas in the United States over the past ten years.

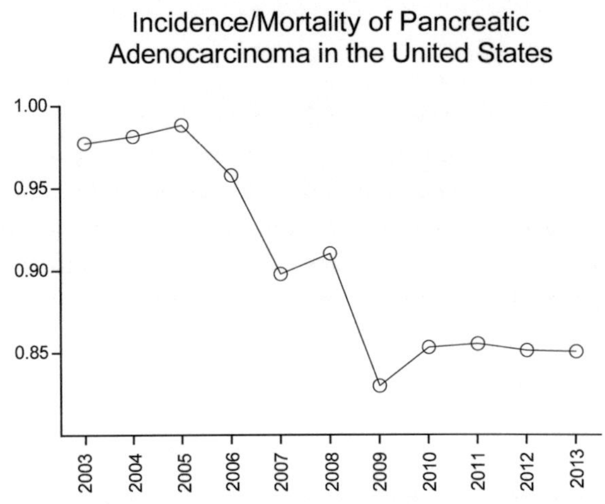

Figure 2. The incidence divided by the mortality in the Unites States over the past.

up to 3.6 compared to non-smokers and smoking is estimated to contribute to 25% as an etiology of pancreatic cancer [14;15]. Other risk factors for pancreatic cancer include: diabetes, obesity, Helicobacter *pylori* infection, non-O blood group and chronic pancreatitis [16-20].

Most forms of pancreatic cancer are sporadic. However, familial pancreatic cancer accounts for 5-10% of all pancreatic cancers [21]. Data from the National Familial Tumor Registry demonstrates that the risk of pancreatic cancer of the pancreas is 18-fold higher if two first-degree relatives are involved and 57-fold higher if three first-degree family members are affected [22]. This risk is conferred by an increased risk in several recognized genetic syndromes caused by germline mutations leading to familial syndromes. For instance Peutz-Jeghers Syndrome results from a germline mutation of the *STK11* gene. Affected individuals have a 132-fold increased risk for pancreatic cancer [23]. Familial Atypical Mole Multiple

http://dx.doi.org/10.5772/60451

Melanoma Syndrome patients with a germline mutation of the *CDKN2A* gene have a 46-fold increased risk for the development of pancreatic cancer. Individuals with mutations of the *PRSS1* gene have an increase in trypsin activity, which in turn causes chronic inflammation of the pancreas. These patients suffer from hereditary pancreatitis and have a 50-fold increase risk of pancreatic cancer [23]. Other genetic syndromes that confer a higher risk include cystic fibrosis (CTFR gene mutation), Fanconi Anemia, familial breast or ovarian cancer (BRCA2 gene mutations), familial adenomatous polyposis (*APC* gene mutations), Li-Fraumeni syndrome (*p53* gene mutation) and Lynch II syndrome (MLH1 gene mutation) [24].

3. Pathology

Pancreatic ductal carcinomas arising from the exocrine pancreas is the most common type accounting for 95% of these tumors. Two-thirds of these tumors occur in the head of the pancreas and have an aggressive behavior [25]. The vast majority of malignancies of the pancreas are infiltrating ductal adenocarcinomas and the term pancreatic cancer generally refers to adenocarcinoma of the pancreas. Pancreatic cancer can originate from each of the cell types that form the pancreas. For instance, neuroendocrine tumors arise from the pancreatic islet cells. Unlike ductal adenocarcinoma, many of the endocrine tumors are benign. Small subsets are endocrine carcinomas and make up around 1% of pancreatic cancers. Pancreatic cystic neoplasms include a group of tumors having varying malignant potential. Uncommonly, extrapancreatic tumors can metastasize to the pancreas and have been reported from renal cell carcinoma, non-small cell lung cancer, sarcoma, melanoma, and bladder cancers (Figure 3) [26].

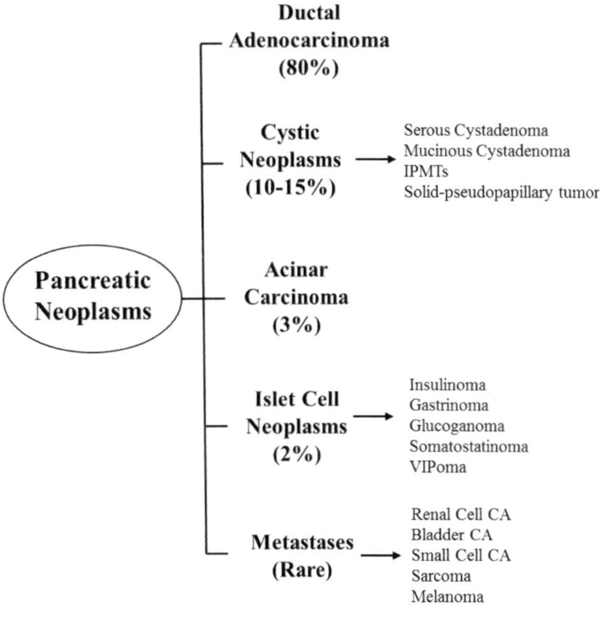

Figure 3. Incidence of malignancies of the pancreas.

Current pancreatic cancer models are similar to that of colon cancer, in which there is a progression from precancerous lesions to invasive carcinomas. Pancreatic cancer evolves from normal ductal epithelium, to pancreatic intraepithelial neoplasms/ductal lesions, to invasive adenocarcinomas [27;28]. The ductal epithelium undergoes changes that are characterized by PanIN-1A. Changes continue to accumulate and lead to PanIN-3, which denotes carcinoma *in situ* (Figure 4). This evolution is associated with the acquisition of a large number of genetic alterations that function through a small number of signaling processes and pathways. The stepwise acquisition of genetic abnormalities leading up to invasive ductal adenocarcinoma is now well characterized and includes mutations in *KRAS2*, inactivation of *p16*, *p53*, *PDX1*, and *SMAD4* [29].

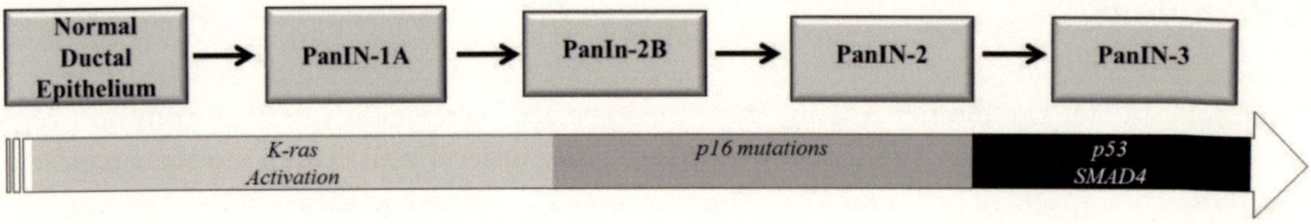

Figure 4. Progression of normal epithelium to pancreatic cancer and genes involved in the pathogenesis of sporadic pancreatic cancer.

Comprehensive genetic analysis of pancreatic cancer specimens demonstrated that the most frequent genetic abnormality in invasive pancreatic adenocarcinomas is activation of KRAS2 oncogene, which was present in more than 90% of pancreatic cancers [28]. *KRAS2* mutations are thought to be acquired early in the development of pancreatic cancer as they are found in a large number of ductal lesions and become more prevalent as these lesions progress to invasive adenocarcinoma [27]. In addition to *KRAS2* mutations, several other pathways in cellular signaling have been found to be altered in 67-100% of the tumors. These pathways include: TGF β, JNK, Integrin, Wnt/Notch, Hedgehog, control of G1/S phase transition, apoptosis, DNA damage control, small GTPase, invasion, and homophilic cell adhesion [30].

Histologically, poorly formed glands are present in a dense fibrotic background within the pancreatic parenchyma and sprinkled inflammatory cells. Some of the tumor cells might show some mucin production. Perineural invasion is often seen and can help with the diagnosis in well-differentiated tumors. Other features of malignancy include nuclear pleomorphism, occasional large nuclei and multiple large nucleoli (Figure 5).

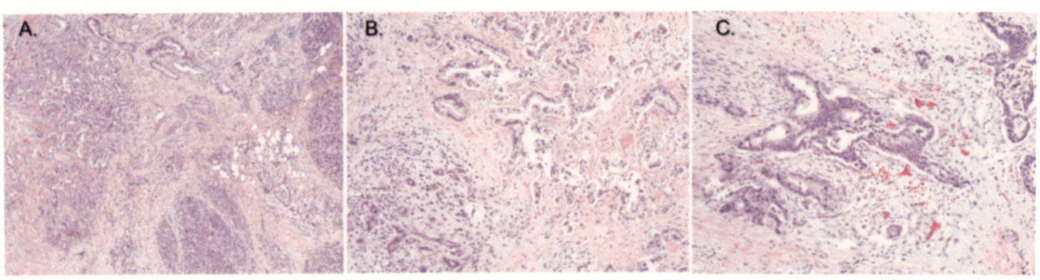

Figure 5. H&E stains of normal and adjacent ductal adenocarcinoma 40X (panel A). Panel B demonstrates invasive adenocarcinoma (100X). Perineural invasion is demonstrated in panel C.

http://dx.doi.org/10.5772/60451

4. Clinical features

4.1. History

Currently there are no established screening tests for pancreatic cancer. The vague and nonspecific symptoms in pancreatic cancer contribute to its delay in diagnosis. The location of the tumor within the pancreas dictates some historical features and clinical presentation. The stage of the disease is also important. Because most pancreatic tumors are located in the head of the pancreas and present at an advanced stage, clinical findings suspicious for pancreatic cancer must be rapidly addressed to exclude this lethal diagnosis.

Patients with lesions of the head of the pancreas present with painless jaundice and weight loss, which might be accompanied with anorexia and weakness [31]. The frequency of presenting symptoms in 1175 patients with adenocarcinoma of the pancreas was: 2/3 painless jaundice, ½ weight loss, and about 1/3 abdominal pain [32]. Obstructive cholestasis might lead to dark urine, light stools and pruritus. Distention of the pancreatic capsule causes vague epigastric and/or back pain that poorly localizes to the location of the tumor. Obstruction of the pancreatic duct or perineural invasion also causes pain, but this is less specific and poorly localized. Ten percent of patients have symptoms attributed to cholelithiasis and will have undergone recent cholecystectomy prior to the diagnosis of pancreatic cancer. Similarly, obstruction of the pancreatic duct might lead to acute pancreatitis [13, 33]. Uncommonly, large tumors might present with symptoms of duodenal obstruction such as nausea and vomiting or symptoms associated with a gastrointestinal bleed [31].

Systemic manifestations are more usual in patients with lesions of the body and tail of the pancreas such as weight loss and anorexia [31]. Constant pain is attributed to tumor invasion of the celiac and mesenteric plexuses and occurs with advanced disease. Eight weeks is a typical mean duration of symptoms. New-onset diabetes mellitus may be an initial presenting symptom in patients with pancreatic cancer and glucose intolerance occurs in 15%-20% of these patients. Depression, increased abdominal girth, and a history of panniculitis are rare, but might accompany a diagnosis of pancreatic cancer [31, 34].

4.2. Physical examination

The physical examination for patients with pancreatic cancer is unyielding. Since two-thirds of pancreatic adenocarcinomas occur in the head of the pancreas, the most common presenting physical finding is evidence of obstructive cholestasis. Painless jaundice in an older patient has been attributed a hallmark of physical findings necessitating careful exclusion of pancreatic cancer. The examiner must investigate for signs of weight loss such as temporal wasting as well as careful interrogation of lymph node basins [31].

Hepatomegaly, ascites or a palpable gallbladder (Courvoisier's sign/law) may be present in some patients with advanced pancreatic cancer. Courvoisier's sign is more likely to be present in patients with pancreatic cancer compared to calculi disease [35]. Physical findings in patients with disseminated disease include supraclavicular lymphadenopathy (Virchow's node). However, pancreatic cancer usually does not metastasize to the supraclavicular nodes and only a few cases have been reported [36]. Cutaneous metastasis in the periumbilical area (Sister

Mary Joseph's nodule) [37] and peritoneal seeding (Blumer's shelf) are also rarely found with pancreatic metastatic disease. Migratory thrombophlebitis (Trousseau's sign), which is evidence of intravascular thrombosis, may occur in patients with advanced pancreatic cancer as well as other advanced cancers resulting from a hypercoagulable state from malignant disease [38].

5. Staging

The AJCC staging system, based on the TNM stage, is most often used staging system for pancreatic cancer. The tumor stage describes the size of the primary tumor, vascular structure involvement and any direct extension of the tumor outside of the pancreas. The nodal stage assesses the presence or absence of any regional lymph node involvement. The metastasis stage describes the presence or absence of any distant disease (Table 1).

(a)	**Primary Tumor (T)**		
Tx	Primary tumor cannot be assessed		
T0	No evidence of primary tumor		
Tis	Carcinoma in situ (includes lesions classified as PanInIII classification)		
T1	Tumor limited to the pancreas, 2 cm or less in greatest dimension		
T2	Tumor limited to the pancreas, more than 2 cm in greatest dimension		
T3	Tumor extends beyond the pancreas but without involvement of the celiac axis or superior mesenteric artery		
T4	Tumor invades the celiac axis or the superior mesenteric artery (unresectable primary tumor)		
(b)	**Regional Lymph Nodes (N)**		
Nx	Regional lymph nodes cannot be assessed		
N0	No regional lymph node metastasis		
N1	Regional lymph node metastasis		
(c)	**Distant Metastasis (M)**		
M0	No distant metastasis		
M1	Distant metastasis		
(d)	**Anatomic Stage/Prognostic Groups**		
Stage 0	Tis	N0	M0
Stage IA	T1	N0	M0
Stage IB	T2	N0	M0
Stage IIA	T3	N0	M0
Stage IIB	T1	N1	M0
	T2	N1	M0
	T3	N1	M0
Stage III	T4	Any N	M0
Stage IV	Any T	Any N	M1

Table 1. TNM staging system for pancreatic cancer

http://dx.doi.org/10.5772/60451

Common sites of metastatic disease often include the liver, peritoneal cavity, and lungs [39]. The anatomic staging roughly correlates with whether or not the tumor is resectable. Those tumors with Stage IA to IIB are considered resectable. Tumors designated as Stage IV are unresectable and those designated as stage III can be borderline resectable or unresectable. The NCCN classification system which divides tumors into resectable, borderline resectable or unresectable categories may be more applicable clinically [40].

6. Diagnostic evaluation

Routine laboratory analyses are rarely abnormal and if abnormal they lack specificity for a diagnosis of pancreatic cancer. Evidence of extrahepatic obstruction may be revealed by increased levels of serum alkaline phosphatase, bilirubin and gamma-glutamyl transferase with possible mild elevations in hepatic aminotransferases [31]. Hypoalbuminemia and anemia may be present in patients with advanced disease. Mild coagulopathy can be seen in patients with obstructive jaundice. Poor flow of bile acids in the small bowel in these patients decreases vitamin K absorption resulting in depletion of vitamin K dependent clotting factors over time. Elevated pancreatic enzymes (elevated amylase and lipase) associated with acute pancreatitis can rarely be the first manifestation of pancreatic cancer [41].

There are no accurate or reliable serum markers to aid in the diagnosis of pancreatic cancer. Low sensitivity and cross-reactivity with other tumors have prevented the clinical use of carcinoembryonic antigen (CEA), fetoprotein, and pancreatic oncofetal antigen in the diagnosis of pancreatic cancer. Carbohydrate antigen 19-9 levels (normal <37 units/mL) has been the most useful commercially available test. However, the sensitivity of CA 19-9 ranges from 70% to 92% and the specificity is poor (68% to 92%) [42]. The accuracy of CA 19-9 in the diagnosis of pancreatic cancer is excellent when combined with ERCP, abdominal CT, or abdominal US [43]. High levels of CA 19-9 have been associated with poor prognosis and tumor unresectability [43]. CA 19-9 is also useful in monitoring the response of therapeutic interventions. As the CA 19-9 requires the presence of Lewis blood group antigen (a glycosyl transferase enzyme) to be expressed, this serum marker is of no value in 10% of the population who is negative for this antigen [44, 45].

7. Conventional imaging modalities

Imaging studies are essential in the management of pancreatic cancer. The most important goal of imaging is to determine tumor resectability. Involvement of adjacent vessels (superior mesenteric vein, portal vein, and superior mesenteric artery), nodal involvement and distant metastatic lesions are paramount in selecting treatment options. The investigation of most patients with pancreatic cancer generally begins with a right upper quadrant ultrasound to evaluate jaundice.

7.1. Abdominal ultrasound

Abdominal ultrasound (US) examination reliably detects extra-hepatic and intra-hepatic ductal dilatation. However, accurate identification of a pancreatic mass may be compromised by operator experience, bowel gas interference, or obesity, and does not provide information regarding tumor involvement of the vascular structures or lymph node involvement. In advanced disease, ascites and liver metastases (>1 cm) may be seen by abdominal US.

7.2. Computed Tomography

Computed tomography (CT) has been used routinely for evaluation of pancreatic cancer over the last few decades. However, since the advent of triple phase (noncontrast, arterial, and portal venous) helical multidetector row CT (MDCT) with thin cuts (1 mm slices) through the pancreas along with coronal three dimensional reconstruction (pancreatic protocol), it has become the gold standard initial test for the diagnosis and staging of all pancreatic cancers. The sensitivity for lesions greater than 2 cm is 100% [46]. While the false positive rate is low, it might occur in the setting of focal chronic pancreatitis or autoimmune pancreatitis. The advantage of CT is its wide availability, non-invasive approach, non-operator dependent and easily reproducible images. It is also deliberately used in conjunction with ^{18}F-fluorodeoxy-glucose positron emission tomography (PET)/CT for surveillance imaging post treatment.

7.3. Endoscopic ultrasound

Endoscopic ultrasound (EUS) transmits high-frequency sound waves through the upper GI tract to detect abnormalities in the pancreas (Figure 6). The accuracy of EUS is operator dependent and it is not yet available at many community hospitals. At experienced centers, EUS has been shown to have a similar (or better) sensitivity and specificity for the diagnosis of pancreatic cancer to that of MDCT [47]. Being a dynamic test, it can distinguish subtle abnormalities such as pancreatic duct strictures and small neuroendocrine tumors. Not uncommonly, it can detect small (<1cm) pancreatic cancers, which would escape detection by MDCT. EUS can also evaluate malignant as well as pre-malignant cystic lesions such as intra-ductal papillary mucinous neoplasms with its characteristic findings of intramural nodules and communication with the main pancreatic duct.

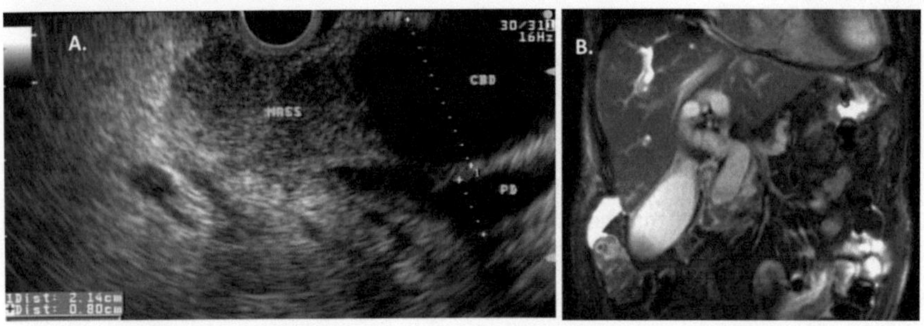

Figure 6. Malignant biliary obstruction from mass in head of pancreas causing CBD and PD dilation (double-duct sign) US (A). MRCP in (B) Note the distended gallbladder, seen in patients with malignant biliary obstruction (Courvoisier's sign)

Due to the high sensitivity of EUS in detecting small lesions, it is widely used to screen patients with familial pancreatic cancer or other hereditary syndromes [48]. EUS has the advantage of allowing sampling of the tumor mass, regional nodes, liver lesions, ascites and malignant cyst fluid, as well as assessing tumor resectability during diagnostic evaluation (Figure 7). In one study, the sensitivity, specificity, and accuracy of EUS-FNA for diagnosis of a pancreatic malignancy were 91%, 100%, and 92%, respectively. No mortalities were reported in this analysis and morbidity was only 2% [49]. Recently, the EUS-FNA needles have been employed to introduce sophisticated probes directly into the pancreatic lesions for diagnostic needs, as well as deliver therapeutic approaches such as local injections of cytotoxic agents and probe based application of radiofrequency ablation.

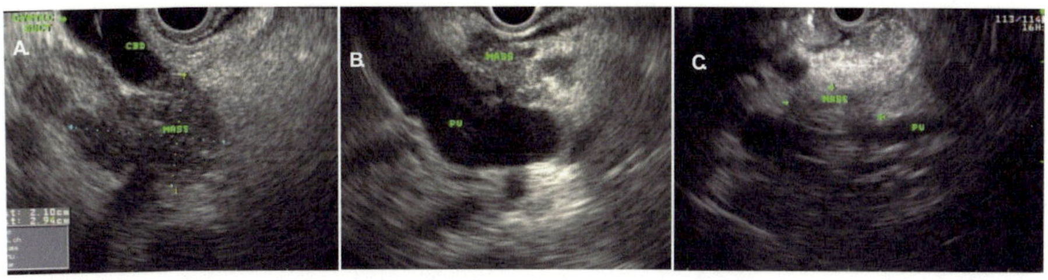

Figure 7. Mass in head of pancreas causing biliary obstruction (note both cystic duct and common bile duct are dilated)-A; The portal Vein PV-B and PV confluence (C).

EUS is not without limitations in the evaluation of patients with pancreatic cancer. In some cases pancreatic cancer might be indistinguishable from focal chronic pancreatitis (with or without focus of ductal adenocarcinoma), pancreatic intraepithelial neoplasms-PanINs, and patients with autoimmune pancreatitis. The ability of EUS alone in differentiating these from malignant lesions can be challenging and thus a multimodality diagnostic evaluation becomes necessary along with the history and physical exam findings. Tissue sampling for pathological evaluation might also be challenging with EUS as fine needle aspiration provides scant aspirate and core biopsies (by pro-core needles) might not give adequate histological architecture needed to make an accurate diagnosis. Further limitations of EUS are the result of anatomical constraints such as tumors located in the uncinate process because the acute angle of the echoendoscope in the second portion of the duodenum makes this location challenging for FNA sampling.

7.4. Endoscopic retrograde cholangiopancreatography

Endoscopic retrograde cholangiopancreatography (ERCP) has been used historically to allow direct visualization of the duodenum and ampulla, as well as delineation of the biliary and pancreatic ductal systems. ERCP may also be used to obtain "brush" samples for cytology and intra-ductal biopsies in order to increase diagnostic yield, especially in situations where EUS-FNA results are inconclusive. However, ERCP remains an invasive test with potential risks such as post ERCP-pancreatitis, which might result from injecting contrast to delineate a suspected malignant pancreatic duct stricture. Hence, the usefulness of ERCP as a primary diagnostic modality for pancreatic cancer has significantly decreased since the introduction of endoscopic ultrasonography. Currently, ERCP is not favored as an initial test for the diagnosis of adenocarcinoma of the pancreas. On the other hand, ERCP is generally reserved for therapeutic indications such as palliating patients with obstructive jaundice from pancreatic cancer with metastatic or locally advanced disease who are not candidates for resection. These patients benefit from biliary sphincterotomy and/or stent placement (Figure 8). Routine stenting of patients with resectable pancreatic cancer, however, has not shown clear benefits in patients that might be considered candidates for resection as this might lead to unjustified complications [50]. A new role of ERCP is evolving as a means to access the pancreatic duct for endoscopic pancreatic imaging and therapeutics.

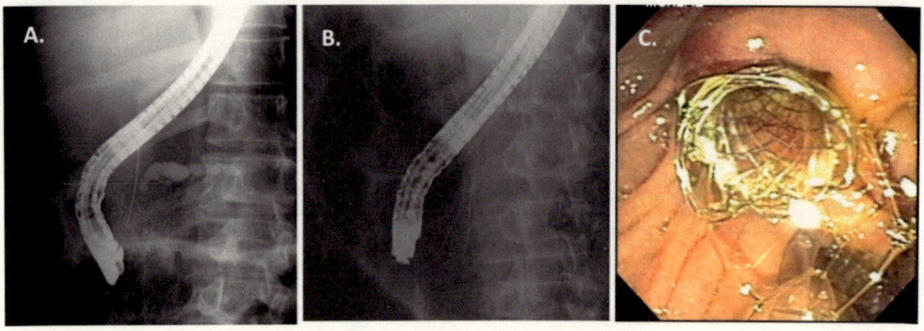

Figure 8. Malignant pancreatic stricture causing upstream pancreatic duct dilation. Note that the wire was advanced into the bile duct during ERCP to place biliary stent for palliation of obstructive jaundice (A). Placement of metallic biliary stent for palliation of obstructive jaundice in a patient with unresectable pancreatic cancer [fluoroscopic picture (B); endoscopic picture (C)]

7.5. Magnetic resonance cholangiopancreatography

Magnetic resonance cholangiopancreatography (MRCP) is better than CT in outlining the anatomy of biliary and pancreatic tree and can provide useful information in patients who have suspected biliary or pancreatic strictures. It can also provide a road map for future endoscopic therapy. MRI of the pancreas can provide valuable information about solid tumors of the pancreas as well as cystic neoplasms, and is generally comparable to MDCT in determining resectability (Figure 6) [51].

Centers without personnel experienced with EUS-FNA rely on percutaneous fine-needle aspiration (FNA) of pancreatic masses to establish a diagnosis. CT-guided percutaneous FNA performed by interventional radiologist carries a theoretical risk of malignant seeding of the needle tract, but no convincing data has proven this theory conclusively. The CT guided approach is technically easier for masses in the tail of the pancreas rather than the head. A negative result on tissue diagnosis with a suspicious mass on CT scan does not preclude surgical intervention. This approach can be helpful in patients who are considered poor candidates for any endoscopic intervention due to underlying co-morbidities and individuals who have unresectable disease.

http://dx.doi.org/10.5772/60451

7.6. Exploratory laparoscopy

Reportedly, 20% to 40% of patients staged by CT, MRI, ERCP or EUS will have undetected disseminated disease during exploratory laparoscopy. The use of laparoscopy has proponents that span usefulness [52-54] to an entirely unnecessary procedure. The main argument against its use emanates from the currently available non-invasive image modalities, which in the view of some clinicians eliminates the need for a further invasive procedure [55]. Laparoscopic exploration for patients with pancreatic lesions is best used selectively rather than routinely and may have a larger role in resectable tumors of the body and tail of the pancreas [56;57]. Selective criteria for patients with pancreatic cancer include tumors larger than 3 cm, a CA 19-9 level above 100 U/ml, and questionable imaging findings.

8. EUS combined modalities

There has been recent interest in mucosal imaging (as discussed below), but none has yet been accepted in the standard of care in diagnosing pancreatic cancer. Narrow band imaging technology uses light of specific blue and green wavelengths to enhance the detail of certain aspects of the surface of the mucosa. This technology has made it possible to visualize the wall of the pancreatic duct with the help of a small catheter inserted into the pancreatic duct ('pancreatoscopy') [58].

Optical endomicroscopy using a small diameter probe advanced into the pancreatic duct, at the time of ERCP or EUS, allows real time microscopic imaging of the epithelial lining of the pancreatic duct and pancreatic cyst wall. This allows direct high yield targeted tissue sampling in the region of interest. Two modalities used in this fashion include confocal laser endomicroscopy (CLE) [59;60] and high resolution microendoscopy [59;61]. On the other hand, optical coherence tomography uses infrared light to scan areas beneath the mucosal lining of the duct but the field of view is limited to only a few millimeters making evaluation of the entire pancreatic duct difficult and time consuming [62].

During intraductal ultrasound (IDUS), a mini-ultrasound probe is advanced into the main pancreatic duct to evaluate the wall of the pancreatic duct in indeterminate pancreatic strictures. This allows diagnosis of early pancreatic cancers and outlines margins of IPMNs before surgical resection [63;64]. IDUS is not widely used in United States due to the risk of pancreatitis associated with the procedure and inability to obtain tissue for pathological examination [65]. Another modality using EUS, contrast enhanced EUS, utilizes intravenous contrast to highlight the echogenicity and enhancement of a lesion [66]. In a recent meta-analysis, the pooled sensitivity of contrast-enhanced EUS for the differential diagnosis of pancreatic adenocarcinomas was 94% (95% CI, 0.91-0.95), and the specificity was 89% (95% CI, 0.85-0.92) [67].

EUS elastography allows quantitative analysis of tissue stiffness and helps differentiate pancreatic cancers from benign conditions such as chronic pancreatitis. In one study, the sensitivity and specificity for detecting pancreatic malignancies was 100% and 92.9% respectively [68]. Three-dimensional reconstruction and spectrum analysis using EUS has shown promising results, and will likely be used more often in the future [69].

9. Novel diagnostic imaging modalities

Because pancreatic cancer might metastasize at an early stage, an ideal imaging modality is one that would predict the biological behavior of the tumor. Understanding the molecular aspects of pancreatic cancer has facilitated use of investigational modalities in this area. Imaging agents such as peptides that bind to specific factors on the surface of pancreatic tumors have been developed and include: plectin 1 (Plec 1), integrin $\alpha_v\beta_6$, cathepsin E and claudin-4 [70-73]. Early studies have shown promising results, but more work is needed before routine clinical use.

A similar approach, but by interrogating normal tissue has also been investigated. Montet *et al.* demonstrated that as pancreatic tumors do not express receptors for bombesin, a bombesin peptide-coupled nanoparticle (BN-CLIO[Cy5.5]) can be used to image normal pancreas and hence, differentiate it from pancreatic tumors [74]. Similarly, a novel concept of microbubbles, small gas –filled microspheres, has been used in preliminary studies to image the peri-tumoral vasculature with the assistance of ultrasound. Moreover, this technology can also be used as a vehicle to deliver anti-cancer therapies [75].

10. Treatment

10.1. Surgical intervention

Surgery offers the only possibility for long term survival, however the majority (>85%) of patients with pancreatic cancer will present with unresectable or metastatic disease [76]. Removal of all disease offers the patient the only chance of long-term survival. Those who undergo surgical resection have a disappointing ~20% 5-year survival. Over the years it has become clear that the indications for surgical intervention have been substantially widened. Typically, the current criteria dictates possible resection for tumors stage I-A to II-B [77]. There are no randomized trials that assess resectability criteria to guide surgical intervention. In the absence of controlled trials, the best recommendations emanate from consensus guidelines [40, 78, 79]. It is practical to classify pancreatic tumors into one of three categories following diagnostic imaging [77]:

i. **Resectable Tumors**: These are tumors localized to the pancreas. In this case, there is no evidence of SMV or portal vein involvement of any kind. A plane of dissection indicated by a fat pad between the SMA, celiac axis, and hepatic artery and the pancreas has to be identified by CT scan as well as absent involvement of the SMV and portal vein [40, 78]. These patients should proceed with surgical intervention.

ii. **Borderline Resectable Tumors**: There is a dynamic criteria for resection of these tumors that continues to change based on the ability of specialized centers to perform complex arterial/venous/portal resection and reconstruction [79]. These tumors include those that have (A) Severe SMV-portal impingement (unilateral or bilateral), (B) SMA/celiac artery involvement, but less than 180°, (C) Hepatic artery involvement with the possibility of reconstruction, and (D) SMV occlusion or involvement with

http://dx.doi.org/10.5772/60451

the possibility of reconstruction [40, 77]. These patients should undergo surgical intervention at the discretion of highly specialized pancreatic cancer centers, undergo neoajuvant treatment, and/or enrollment in clinical trials.

iii. **Unresectable Tumors**: These are tumors in which distant or extensive lymph node metastatic disease has been identified. Involvement of vasculature beyond resection or malignant ascites are also considered contra-indications for resection (i.e. major venous thrombosis of the portal vein or SMA that extends for several centimeters or circumferential encasement of the SMA) [78]. Resectability is best determined preoperatively rather than intraoperatively. These patients are candidates for chemotherapeutic interventions and enrollment in clinical trials as well as palliative interventions depending on degree of the disease.

According to a consensus statement by the American Hepato-Pancreato-Biliary Association, tissue obtained via EUS guided FNA is only required prior to surgery if neoadjuvant chemoradiation is indicated. However, if there is sufficient evidence for pancreatic adenocarcinoma based on history, physical exam, and diagnostic modalities; no tissue is required in good surgical candidates prior to surgical intervention [78].

11. Surgical intervention for tumors of the pancreatic head

Extirpation of pancreatic tumors at the head of the pancreas require pancreatic and duodenal resection as well as common bile duct re-implantation with reconstruction. The pacreaticoduodenectomy procedure (Figure 9) was first described in 1909 by Walter Kausch. Twenty six years later, the success with the procedure in three patients was reported at the American Surgical Association by Allen O. Whipple and Parson. The pancreaticodudenectomy procedure then became widely performed and it is commonly referred to as the Whipple procedure. Although, it's original description was a two-stage operative approach, it was rapidly modified [80]. The commonly known one-stage Whipple operation is credited to Trimble's group from John Hopkins in 1941 [81]. The drastic increase in the number of operations performed today is represented by the experience at Mass General where between 1940 and 1950, twenty pancreaticoduodenectomies were performed; while, between 2005-2011 813 were described (~125 per year) [82].

Technical considerations for standard pancreaticoduodenectomy (PD) have been reviewed extensively [83]. The proposed lines of resection are shown in (Figure 9). The general exploration of the abdomen includes careful inspection of the peritoneal surfaces and liver for metastases, which can be more accurately determined by intra-operative liver ultrasonography. Suspicious lymph nodes need to be submitted for frozen section histology to evaluate for metastatic disease. The presence of peritoneal implants and liver metastases render the patient incurable. Similarly, histologically proven metastases in lymph nodes accessible during the initial abdominal exploration makes the chance of cure highly remote.

Following abdominal exploration, the right colon is mobilized and retracted medially; a technique known as the Cattell-Braasch maneuver. The lesser sac is entered and posterior attachments of the stomach are divided. The superior mesenteric vein is identified by tracing the middle colic vein proximally, or after Kocherization by following the sweep of the duodenum medially. The gallbladder is mobilized and the common hepatic duct and gastroduodenal arteries are divided. These maneuvers allow exposure of the anterior surface of the portal vein. The portal vein and superior mesenteric vein are carefully separated from the overlying pancreas. The stomach (or duodenum in cases of pylorus-preserving pancreaticoduodenectomy [PPPD]), small bowel, and pancreas are then divided sequentially. The uncinate process is liberated from its retroperitoneal attachments to complete the dissection. Gastrointestinal continuity is re-established by a pancraticojejunostomy (or pancreaticogastrostomy), choledocojejunostomy, and gastrojejunostomy (or duodenojejunostomy in the case of PPPD). Anastomoses are done in sequence: pancreas, then bile duct, then stomach (or duodenum in the case of PPPD) (Figure 9).

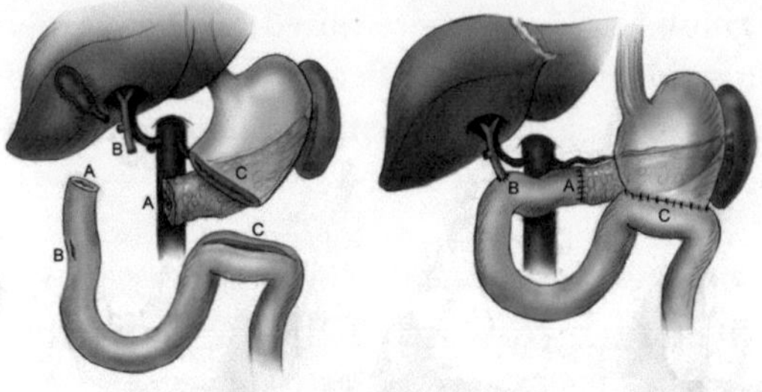

Figure 9. Lines of resection of the typical pancreaticodoudenectomy. Reconstruction is performed in order from A to C.

PPPD is a modification of the standard Whipple procedure in which the entire stomach, including the pylorus, and 2 cm to 3 cm of the duodenal cuff, are preserved. This modification retains the entire stomach as a reservoir and may prevent the development of postgastrectomy syndromes, marginal ulceration, and enterogastric reflux. PPPD is touted to result in shorter operative times, less blood loss, and fewer transfusions. PPPD was first described by Dr. Warshaw in 1981 and has been the largest variation of the procedure since the one-stage approach was introduced in clinical practice [83]. However, delayed gastric emptying without much further benefit has led to a change back to the gastrojejunostomy approach in some centers, but this remains a point of controversy [84, 85].

Pancreaticojejunostomy may be performed as an end to-end "dunking" procedure, an end-to-side anastomosis between pancreas and jejunum, or an end-to-side duct-to-mucosa anastomosis. A duct-to mucosa anastomosis may be performed over a stent and left in place for pancreatic ducts less than 5 mm. The primary theoretical advantage of duct-to-mucosa pancreaticojejunostomy is long-term patency. Pancreaticogastrostomy (PG) is performed in an end-to-side fashion. There is no evidence that the type of pancreatic-enteric anastomosis affects the rate of pancreatic fistula. Because pancreatic fistulas remain the most serious complication of the operation, a pancreaticogastrostomy (PG) instead of a pancreaticojejunostomy (PJ) has been performed by some surgeons. Randomized controlled trials (n=3) have not shown a difference in complications with these two approaches. However, thirteen non-randomized observational clinical studies have been in favor of PG [86]. Further studies are needed to clarify these findings.

http://dx.doi.org/10.5772/60451

The biliary and pancreatic anastomoses are drained and jejunostomy (for feeding) and gastrostomy (for decompression) tubes are placed prior to closure. Routine placement of feeding and decompression tubes is paramount in the postoperative management of patients following a pancreaticodudodenectomy.

Total pancreatectomy for pancreatic cancer is rarely performed. Total pancreatectomy had been proposed to obtain superior tumor margins and provide a more extensive lymph node dissection. In practice, total pancreatectomy is associated with increased postoperative mortality and no change in survival compared to standard pancreaticodudenectomy. Postoperative diabetes is extremely difficult to manage in patients undergoing total pancreatectomy. Similarly, extensive lymph node dissection does not improve survival and leads to a higher complication rate [87].

Fifteen percent of pancreatic adenocarcinomas occur in the body and the tail of the pancreas. Because these tumors typically do not cause biliary obstruction, its diagnosis is not made until the disease is advanced and unresectable. Only 5% to 7% of individuals with adenocarcinoma of the body or the tail of the pancreas undergo resection and their survival is much worse compared to patients with adenocarcinoma of the head of the pancreas [77]. Distal pancreatectomy with splenectomy is reserved for rare instances when the tumor located in the body or the tail of the pancreas is resectable.

11.1. Laparoscopic Pancreaticoduodenectomy

While the formidable Whipple remains one of the most complex abdominal operations performed today, at some centers it has become common practice where several open operations are performed in a week at Johns Hopkins or Mass General. With the continued advancement in laparoscopic technique and popularity of this approach to surgical intervention, there has been a rapid acceptance of more advanced laparoscopic approaches to patients with cancer. The first total laparoscopic pancreaticoduedenectomy was described by Gagner and Pomp in 1994 and constitutes one of the most advanced laparoscopic procedures today [88;89]. Between the time it was first described to 2009, 146 laparoscopic pancreaticoduodenectomies were performed worldwide. A large series has been reported by Palanivelu and colleagues which included 45 pancreaticoduodenectomies between 1998 and 2010 of which 18 were for pancreatic adenocarcinoma [90]. Another large report from the U.S. included 65 cases of laparoscopic pancreaticoduodenectomy and documented a morbidity of 42% and a mortality of 1.5% [89]. A more recent review reported 10 case series totaling 150 totally laparoscopic pancreaticoduodenectomies. In this review, mortality and morbidity have been comparable to the open approach. Operative time for this cohort has been 483 minutes and length of hospital stay 14.1 days [91]. The leading authors on these studies have concluded that the laparoscopic Whipple is feasible and safe. However, in the absence of controlled trials this approach remains experimental.

11.2. Robotic pancreaticoduodenectomy

The first pancreaticoduodenectomy was described in 1909 by Kausch. In 1935 AO Whipple described three successful cases via a two-stage approach [80]. One-stage Whipple was introduced in 1941 by Trimble [81]. No major variations occurred in technique until preservation of the pylorus was introduced by Warshaw in 1981 [85]. These changes in operative technique were not as radical as the introduction of the minimally invasive approach. The laparoscopic pancreaticoduodenectomy was introduced by Gagner and Pomp in 1994 [88]. Almost 100 years later, the first human robotic surgery was described by Himpens in 1997 [92] and the first robotic pancreaticoduodenectomy is credited to Giulianotti in 2000 [93]. While several limitations still exist, robotic surgery is the most innovative technology brought to the operating room in the last century.

A recent systematic review of the robotic approach demonstrated that up to date, 203 patients have had an intention to treat approach to a pancreaticoduodenectomy [94]. While the technical approach is wide and not clearly defined, the number of reported cases appears to be increasing over the past few years. In Cirocchi's review, the conversion rate was 14%, overall morbidity 58% and reoperation occurred in 7.3% of the cases [94]. Totally robotic technique has been reported by several surgeons [93;95-98]. While oncologic operations (R0) have been performed with similar morbidity and mortality to the open Whipple, the innovative nature of this approach makes it highly experimental and should only be undertaken in specialized centers. Similarly, cost analysis must be addressed in subsequent studies.

12. Outcomes

In the United States, there has been a substantial increase in the number of pancreaticoduodenectomies performed. The average age of patients undergoing surgical intervention has also increased from 1991 to 2005. Similarly, more patients with a higher index of comorbidities underwent Whipples during this time. In spite of this, perioperative morbidity remained unchanged (53%) and 30-day mortality decreased from 6% to 3% in this cohort of patients [1].

The mortality rate in high volume centers performing pancreaticoduodenectomies is 2-4% [99]. However, perioperative morbidity remains substantially high (15% to 50%) even at high volume centers [100]. In patients undergoing resection for cure and treated with neoadjuvant chemoradiation, the 5-year survival is still disappointingly low (10% to 20%) [101-106]. In a study using the Surveillance, Epidemiology, and End Results-Medicare data inclusive of 2,461 patients investigating outcomes and use of adjuvant therapy between 1991 and 2005 in the USA, the median survival of patients treated for cure was 14 months, the 1-, 3-, and 5- year survival was 53.2%, 19.7%, and 12.6%, respectively. This study, demonstrated that the use of adjuvant chemoradiotherapy led to a 2 month increase in overall survival [1]. A study from Johns Hopkins examining temporal variation in morbidity and mortality following pancreaticoduodenectomy found a magnificent decrease in mortality to 4% (1981-1986) from 24% (1969-1980) with an accompanying decrease in morbidity from 59% to 36% during the same periods. The 5-year survival in patients with pancreatic cancer was 18% [107]. Thus, while the number of patients undergoing pancreaticoduodenectomy has increased with a variable decrease in complications, the overall mortality has not improved in most high volume centers [108].

http://dx.doi.org/10.5772/60451

13. Morbidity

Postoperative complications occur in 25-50% of patients following this operation. Delayed gastric emptying, even with standard definitions by the International Study Group of Pancreatic Surgery, occurs in a wide range of 14% to 45% and constitutes the most common complication following pancreaticoduodenectomy [109-111]. Erythromycin or metoclopramide may reduce the incidence of gastric emptying by only 37% [112]. Thus, a jejunostomy tube for prolonged postoperative feeding as well as a gastrostomy tube for postoperative decompression should be routinely employed during pancreaticoduodenectomy.

Pancreatic fistula (defined as the output of more than 50 cc of amylase-rich fluid) accompanies 5%-30% of cases [113-117] and is directly responsible for up to 20% of postoperative deaths [115;117], which constitutes the most serious complication of pancreaticoduodenectomy. Pancreatic fistula indicates disruption of the pancreatic-enteric anastomosis and occurs at the same rate regardless of anastomosis (i.e. pancreaticogastrostomy *vs.* pancreaticojejunostomy), modified drainage strategies, or somatostatin administration [118].

Disruption of biliary and gastric anastomoses are rare and less serious. Patients with pancreatic fistula may be completely asymptomatic if it is a controlled fistula and the output is well captured by the drain. These patients do well with a clear liquid diet, enteral nutrition through a jejunostomy tube, or parenteral nutrition. A CT scan should be performed to exclude abdominal fluid collections. The benefits of somatostatin in this setting are unclear. Diet may be progressively advanced as output decreases. Eighty percent of patients can be managed conservatively. An additional 10%-15% of patients with this complication respond well to percutaneous drainage.

Patients with sepsis or hemorrhage related to pancreaticoenteric anastomotic disruption necessitate immediate and aggressive intervention. Septic patients who do not respond to aggressive medical management within 48 hours should be explored. Hemorrhage associated with pancreatic fistulas can be managed with angiographic embolization. Patients who require operative exploration and have diffuse retroperitoneal hemorrhage and necrosis require completion pancreatectomy. The rare cases of hemobilia and hemopancreaticus are best diagnosed and treated angiographically.

Endocrine pancreatic function is rarely impaired and diabetes is unusual following pancreaticoduodenectomy. Exocrine pancreatic function, on the other hand, is affected to various degrees and in severe cases may require lifelong exogenous enzyme supplementation.

14. Neoadjuvant therapy

There are no randomized controlled trials that compare neoadjuvant to adjuvant therapy for patients with resectable disease. Potential benefits of neoadjuvant therapy include identifying those patients with occult metastatic disease thereby selecting patients who would probably not benefit from surgery. Another potential benefit is avoiding delay in chemotherapy for those patients who have postoperative complications or prolonged recovery. Conversely, the response rates to neoadjuvant therapy are low (9-12%) which may allow for disease progression with the delay of surgery [119;120]. Since there is stronger data supporting adjuvant therapy, most centers prefer this approach over neoadjuvant therapy for patients with resectable disease.

Patients with borderline resectable cancer or locally advanced disease can be treated with neoadjuvant therapy with the goal of down-staging allowing for possible resection. Currently, there is no defined optimal neoadjuvant therapy for this population of patients supported by randomized controlled trials. The National Comprehensive Cancer Network recommends that patients with borderline resectable disease undergo a laparotomy followed by resection if possible or upfront neoadjuvant therapy. Available options for neoadjuvant therapy include FOLFIRINOX, gemcitabine, gemcitabine-based combination therapy, capecitabine or continuous infusion 5-FU [40]. It is suggested that chemoradiation should be reserved for patients who do not develop metastatic disease while receiving chemotherapy [40]. A meta-analysis showed that 31.6% of patients with initially borderline/unresectable tumors treated with neoadjuvant therapy were able to undergo resections. These patients had a median survival of 22 months which appears comparable to those patients with initially resectable disease [120].

15. Adjuvant therapy

Only about 15-20% of cases of pancreatic cancer are considered resectable. Even after resection the prognosis is poor with 5-year survival rates approximating 20% [121]. Systemic chemotherapy and radiation have been used adjuvantly to improve the survival rates. However the optimal choice of adjuvant therapy remains quite controversial. There have been several phase III studies evaluating therapy in the adjuvant setting; these are summarized in Table 2. The GITSG Trial compared concurrent 5-FU based chemoradiation with observation alone after resection. This study was closed early due to slow accrual and only had 49 patients enrolled at the time of analysis. The GITSG Trial showed an improved survival benefit (median survival 20 months *vs.* 11 months, p=0.03) favoring the concurrent chemoradiation group [122]. The GITSG study was followed up by the EORTC study which was similar in design, comparing 5-FU based concurrent chemoradiation to observation. The EORTC study demonstrated no survival advantage with adjuvant therapy. The 2-year survival was 26% *vs.* 34% for the observation and treatment arms respectively; this difference was not statistically significant [123]. The ESPAC-1 Trial had a 2 x 2 factorial design in which they compared concurrent chemoradiation, chemotherapy, chemoradiation followed by chemotherapy or observation. This study was only powered to compare the chemotherapy *vs.* no chemotherapy group and the chemoradiotherapy *vs.* no chemoradiotherapy group. The results showed a statistically significant improved median survival for those patients who received chemotherapy (20.1 months) compared to those patients who did not receive chemotherapy (15.5 months). Interestingly this study demonstrated a worse median survival for patients receiving chemoradiotherapy (15.9 months) compared to those patients that did not receive chemoradiotherapy (17.9 months) [124]. Three trials were done evaluating the efficacy of gemcitabine. The CONKO-001 trial compared adjuvant gemcitabine to observation. The trial showed a statistically significant improvement in median disease free survival of 13.4 months (gemcitabine

http://dx.doi.org/10.5772/60451

arm) compared to 6.9 months (observation arm). There was no difference in overall survival, but this was attributed to the fact that most patients in the observation arm received gemcitabine on relapse [104]. Two trials compared 5-FU with gemcitabine. In the RTOG 9704 study all patients received concurrent 5-FU based chemoradiation with either 5-FU or gemcitabine given before and after. The ESPAC-3 trial compared adjuvant 5-FU to gemcitabine without the use of radiation. Both of these studies showed no survival advantage for one arm over the other. However in the RTOG 9704 study those patients stratified to the gemcitabine arm did have a greater proportion of T3 or T4 disease which may account for no improvement in survival. The ESPAC-3 trial did demonstrate that gemcitabine was associated with fewer adverse events [104;124]. The treatment practice for these patients can be quite variable. Some advocate for adjuvant chemotherapy alone without radiotherapy based on the EORTC and ESPAC-1 trials. Others continue to advocate for radiotherapy given the high risk of local failure and the benefit seen in the GITSG study. The dose of radiation given in these studies would be considered suboptimal by today's standards which the supporters of radiotherapy argue explains why the benefit was not seen in the EORTC and ESPAC-1 studies.

Trial	Intervention	Results	Conclusions
GITSG	Concurrent CRT (5-FU) ->maintenance 5-FU Observation	**Median Survival** 20 mos vs. 11 mos P=0.03	-Survival benefit of CRT followed by maintenance chemo
EORTC	Concurrent CRT (5-FU, 40Gy) Observation	**2-yr Survival** 34% vs. 26% P=0.099	-No statistically survival benefit observed
ESPAC-1	Observation Chemotherapy (5-FU/L) CRT (5-FU/L) CRT -> Chemo (5-FU/L)	**5-yr Survival** 10% (CRT) vs. 20% (no CRT) P=0.05 21% (chemo) vs. 8%(no chemo) P=0.009	-Adjuvant chemo has a survival benefit -CRT with a deleterious effect on survival
RTOG 9704	5-FU pre and post CRT Gemcitabine pre and post CRT	**Median Survival** 17.1 mos vs. 20.5 mos P=0.08	-No improvement of Gemcitabine over 5-FU
CONKO-001	Gemcitabine Observation	**Median DFS** 13.4 mos vs. 6.9 mos P<0.001 **Median Survival** 22.8 mos vs. 20.2 mos. P=0.005 (update from 2008)	-Gemcitabine improved DFS. -Updated survival data shows a benefit with Gemcitabine
ESPAC-3	5-FU Gemcitabine	**Median Survival** 23 mos vs. 23.6 mos P=0.39 **Serious Adverse Events** 14% vs. 7.5% P<0.001	-No difference in survival -Gemcitabine associated with less toxicity

Table 2. Phase III Adjuvant Therapy Trials

16. Metastatic disease

Systemic therapy for metastatic pancreatic cancer is aimed at minimizing disease-related symptoms and prolonging survival. For several years the standard of care was 5-fluorouracil (5-FU)-based combinations with an observed survival benefit over best supportive care. The median survival with 5-FU-based combinations on average approximates 6 months versus 3 to 4 months with best supportive care [125]. In 1996, gemcitabine was approved for treatment of metastatic pancreatic cancer after a phase III trial demonstrated a clinical benefit response of 23.8% for those in the gemcitabine group compared to only 4.8% in the 5-FU group (P=0.0022). Secondary endpoints evaluated in the trial included survival rate, which at 12 months was 18% for the gemcitabine arm and 2% for the 5-FU arm [126]. Several gemcitabine-based combinations have been investigated with the goal of further improving its therapeutic efficacy. Sun *et al.* performed a meta-analysis investigating gemcitabine-based combinations compared with gemcitabine monotherapy. The meta-analysis found that combination therapy provided a modest 1-year overall survival with a RR of 0.90 (P=0.04). However, this benefit with combination therapy was associated with more grade 3-4 toxicities including vomiting, diarrhea, neutropenia, anemia and thrombocytopenia. Based on subgroup analyses patients with a good performance status appeared to derive the most survival benefit from combination therapy [127]. The combination of gemcitabine and erlotinib was compared to gemcitabine alone in a phase III trial where a very modest improvement in median survival was observed (6.24 months *vs.* 5.91 months). In this study, 53% of samples were classified as EGFR positive. Interestingly EGFR status did not have any association with response or disease stability [128]. In 2011, Conroy *et al.* reported results of a randomized controlled trial of FOLFIRINOX compared to gemcitabine. The combination chemotherapy regimen improved the objective response rate from 9.4% in the gemcitabine group to 31.6% in the FOLIRINOX group (P<0.001). Median survival was also improved to 11.1 months in the FOLFIRNOX arm compared to 6.8 months in the gemcitabine arm (P<0.001). The combination chemotherapy, as seen with prior combination regimens, was associated with more adverse events [129]. Recently, the combination of nab-paclitaxel and gemcitabine was approved for first-line therapy in metastatic adenocarcinoma of the pancreas. Objective response rates were 23% and 7% in the nab-paclitaxel plus gemcitabine arm and single agent gemcitabine arms, respectively (P<0.0001). Progression free survival was also improved with a median PFS of 5.5 months in the combination arms compared with 3.7 months in the single agent arm (P<0.0001). There was also an observed median survival benefit of 8.5 months for the nab-paclitaxel plus gemcitabine arm while the single agent gemcitabine arm only had a median survival of 6.7 months (P<0.0001) [130] (Table 3).

17. Palliation

Palliation of pancreatic cancer patients may be the goal of operative exploration or may result from operative findings indicating unresectablility. Palliation can be performed

http://dx.doi.org/10.5772/60451

Study	Intervention	Results
Burris et al. 1997 Phase III	Gemcitabine 5-FU	**Clinical Benefit Response** 23.8% vs. 4.8% P=0.0022 **Median Survival** 5.65 mos vs. 4.41 mos P=0.0025
Moore et al. 2007 Phase III	Gemcitabine + Erlotinib Gemcitabine + Placebo	**Median Survival** 6.24 mos vs. 5.91 mos P=0.038
Sun et al. 2012 Meta-analysis	Gemcitabine monotherapy Gemcitabine combination therapy	**Objective Response Rate** RR, 0.72; 95% CI: 0.63-0.83 P<0.001 **1-yr Overall Survival** RR, 0.90; 95% CI: 0.82-0.99 P=0.04
Conroy et al. 2011 Phase III	FOLFIRINOX Gemcitabine	**Median Survival** 11.1 mos vs. 6.8 mos P<0.001 **Median PFS** 6.4 mos vs. 3.3 mos P<0.001
Von Hoff et al. 2013 Phase III	Nab-Paclitaxel + Gemcitabine Gemcitabine	**Median Survival** 8.5 mos vs. 6.7 mos P<0.0001 **PFS** 5.5 mos vs. 3.7 mos P<0.0001

Table 3. Selected studies for palliative chemotherapy in the metastatic setting

operatively and nonoperatively and this decision should be individualized depending on the overall status of the patient. Whether palliation is accomplished operatively or nonoperatively, relief of obstructive jaundice, duodenal obstruction, and back pain are the primary goals. About 65% to 75% of patients with pancreatic cancer will develop symptoms of obstructive jaundice [131]. In patients with obstructive jaundice endoscopic biliary stenting and surgical biliary bypass are palliative options. Endoscopic biliary stenting is associated with lower complication rates and shorter hospital stays while maintaining similar efficacy and overall survival compared with surgical bypass [132]. In the event that endoscopic management is not successful, external biliary drainage can be attempted. Duodenal obstruction develops in about 15% to 20% of patients with pancreatic cancer [133]. Traditionally duodenal obstruction had been palliated with gastrojejunostomy, but with data showing similar efficacy with enteral stents, improved cost-effectiveness and shorter hospitalizations this option has become a viable alternative [134].

Most patients with pancreatic cancer, at some point in their disease course, will experience severe cancer-related pain. This pain can be a severely debilitating symptom leading to poor quality of life and decreasing performance status. In addition to systemic analgesics, regional celiac plexus nerve block is effective at alleviating pain [135]. In general, endoscopic palliative measures are preferred for those patients with known unresectable disease or those with a poor performance status. For patients who are discovered to have unresectable or metastatic disease on open exploration and expected to have a life expectancy of at least 3 to 6 months operative palliative measures (choledochojejunostomy, gastrojejunostomy and intraoperative chemical splanchnicectomy) can be considered for symptoms of obstruction and pain [136].

18. Conclusions

Multiple diagnostic and therapeutic modalities in the evaluation and treatment of pancreatic cancer have not resulted in a meaningful survival advantage in patients with pancreatic cancer. This dismal performance is primarily related to the inherent aggressive tumor biology of pancreatic adenocarcinoma. Early diagnosis and curative resection, when possible, holds promise for better survival but surgery in itself carries a definite morbidity and mortality, even in specialized centers. Hence, pancreatic adenocarcinoma should be managed at high volume centers in a multi-disciplinary setting and in light of proposed guidelines, until better treatment options are available in the future.

Author details

Zeeshan Ramzan, Phat Le, Payal Kapur and Sergio Huerta*

*Address all correspondence to: Sergio.Huerta@UTSouthwestern.edu

University of Texas Southwestern Medical Center / VA North Texas Health Care System, USA

References

[1] Mayo SC, Gilson MM, Herman JM, Cameron JL, Nathan H, Edil BH et al. Management of patients with pancreatic adenocarcinoma: national trends in patient selection, operative management, and use of adjuvant therapy. J Am Coll Surg 2012; 214(1):33-45.

http://dx.doi.org/10.5772/60451

[2] Siegel R, Naishadham D, Jemal A. Cancer statistics, 2012. CA Cancer J Clin 2012; 62(1):10-29.

[3] Jemal A, Murray T, Samuels A, Ghafoor A, Ward E, Thun MJ. Cancer statistics, 2003. CA Cancer J Clin 2003; 53(1):5-26.

[4] Jemal A, Tiwari RC, Murray T, Ghafoor A, Samuels A, Ward E et al. Cancer statistics, 2004. CA Cancer J Clin 2004; 54(1):8-29.

[5] Jemal A, Murray T, Ward E, Samuels A, Tiwari RC, Ghafoor A et al. Cancer statistics, 2005. CA Cancer J Clin 2005; 55(1):10-30.

[6] Jemal A, Siegel R, Ward E, Murray T, Xu J, Smigal C et al. Cancer statistics, 2006. CA Cancer J Clin 2006; 56(2):106-130.

[7] Jemal A, Siegel R, Ward E, Murray T, Xu J, Thun MJ. Cancer statistics, 2007. CA Cancer J Clin 2007; 57(1):43-66.

[8] Jemal A, Siegel R, Ward E, Hao Y, Xu J, Murray T et al. Cancer statistics, 2008. CA Cancer J Clin 2008; 58(2):71-96.

[9] Jemal A, Siegel R, Ward E, Hao Y, Xu J, Thun MJ. Cancer statistics, 2009. CA Cancer J Clin 2009; 59(4):225-249.

[10] Jemal A, Siegel R, Xu J, Ward E. Cancer statistics, 2010. CA Cancer J Clin 2010; 60(5): 277-300.

[11] Siegel R, Ward E, Brawley O, Jemal A. Cancer statistics, 2011: the impact of eliminating socioeconomic and racial disparities on premature cancer deaths. CA Cancer J Clin 2011; 61(4):212-236.

[12] Siegel R, Naishadham D, Jemal A. Cancer statistics, 2013. CA Cancer J Clin 2013; 63(1):11-30.

[13] Yeo TP, Hruban RH, Leach SD, Wilentz RE, Sohn TA, Kern SE et al. Pancreatic cancer. Curr Probl Cancer 2002; 26(4):176-275.

[14] Hassan MM, Bondy ML, Wolff RA, Abbruzzese JL, Vauthey JN, Pisters PW et al. Risk factors for pancreatic cancer: case-control study. Am J Gastroenterol 2007; 102(12):2696-2707.

[15] Fuchs CS, Colditz GA, Stampfer MJ, Giovannucci EL, Hunter DJ, Rimm EB et al. A prospective study of cigarette smoking and the risk of pancreatic cancer. Arch Intern Med 1996; 156(19):2255-2260.

[16] Ben Q, Xu M, Ning X, Liu J, Hong S, Huang W et al. Diabetes mellitus and risk of pancreatic cancer: A meta-analysis of cohort studies. Eur J Cancer 2011; 47(13): 1928-1937.

[17] Michaud DS, Giovannucci E, Willett WC, Colditz GA, Stampfer MJ, Fuchs CS. Physical activity, obesity, height, and the risk of pancreatic cancer. JAMA 2001; 286(8): 921-929.

[18] Stolzenberg-Solomon RZ, Blaser MJ, Limburg PJ, Perez-Perez G, Taylor PR, Virtamo J et al. Helicobacter pylori seropositivity as a risk factor for pancreatic cancer. J Natl Cancer Inst 2001; 93(12):937-941.

[19] Lowenfels AB, Maisonneuve P, Cavallini G, Ammann RW, Lankisch PG, Andersen JR et al. Pancreatitis and the risk of pancreatic cancer. International Pancreatitis Study Group. N Engl J Med 1993; 328(20):1433-1437.

[20] Wolpin BM, Chan AT, Hartge P, Chanock SJ, Kraft P, Hunter DJ et al. ABO blood group and the risk of pancreatic cancer. J Natl Cancer Inst 2009; 101(6):424-431.

[21] Shi C, Hruban RH, Klein AP. Familial pancreatic cancer. Arch Pathol Lab Med 2009; 133(3):365-374.

[22] Tersmette AC, Petersen GM, Offerhaus GJ, Falatko FC, Brune KA, Goggins M et al. Increased risk of incident pancreatic cancer among first-degree relatives of patients with familial pancreatic cancer. Clin Cancer Res 2001; 7(3):738-744.

[23] Klein AP, Hruban RH, Brune KA, Petersen GM, Goggins M. Familial pancreatic cancer. Cancer J 2001; 7(4):266-273.

[24] Raimondi S, Maisonneuve P, Lowenfels AB. Epidemiology of pancreatic cancer: an overview. Nat Rev Gastroenterol Hepatol 2009; 6(12):699-708.

[25] Kloppel G. Mixed exocrine-endocrine tumors of the pancreas. Semin Diagn Pathol 2000; 17(2):104-108.

[26] Hiotis SP, Klimstra DS, Conlon KC, Brennan MF. Results after pancreatic resection for metastatic lesions. Ann Surg Oncol 2002; 9(7):675-679.

[27] Hruban RH, Goggins M, Parsons J, Kern SE. Progression model for pancreatic cancer. Clin Cancer Res 2000; 6(8):2969-2972.

[28] Hruban RH, van Mansfeld AD, Offerhaus GJ, van Weering DH, Allison DC, Goodman SN et al. K-ras oncogene activation in adenocarcinoma of the human pancreas. A study of 82 carcinomas using a combination of mutant-enriched polymerase chain reaction analysis and allele-specific oligonucleotide hybridization. Am J Pathol 1993; 143(2):545-554.

[29] Wilentz RE, Iacobuzio-Donahue CA, Argani P, McCarthy DM, Parsons JL, Yeo CJ et al. Loss of expression of Dpc4 in pancreatic intraepithelial neoplasia: evidence that DPC4 inactivation occurs late in neoplastic progression. Cancer Res 2000; 60(7): 2002-2006.

[30] Jones S, Zhang X, Parsons DW, Lin JC, Leary RJ, Angenendt P et al. Core signaling pathways in human pancreatic cancers revealed by global genomic analyses. Science 2008; 321(5897):1801-1806.

[31] Hidalgo M. Pancreatic cancer. N Engl J Med 2010; 362(17):1605-1617.

[32] Winter JM, Cameron JL, Campbell KA, Arnold MA, Chang DC, Coleman J et al. 1423 pancreaticoduodenectomies for pancreatic cancer: A single-institution experience. J Gastrointest Surg 2006; 10(9):1199-1210.

[33] Murr MM, Sarr MG, Oishi AJ, van Heerden JA. Pancreatic cancer. CA Cancer J Clin 1994; 44(5):304-318.

[34] Huerta S, Arteaga J, Li Z, Livingston EH. Acinar cell carcinoma of the pancreas in a morbidly obese patient. Pancreas 2002; 25(4):414-415.

[35] Memon AA, Soomro MI, Soomro QA. Courvoisier's law revisited. J Coll Physicians Surg Pak 2012; 22(6):392-394.

[36] Soman AD, Collins JM, DePetris G, Decker GA, Silva A, Moss A et al. Isolated supraclavicular lymph node metastasis in pancreatic adenocarcinoma: a report of three cases and review of the literature. JOP 2010; 11(6):604-609.

[37] Shimizu H, Maegawa J, Ho T, Yamamoto Y, Mikami T, Nagahama K. Cutaneous metastasis of pancreatic carcinoma as an initial symptom in the lower extremity with obstructive lymphedema treated by physiotherapy and lymphaticovenous shunt: a case report, review, and pathophysiological implications. Lymphology 2010; 43(1): 19-24.

[38] Bjersing L, Lundmark F. Multiple thrombophlebitis with cancer-Trousseau's sign. Sven Lakartidn 1960; 57:466-475.

[39] Edge SB, Compton CC. The American Joint Committee on Cancer: the 7th edition of the AJCC cancer staging manual and the future of TNM. Ann Surg Oncol 2010; 17(6): 1471-1474.

[40] NCCN Guidelines Version 1.2013 Pancreatic Adenocarcinoma. 2013. Ref Type: Online Source

[41] Enweluzo C, Dutta S, Aziz F, Lenfest S. From Acute Pancreatitis to Stage IV Pancreatic Cancer in 12 Weeks. Case Rep Gastroenterol 2013; 7(2):287-292.

[42] Cwik G, Wallner G, Skoczylas T, Ciechanski A, Zinkiewicz K. Cancer antigens 19-9 and 125 in the differential diagnosis of pancreatic mass lesions. Arch Surg 2006; 141(10):968-973.

[43] Ritts RE, Jr., Nagorney DM, Jacobsen DJ, Talbot RW, Zurawski VR, Jr. Comparison of preoperative serum CA19-9 levels with results of diagnostic imaging modalities in patients undergoing laparotomy for suspected pancreatic or gallbladder disease. Pancreas 1994; 9(6):707-716.

[44] Lamerz R. Role of tumour markers, cytogenetics. Ann Oncol 1999; 10 Suppl 4:145-149.

[45] Tempero MA, Uchida E, Takasaki H, Burnett DA, Steplewski Z, Pour PM. Relationship of carbohydrate antigen 19-9 and Lewis antigens in pancreatic cancer. Cancer Res 1987; 47(20):5501-5503.

[46] Bronstein YL, Loyer EM, Kaur H, Choi H, David C, DuBrow RA et al. Detection of small pancreatic tumors with multiphasic helical CT. AJR Am J Roentgenol 2004; 182(3):619-623.

[47] Soriano A, Castells A, Ayuso C, Ayuso JR, de Caralt MT, Gines MA et al. Preoperative staging and tumor resectability assessment of pancreatic cancer: prospective study comparing endoscopic ultrasonography, helical computed tomography, magnetic resonance imaging, and angiography. Am J Gastroenterol 2004; 99(3):492-501.

[48] Canto MI, Hruban RH, Fishman EK, Kamel IR, Schulick R, Zhang Z et al. Frequent detection of pancreatic lesions in asymptomatic high-risk individuals. Gastroenterology 2012; 142(4):796-804.

[49] Raut CP, Grau AM, Staerkel GA, Kaw M, Tamm EP, Wolff RA et al. Diagnostic accuracy of endoscopic ultrasound-guided fine-needle aspiration in patients with presumed pancreatic cancer. J Gastrointest Surg 2003; 7(1):118-126.

[50] van der Gaag NA, Rauws EA, van Eijck CH, Bruno MJ, van der Harst E, Kubben FJ et al. Preoperative biliary drainage for cancer of the head of the pancreas. N Engl J Med 2010; 362(2):129-137.

[51] Lee JK, Kim AY, Kim PN, Lee MG, Ha HK. Prediction of vascular involvement and resectability by multidetector-row CT versus MR imaging with MR angiography in patients who underwent surgery for resection of pancreatic ductal adenocarcinoma. Eur J Radiol 2010; 73(2):310-316.

[52] Conlon KC, Dougherty E, Klimstra DS, Coit DG, Turnbull AD, Brennan MF. The value of minimal access surgery in the staging of patients with potentially resectable peripancreatic malignancy. Ann Surg 1996; 223(2):134-140.

[53] Holzman MD, Reintgen KL, Tyler DS, Pappas TN. The role of laparoscopy in the management of suspected pancreatic and periampullary malignancies. J Gastrointest Surg 1997; 1(3):236-243.

[54] Jimenez RE, Warshaw AL, Rattner DW, Willett CG, McGrath D, Fernandez-del CC. Impact of laparoscopic staging in the treatment of pancreatic cancer. Arch Surg 2000; 135(4):409-414.

[55] Zamboni GA, Kruskal JB, Vollmer CM, Baptista J, Callery MP, Raptopoulos VD. Pancreatic adenocarcinoma: value of multidetector CT angiography in preoperative evaluation. Radiology 2007; 245(3):770-778.

[56] Lowy AM, Mansfield PF, Leach SD, Ajani J. Laparoscopic staging for gastric cancer. Surgery 1996; 119(6):611-614.

[57] Nieveen van Dijkum EJ, Romijn MG, Terwee CB, de Wit LT, van der Meulen JH, Lameris HS et al. Laparoscopic staging and subsequent palliation in patients with peripancreatic carcinoma. Ann Surg 2003; 237(1):66-73.

[58] Yelamali A, Mansard MJ, Dama R, Rebela P, Rao GV, Reddy DN. Intraoperative pancreatoscopy with narrow band imaging: a novel method for assessment of resection margins in case of intraductal papillary mucinous neoplasm. Surg Endosc 2012; 26(12):3682-3685.

[59] Giovannini M, Bories E, Monges G, Pesenti C, Caillol F, Delpero JR. Results of a phase I-II study on intraductal confocal microscopy (IDCM) in patients with common bile duct (CBD) stenosis. Surg Endosc 2011; 25(7):2247-2253.

[60] Konda VJ, Aslanian HR, Wallace MB, Siddiqui UD, Hart J, Waxman I. First assessment of needle-based confocal laser endomicroscopy during EUS-FNA procedures of the pancreas (with videos). Gastrointest Endosc 2011; 74(5):1049-1060.

[61] Regunathan R, Woo J, Pierce MC, Polydorides AD, Raoufi M, Roayaie S et al. Feasibility and preliminary accuracy of high-resolution imaging of the liver and pancreas using FNA compatible microendoscopy (with video). Gastrointest Endosc 2012; 76(2):293-300.

[62] Testoni PA, Mariani A, Mangiavillano B, Arcidiacono PG, Di PS, Masci E. Intraductal optical coherence tomography for investigating main pancreatic duct strictures. Am J Gastroenterol 2007; 102(2):269-274.

[63] Cheon YK, Cho YD, Jeon SR, Moon JH, Jeong SW, Hur KY et al. Pancreatic resection guided by preoperative intraductal ultrasonography for intraductal papillary mucinous neoplasm. Am J Gastroenterol 2010; 105(9):1963-1969.

[64] Hara T, Yamaguchi T, Ishihara T, Tsuyuguchi T, Kondo F, Kato K et al. Diagnosis and patient management of intraductal papillary-mucinous tumor of the pancreas by using peroral pancreatoscopy and intraductal ultrasonography. Gastroenterology 2002; 122(1):34-43.

[65] Varadarajulu S, Eloubeidi MA, Wilcox CM. Prospective evaluation of indeterminate ERCP findings by intraductal ultrasound. J Gastroenterol Hepatol 2007; 22(12): 2086-2092.

[66] Kitano M, Kudo M, Yamao K, Takagi T, Sakamoto H, Komaki T et al. Characterization of small solid tumors in the pancreas: the value of contrast-enhanced harmonic endoscopic ultrasonography. Am J Gastroenterol 2012; 107(2):303-310.

[67] Gong TT, Hu DM, Zhu Q. Contrast-enhanced EUS for differential diagnosis of pancreatic mass lesions: a meta-analysis. Gastrointest Endosc 2012; 76(2):301-309.

[68] Iglesias-Garcia J, Larino-Noia J, Abdulkader I, Forteza J, Dominguez-Munoz JE. Quantitative endoscopic ultrasound elastography: an accurate method for the differentiation of solid pancreatic masses. Gastroenterology 2010; 139(4):1172-1180.

[69] Kumon RE, Repaka A, Atkinson M, Faulx AL, Wong RC, Isenberg GA et al. Characterization of the pancreas in vivo using EUS spectrum analysis with electronic array echoendoscopes. Gastrointest Endosc 2012; 75(6):1175-1183.

[70] Bausch D, Thomas S, Mino-Kenudson M, Fernandez-del CC, Bauer TW, Williams M et al. Plectin-1 as a novel biomarker for pancreatic cancer. Clin Cancer Res 2011; 17(2):302-309.

[71] Cruz-Monserrate Z, Abd-Elgaliel WR, Grote T, Deng D, Ji B, Arumugam T et al. Detection of pancreatic cancer tumours and precursor lesions by cathepsin E activity in mouse models. Gut 2012; 61(9):1315-1322.

[72] Hausner SH, Abbey CK, Bold RJ, Gagnon MK, Marik J, Marshall JF et al. Targeted in vivo imaging of integrin alphavbeta6 with an improved radiotracer and its relevance in a pancreatic tumor model. Cancer Res 2009; 69(14):5843-5850.

[73] Neesse A, Hahnenkamp A, Griesmann H, Buchholz M, Hahn SA, Maghnouj A et al. Claudin-4-targeted optical imaging detects pancreatic cancer and its precursor lesions. Gut 2013; 62(7):1034-1043.

[74] Montet X, Weissleder R, Josephson L. Imaging pancreatic cancer with a peptide-nanoparticle conjugate targeted to normal pancreas. Bioconjug Chem 2006; 17(4): 905-911.

[75] Korpanty G, Carbon JG, Grayburn PA, Fleming JB, Brekken RA. Monitoring response to anticancer therapy by targeting microbubbles to tumor vasculature. Clin Cancer Res 2007; 13(1):323-330.

[76] Maithel SK, Maloney S, Winston C, Gonen M, D'Angelica MI, Dematteo RP et al. Preoperative CA 19-9 and the yield of staging laparoscopy in patients with radiographically resectable pancreatic adenocarcinoma. Ann Surg Oncol 2008; 15(12):3512-3520.

[77] Jesen E, Borja-Cacho D, Al-Rafaie W, Vickers S. Exocrine Pancreas. In: Townsend C, Beauchamp R, Evers B, Mattox K, editors. Sabiston Textbook of Surgery. 19 ed. Elsevier; 2013. p. 1515-1547.

[78] Callery MP, Chang KJ, Fishman EK, Talamonti MS, William TL, Linehan DC. Pretreatment assessment of resectable and borderline resectable pancreatic cancer: expert consensus statement. Ann Surg Oncol 2009; 16(7):1727-1733.

[79] Varadhachary GR, Tamm EP, Abbruzzese JL, Xiong HQ, Crane CH, Wang H et al. Borderline resectable pancreatic cancer: definitions, management, and role of preoperative therapy. Ann Surg Oncol 2006; 13(8):1035-1046.

[80] Whipple AO, Parsons WB, Mullins CR. Treatment of Carcinoma of the Ampulla of Vater. Ann Surg 1935; 102(4):763-779.

[81] Trimble I, Parsons J, Sherman C. A one-stage operation for the cure of carcinoma of the ampulla of Vater and the head of the pancreas. Surg Gynecol Obstet 1941; 73:711-722.

[82] Fernandez-del CC, Morales-Oyarvide V, McGrath D, Wargo JA, Ferrone CR, Thayer SP et al. Evolution of the Whipple procedure at the Massachusetts General Hospital. Surgery 2012; 152(3 Suppl 1):S56-S63.

[83] Tyler DS, Evans DB. Reoperative pancreaticoduodenectomy. Ann Surg 1994; 219(2): 211-221.

[84] Jimenez RE, Fernandez-del CC, Rattner DW, Chang Y, Warshaw AL. Outcome of pancreaticoduodenectomy with pylorus preservation or with antrectomy in the treatment of chronic pancreatitis. Ann Surg 2000; 231(3):293-300.

[85] Warshaw AL, Torchiana DL. Delayed gastric emptying after pylorus-preserving pancreaticoduodenectomy. Surg Gynecol Obstet 1985; 160(1):1-4.

[86] Wente MN, Shrikhande SV, Muller MW, Diener MK, Seiler CM, Friess H et al. Pancreaticojejunostomy versus pancreaticogastrostomy: systematic review and meta-analysis. Am J Surg 2007; 193(2):171-183.

[87] Farnell MB, Aranha GV, Nimura Y, Michelassi F. The role of extended lymphadenectomy for adenocarcinoma of the head of the pancreas: strength of the evidence. J Gastrointest Surg 2008; 12(4):651-656.

[88] Gagner M, Palermo M. Laparoscopic Whipple procedure: review of the literature. J Hepatobiliary Pancreat Surg 2009; 16(6):726-730.

[89] Kendrick ML, Cusati D. Total laparoscopic pancreaticoduodenectomy: feasibility and outcome in an early experience. Arch Surg 2010; 145(1):19-23.

[90] Palanivelu C, Jani K, Senthilnathan P, Parthasarathi R, Rajapandian S, Madhankumar MV. Laparoscopic pancreaticoduodenectomy: technique and outcomes. J Am Coll Surg 2007; 205(2):222-230.

[91] Jacobs MJ, Kamyab A. Total laparoscopic pancreaticoduodenectomy. JSLS 2013; 17(2):188-193.

[92] Himpens J, Leman G, Cadiere GB. Telesurgical laparoscopic cholecystectomy. Surg Endosc 1998; 12(8):1091.

[93] Giulianotti PC, Coratti A, Angelini M, Sbrana F, Cecconi S, Balestracci T et al. Robotics in general surgery: personal experience in a large community hospital. Arch Surg 2003; 138(7):777-784.

[94] Cirocchi R, Partelli S, Trastulli S, Coratti A, Parisi A, Falconi M. A systematic review on robotic pancreaticoduodenectomy. Surg Oncol 2013.

[95] Chan OC, Tang CN, Lai EC, Yang GP, Li MK. Robotic hepatobiliary and pancreatic surgery: a cohort study. J Hepatobiliary Pancreat Sci 2011; 18(4):471-480.

[96] Horiguchi A, Uyama I, Ito M, Ishihara S, Asano Y, Yamamoto T et al. Robot-assisted laparoscopic pancreatic surgery. J Hepatobiliary Pancreat Sci 2011; 18(4):488-492.

[97] Lai EC, Yang GP, Tang CN. Robot-assisted laparoscopic pancreaticoduodenectomy versus open pancreaticoduodenectomy--a comparative study. Int J Surg 2012; 10(9): 475-479.

[98] Zhou NX, Chen JZ, Liu Q, Zhang X, Wang Z, Ren S et al. Outcomes of pancreatoduodenectomy with robotic surgery versus open surgery. Int J Med Robot 2011; 7(2): 131-137.

[99] Sohn TA, Yeo CJ, Cameron JL, Koniaris L, Kaushal S, Abrams RA et al. Resected adenocarcinoma of the pancreas-616 patients: results, outcomes, and prognostic indicators. J Gastrointest Surg 2000; 4(6):567-579.

[100] Fischer M, Matsuo K, Gonen M, Grant F, Dematteo RP, D'Angelica MI et al. Relationship between intraoperative fluid administration and perioperative outcome after pancreaticoduodenectomy: results of a prospective randomized trial of acute normovolemic hemodilution compared with standard intraoperative management. Ann Surg 2010; 252(6):952-958.

[101] Davila JA, Chiao EY, Hasche JC, Petersen NJ, McGlynn KA, Shaib YH. Utilization and determinants of adjuvant therapy among older patients who receive curative surgery for pancreatic cancer. Pancreas 2009; 38(1):e18-e25.

[102] Hazard L, Tward JD, Szabo A, Shrieve DC. Radiation therapy is associated with improved survival in patients with pancreatic adenocarcinoma: results of a study from the Surveillance, Epidemiology, and End Results (SEER) registry data. Cancer 2007; 110(10):2191-2201.

[103] Mayo SC, Austin DF, Sheppard BC, Mori M, Shipley DK, Billingsley KG. Adjuvant therapy and survival after resection of pancreatic adenocarcinoma: a population-based analysis. Cancer 2010; 116(12):2932-2940.

[104] Oettle H, Post S, Neuhaus P, Gellert K, Langrehr J, Ridwelski K et al. Adjuvant chemotherapy with gemcitabine vs observation in patients undergoing curative-intent resection of pancreatic cancer: a randomized controlled trial. JAMA 2007; 297(3): 267-277.

[105] Regine WF, Winter KA, Abrams R, Safran H, Hoffman JP, Konski A et al. Fluorouracil-based chemoradiation with either gemcitabine or fluorouracil chemotherapy after resection of pancreatic adenocarcinoma: 5-year analysis of the U.S. Intergroup/RTOG 9704 phase III trial. Ann Surg Oncol 2011; 18(5):1319-1326.

[106] Slidell MB, Chang DC, Cameron JL, Wolfgang C, Herman JM, Schulick RD et al. Impact of total lymph node count and lymph node ratio on staging and survival after pancreatectomy for pancreatic adenocarcinoma: a large, population-based analysis. Ann Surg Oncol 2008; 15(1):165-174.

[107] Crist DW, Sitzmann JV, Cameron JL. Improved hospital morbidity, mortality, and survival after the Whipple procedure. Ann Surg 1987; 206(3):358-365.

[108] He J, Ahuja N, Makary MA, Cameron JL, Eckhauser FE, Choti MA et al. 2564 resected periampullary adenocarcinomas at a single institution: trends over three decades. HPB (Oxford) 2013.

http://dx.doi.org/10.5772/60451

[109] Malleo G, Crippa S, Butturini G, Salvia R, Partelli S, Rossini R et al. Delayed gastric emptying after pylorus-preserving pancreaticoduodenectomy: validation of International Study Group of Pancreatic Surgery classification and analysis of risk factors. HPB (Oxford) 2010; 12(9):610-618.

[110] Tan WJ, Kow AW, Liau KH. Moving towards the New International Study Group for Pancreatic Surgery (ISGPS) definitions in pancreaticoduodenectomy: a comparison between the old and new. HPB (Oxford) 2011; 13(8):566-572.

[111] Welsch T, Borm M, Degrate L, Hinz U, Buchler MW, Wente MN. Evaluation of the International Study Group of Pancreatic Surgery definition of delayed gastric emptying after pancreatoduodenectomy in a high-volume centre. Br J Surg 2010; 97(7): 1043-1050.

[112] Yeo CJ, Barry MK, Sauter PK, Sostre S, Lillemoe KD, Pitt HA et al. Erythromycin accelerates gastric emptying after pancreaticoduodenectomy. A prospective, randomized, placebo-controlled trial. Ann Surg 1993; 218(3):229-237.

[113] Cullen JJ, Sarr MG, Ilstrup DM. Pancreatic anastomotic leak after pancreaticoduodenectomy: incidence, significance, and management. Am J Surg 1994; 168(4):295-298.

[114] Kollmar O, Moussavian MR, Bolli M, Richter S, Schilling MK. Pancreatojejunal leakage after pancreas head resection: anatomic and surgeon-related factors. J Gastrointest Surg 2007; 11(12):1699-1703.

[115] Strasberg SM, Drebin JA, Soper NJ. Evolution and current status of the Whipple procedure: an update for gastroenterologists. Gastroenterology 1997; 113(3):983-994.

[116] Trede M, Schwall G. The complications of pancreatectomy. Ann Surg 1988; 207(1): 39-47.

[117] Yang YM, Tian XD, Zhuang Y, Wang WM, Wan YL, Huang YT. Risk factors of pancreatic leakage after pancreaticoduodenectomy. World J Gastroenterol 2005; 11(16): 2456-2461.

[118] El NA, Salah T, Sultan A, El HM, Askr W, Ezzat H et al. Pancreatic anastomotic leakage after pancreaticoduodenectomy. risk factors, clinical predictors, and management (single center experience). World J Surg 2013; 37(6):1405-1418.

[119] Andriulli A, Festa V, Botteri E, Valvano MR, Koch M, Bassi C et al. Neoadjuvant/preoperative gemcitabine for patients with localized pancreatic cancer: a meta-analysis of prospective studies. Ann Surg Oncol 2012; 19(5):1644-1662.

[120] Assifi MM, Lu X, Eibl G, Reber HA, Li G, Hines OJ. Neoadjuvant therapy in pancreatic adenocarcinoma: a meta-analysis of phase II trials. Surgery 2011; 150(3):466-473.

[121] Yeo CJ, Cameron JL, Lillemoe KD, Sitzmann JV, Hruban RH, Goodman SN et al. Pancreaticoduodenectomy for cancer of the head of the pancreas. 201 patients. Ann Surg 1995; 221(6):721-731.

[122] Kalser MH, Ellenberg SS. Pancreatic cancer. Adjuvant combined radiation and chemotherapy following curative resection. Arch Surg 1985; 120(8):899-903.

[123] Klinkenbijl JH, Jeekel J, Sahmoud T, van PR, Couvreur ML, Veenhof CH et al. Adjuvant radiotherapy and 5-fluorouracil after curative resection of cancer of the pancreas and periampullary region: phase III trial of the EORTC gastrointestinal tract cancer cooperative group. Ann Surg 1999; 230(6):776-782.

[124] Neoptolemos JP, Stocken DD, Friess H, Bassi C, Dunn JA, Hickey H et al. A randomized trial of chemoradiotherapy and chemotherapy after resection of pancreatic cancer. N Engl J Med 2004; 350(12):1200-1210.

[125] Fung MC, Takayama S, Ishiguro H, Sakata T, Adachi S, Morizane T. [Chemotherapy for advanced or metastatic pancreatic cancer: analysis of 43 randomized trials in 3 decades (1974-2002)]. Gan To Kagaku Ryoho 2003; 30(8):1101-1111.

[126] Burris HA, III, Moore MJ, Andersen J, Green MR, Rothenberg ML, Modiano MR et al. Improvements in survival and clinical benefit with gemcitabine as first-line therapy for patients with advanced pancreas cancer: a randomized trial. J Clin Oncol 1997; 15(6):2403-2413.

[127] Sun C, Ansari D, Andersson R, Wu DQ. Does gemcitabine-based combination therapy improve the prognosis of unresectable pancreatic cancer? World J Gastroenterol 2012; 18(35):4944-4958.

[128] Moore MJ, Goldstein D, Hamm J, Figer A, Hecht JR, Gallinger S et al. Erlotinib plus gemcitabine compared with gemcitabine alone in patients with advanced pancreatic cancer: a phase III trial of the National Cancer Institute of Canada Clinical Trials Group. J Clin Oncol 2007; 25(15):1960-1966.

[129] Conroy T, Desseigne F, Ychou M, Bouche O, Guimbaud R, Becouarn Y et al. FOLFIRINOX versus gemcitabine for metastatic pancreatic cancer. N Engl J Med 2011; 364(19):1817-1825.

[130] Von Hoff DD, E. TJ, A.F.P. Randomized phase III study of weekly nab-paclitaxel plus gemcitabine versus gemcitabine alone in patients with metastatic adenocarcinoma of the pancreas (MPACT). ASCO Meeting Abstracts [31], 148. 2013. Ref Type: Abstract

[131] House MG, Choti MA. Palliative therapy for pancreatic/biliary cancer. Surg Clin North Am 2005; 85(2):359-371.

[132] Smith AC, Dowsett JF, Russell RC, Hatfield AR, Cotton PB. Randomised trial of endoscopic stenting versus surgical bypass in malignant low bileduct obstruction. Lancet 1994; 344(8938):1655-1660.

[133] Singh SM, Longmire WP, Jr., Reber HA. Surgical palliation for pancreatic cancer. The UCLA experience. Ann Surg 1990; 212(2):132-139.

http://dx.doi.org/10.5772/60451

[134] Yim HB, Jacobson BC, Saltzman JR, Johannes RS, Bounds BC, Lee JH et al. Clinical outcome of the use of enteral stents for palliation of patients with malignant upper GI obstruction. Gastrointest Endosc 2001; 53(3):329-332.

[135] Lillemoe KD, Cameron JL, Kaufman HS, Yeo CJ, Pitt HA, Sauter PK. Chemical splanchnicectomy in patients with unresectable pancreatic cancer. A prospective randomized trial. Ann Surg 1993; 217(5):447-455.

[136] Shahrokni A, Saif MW. Metastatic pancreatic cancer: the dilemma of quality vs. quantity of life. JOP 2013; 14(4):391-394.

Chapter 11

Recent Advances in the Management of Rectal Cancer

Jeffrey Meyer, Jie J. Yao and Sergio Huerta

Additional information is available at the end of the chapter

http://dx.doi.org/10.5772/60210

1. Introduction

Rectal cancer continues to affect many patients in the United States and world-wide. For instance, in 2012, rectal cancer affected 40,290 Americans [1]. Patients affected with rectal cancer who have a clinical stage II (T3-T4, NO, MO) or III (Any T, N1-N3, M0) tumor are treated with pre-operative chemoradiation (CRT) followed by surgical intervention [total mesorectal excision (TME)]. In up to 40% of patients treated with CRT, the tumor becomes clinically undetectable (cCR) [2]. Clearly, this is a desirable outcome in oncology. Adding novel radiosanitizing agents, prolonging the period from CRT to TME, increasing the radiation dose, adding chemotherapy before CRT are few modalities that have been investigated to increase the number of patients achieving a complete response. The following chapter reviews current strategies in recent attempts at maximizing the ratio of patients who achieve a cCR. Current margins are resection following TME in the era of CRT are also reviewed.

2. Recent status of pre-operative biomarkers to determine a response to neoadjuvant chemoradiation

Neoadjuvant chemoradiation for the management of patients with stage II and III rectal cancer results in a clinical complete response (cCR), the absence of detectable rectal tumor with diagnostic modalities [i.e. endorectal ultrasound (EUS), magnetic resonance imaging (MRI), digital rectal exam (DRE), or proctoscopy], in 10-40% of patients [2].

The fundamental pre-clinical and clinical question is to determine whether there are markers that can detect tumors that will respond well to neoadjuvant treatment such that these patients could be potential candidates for observation without operative intervention. Conversely, if a patient is not likely to respond to neoadjuvant chemoradiation, they should submit to surgical intervention sooner. Therefore, a myriad of pathways and molecules ranging from DNA-repair molecules to molecules that mediate cell cycle dynamics to apoptotic mediators as well as hypoxic mechanisms have been investigated with a wide range of results, which are summarized by Ramzan et al [3]. Currently, there is no unifying pathway that can reliably predict responses to chemoradiation in patients with rectal cancer.

2.1. DNA repair molecules

One of three pathways is responsible for the repair of DNA double-strand breaks (DSB) induced by ionizing radiation: homologous recombination (HR), non-homologous end-joining (NHEJ) pathway, or an alternate NHEJ pathway [3]. Of these, the non-homologous end-joining (NHEJ) pathway is fundamental for DSB repair. The catalytic subunit of DNA-dependent protein kinase (DNA-PKcs) is an integral part of the NHEJ pathway. This mechanism can be broadly classified into three steps: (1) Ku 70/80 heterodimer identifies DSB and stick to DNA broken ends, facilitates the activation and recruitment of DNA-PKcs; (2) enzymatic processing of the DNA ends; and (3) ligation by DNA ligase IV. Ku 70/80 proteins play a fundamental role as they recruit DNA-PKcs which then set the cascade of DNA repair. Recent data demonstrate that DNA-PKcs and Ku proteins may have a central role in radiation induced cell death and might predict the response to radiation. However this is an area that is still under investigation.

2.2. Apoptosis

In the central mediators of apoptosis pathway in response to ionizing radiation, the initial response begins with an up-regulation of p53 (Figure 1). p53 then directly activates the cyclin dependent kinase inhibitors (such as p21). Cell cycle progression stops until the cell repairs the damage induced by ionizing radiation. If the cell is unable to repair itself, it undergoes apoptosis. The anti-apoptotic Bcl-2 inhibits p53, while p53 inhibits the inhibitor of apoptosis (survivin). All of these molecules have been investigated to determine if their up-regulation or down-regulation could predict a response to ionizing radiation. Mutations and manner of detection have to be considered in these studies. Additionally, contrary to expectations, p21 or Bax deficient cells lead to a more radiosensitive rather than a more radioresistant phenotype [4]. Thus, analyses of these molecules in predicting a response to ionizing radiation have been largely unyielding [5].

A recent systematic review analyzing the role of p53 as a predictor of a response to ionizing radiation included 30 studies of which 25 used p53 protein status, 7 used gene analysis detection and two used both. The results revealed that patients that demonstrated a p53 wild-type (and/or low expression) had a good response risk of 1.3 [CI=1.14 to 1.49], complete response RR was 1.65 [CI=1.19 to 2.30] and poor response RR 0.85 [CI = 0.75 to 0.96] [6].

http://dx.doi.org/10.5772/60210

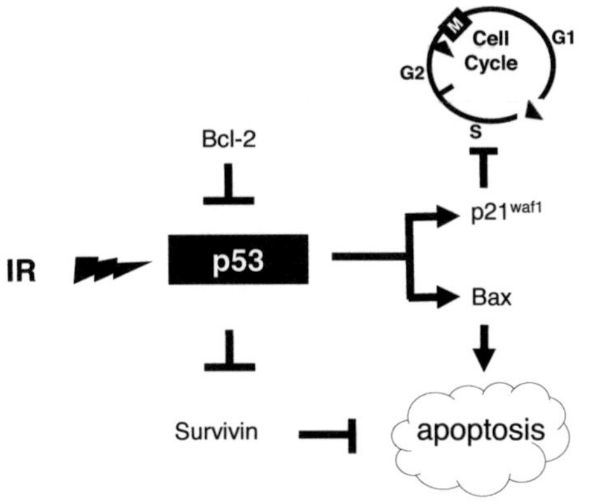

Figure 1. Central mediators of apoptosis. Ionizing radiation (IR) leads to an increase of p53, which in turn activates p21 and causes cell cycle arrest. P53 also activates Bax, which results in apoptosis

2.3. Gene modifications and polymorphisms

It is possible that with standardized techniques, we might be able to utilize other molecules in the apoptotic pathway alone or in combination to better predict neoadjuvant chemotherapeutic responses in patient affected with rectal cancer. Another area that is gaining momentum is that of epigenetic changes. For instance methylation of the retinoic acid receptor gene (RARB) and the checkpoint with forkhead and ring finger gene (CHFR) discriminated between TI-2 *vs.* T2-3 un-irradiated tumors. RARB methylation was also associated with nodal metastasis and lymphovascular invasion (LVI). Methylation of other genes have also predicted nodal metastasis [7]. Thus, methylation can predict aggressiveness and in combination with the mutation status of other molecules, a predictive panel of a response to ionizing radiation can then be constructed. In a separate study, DNA analysis of biopsies of patients prior to radiation demonstrated a gene mutation and two gene polymorphisims to be associated with resistance to radiation as measured by pCR [8].

3. Novel strategies in neoadjuvant therapy for locally advanced rectal cancer

The trimodal approach of neoadjuvant chemoradiotherapy and surgery is generally associated with high rates of local-regional control for patients with locally advanced rectal cancer [9]. However, there is room for improvement in the oncologic outcomes of the most locally advanced tumors, and also great interest in increasing the rate of complete pathologic responses to chemoradiotherapy, which may allow for increased utilization of non-operative management.

A variety of chemotherapy and targeted agents have been studied as part of novel neoadjuvant regimens in an attempt to improve on results obtained with fluoropyrimidine-based chemoradiation. Although early-phase studies have shown modest improvements in tumor responses; this has often been at the expense of increased toxicity.

3.1. Oxaliplatin

There has been much interest in particular in the use of oxaliplatin concurrent with radiation. The ACCORD 12/0405 PRODIGE 1 study randomized patients with locally advanced rectal cancer to preoperative treatment with radiation (45 Gy in 25 fractions) plus capecitabine or radiation (50 Gy in 25 fractions) plus capecitabine and oxaliplatin [10;11]. High-grade toxicity rates were higher in the oxaliplatin-treated patients (25 versus 11%), and there were no significant differences between the two arms with respect to rates of pCR, local control, and overall survival. In the STAR-01 trial, over 700 patients with locally advanced rectal cancer were randomized to neoadjuvant treatment with radiation (50.4 Gy total dose) plus infusional 5-FU with or without weekly oxaliplatin, followed by surgery [12]. The addition of oxaliplatin increased the rate of high grade toxicity (24% versus 8%) but did not improve the pathologic complete response rate (equal in the two arms at 16%). In the PETACC-6 trial, 1094 patients with locally advanced rectal cancer were randomized to preoperative radiation plus capecitabine followed by surgery and adjuvant chemotherapy versus the same regimen with oxaliplatin delivered during the chemoradiation course as well as the adjuvant course [13]. The use of oxaliplatin again increased toxicity rates, with no disease-free survival benefit.

The NSABP R-04 trial is a four-arm study that compared infusional 5-FU and capecitabine, with and without the use of oxaliplatin, during neoadjuvant chemoradiotherapy for rectal cancer [14]. Capecitabine in place of 5-FU yielded a different toxicity profile with similar rates of pCR, local-regional control, and overall survival. Patients treated with oxaliplatin had higher rates of high-grade toxicity without significant improvements in local-regional control or overall survival. Finally, in the CAO/ARO/AIO-04 trial, patients with locally advanced rectal cancer were randomized to treatment with radiation with concurrent 5-FU, surgery, and adjuvant bolus 5-FU versus radiation plus 5-FU, oxaliplatin, surgery, and adjuvant mFOLFOX6 [15]. There were no substantial differences in rates of pathologic complete response or margin-negative surgery. However, 3-year disease-free survival was higher in the oxaliplatin group (75.9% versus 71.2%). The independent contribution of the oxaliplatin delivered in the neoadjuvant setting is unclear.

3.2. Targeted therapies

Incorporation of novel targeted drug agents into trimodality regimens is also an area of dynamic clinical investigation. Bevacizumab is an anti-VEGF antibody. Willett et al. reported on 32 patients who underwent one cycle of bevacizumab followed by radiation, infusional 5-FU, further bevacizumab and subsequent surgery [16]. Local control was 100% at 5 years; disease-free survival was 75% at 5 years. Landry et al. reported on the phase 2 ECOG 3204 study, which combined capecitabine, oxaliplatin, and bevacizumab for patients with operable T3 and T4 rectal cancer [17]. Of the 49 patients who proceeded to surgery, 17% had a pathologic complete response. Surgical complications were common and may have been related to the addition of bevacizumab. Bevacizumab has also been associated with delayed wound healing in other studies [18;19].

Work is also underway evaluating combinations of the anti-EGFR agents panitumumab and cetuximab with chemoradiation. When combining such agents with conventional chemother-

http://dx.doi.org/10.5772/60210

apy and radiation therapy, appropriate sequencing of these treatments may be of critical importance to optimize oncologic efficacy [17;20].

3.3. Novel scheduling modalities

A more recent area of clinical study has been to incorporate systemic therapy prior to chemoradiation or to eliminate radiation as a component of neoadjuvant therapy for selected patients with locally advanced disease (Figure 2). Chua et al. reported, on a phase 2 study, incorporating induction chemotherapy prior to neoadjuvant chemoradiotherapy [21]. Patients had locally advanced rectal cancers that were considered high-risk by MRI criteria (including tumors with threatened mesorectal resection margin, extensive mesorectal fat involvement, and T4 and/or N2 tumors). Patients were treated with 12 weeks of capecitabine and oxaliplatin. This was followed by radiation (total dose of 54 Gy) and concurrent capecitabine for six weeks and finally total mesorectal excision (Figure 2 B). One hundred and five patients were enrolled. Twenty percent of the patients had a pathological complete response, and 3-year progression-free and overall survival were 68% and 83% respectively. In a similar approach, a recent randomized phase II trial incorporating induction capecitabine and oxaliplatin showed no difference in histopathologic downstaging compared to patients treated with chemoradiation alone [22]. The authors of these studies suggest that more data is needed before approaching induction chemotherapy as a standard of care for high risk patients.

Schrag et al. recently reported on 32 patients with stage II or III rectal cancer treated with 6 cycles of FOLFOX, with bevacizumab delivered during cycles 1-4, without planned radiation therapy (Figure 2 C) [23]. Thirty of the 32 patients proceeded to surgery without undergoing preoperative irradiation. Of the 32 patients, 25% had a pathologic complete response. The 4-year local recurrence rate was 0% and the 4-year disease-free survival rate was 84%. This strategy of neoadjuvant chemotherapy without planned use of radiation therapy (without use of bevacizumab) is under further study in the randomized N1048 study. However, these studies are in the initial stages of assessment at this time.

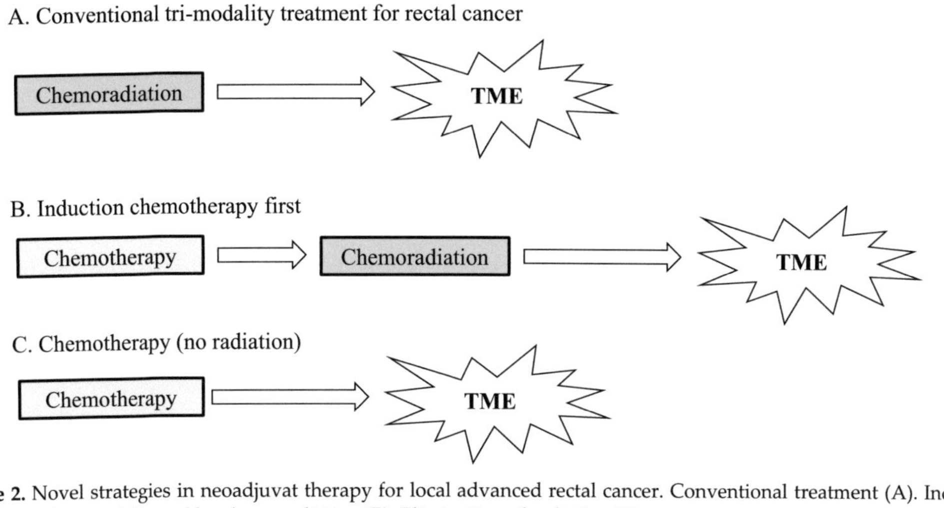

Figure 2. Novel strategies in neoadjuvat therapy for local advanced rectal cancer. Conventional treatment (A). Induction chemotherapy followed by chemoradiation (B). Elimination of radiation (C).

4. What is the appropriate length of the "waiting period" between completion of neoadjuvant chemoradiation and surgery?

Initially, the waiting period following CRT was based on sufficient time to allow the acute radiation reaction to subside. Thus, an interval between 3-5 weeks was selected based on empirical experience. Favorable outcomes in patients who achieve a pCR and the desire to obtain a cCR have led to an increase of the radiation dose to the tumor center, increased intervals between CRT and TME, addition of chemotherapy during the waiting time, or starting with induction chemotherapy [24].

Allowing for a "waiting period" without active treatment of many weeks between the completion of neoadjuvant long-course therapy and surgery is common in the management of rectal cancer. Delaying surgery may allow for continued volume reduction of the treated tumor, potentially increasing the ultimate likelihood of a sphincter-preserving surgery for low-lying tumors and facilitating ease of the operation. However, too long of a delay in proceeding to surgery, especially in patients with poor response to neoadjuvant treatment, may allow for growth of the primary tumor with an increased risk of margin-positive surgery and increased risk of distant dissemination of cancer [25]. Further, there is a perception that waiting too long after the end of CRT (> 12 weeks) might lead to radiation fibrosis, making surgical intervention more difficult. However, this has not been substantiated in the literature [24].

The Lyon R90-01 trial randomized patients with T2-3 (N-any) rectal carcinoma to treatment with preoperative radiation (39 Gy in 13 fractions, without concurrent chemotherapy) followed by either a "short interval" to surgery (surgery performed within 2 weeks of completion of radiation) or a "long interval" to surgery (surgery performed within 6-8 weeks of completion of radiation) [26]. Tumors had to be low enough in the rectum to be palpable on digital examination. The primary endpoint of the study was the rate of sphincter-preserving surgery. The decision regarding the type of surgery was made by the surgeon at the time of the operation. Of the enrolled patients, 201 were assessable. Patients in the long-interval group had improved clinical and pathologic responses compared to the short-interval group. Twenty-six percent of the patients in the long-interval group had either a complete or near-complete pathologic response compared to 10.3% in the short-interval group, likely a reflection of the increased amount of time for lethally injured tumor cells to manifest their injury as death. Ultimately, however, 75.5% of the patients in the long-interval group as opposed to 67.7% in the short-interval group underwent a sphincter-preserving operation, a difference that was not statistically significant. There were no differences in the post-operative toxicity and mortality rates between the two groups. There were also no differences in overall survival or local control rates to a median follow-up of 33 months.

Integrating systemic therapy during the waiting period may have potential benefits for patients with rectal cancer, including improved downstaging of the primary tumor as well as potentially more effective treatment (relative to delayed postoperative treatment) of distant micrometastatic disease, a major cause of the poor disease-free survival rates seen in patients with locally advanced rectal cancer. Garcia-Aguilar and colleagues performed a phased II non-randomized trial investigating the use of chemotherapy with modified FOLFOX-6 delivered

http://dx.doi.org/10.5772/60210

during the waiting period following standard long-course chemoradiotherapy, with successively more administrations of chemotherapy (and thus longer overall waiting periods) [27]. In a preliminary analysis of patients treated with two cycles of mFOLFOX-6 during the waiting period, with a mean time of 11 weeks from completion of neoadjuvant therapy to surgery, the pathologic complete response was 25%. In a comparison group of patients treated with neoadjuvant chemoradiation and no intervening systemic therapy, with a mean time to surgery of 6 weeks, the pCR was 18%. There was no substantial difference between the two arms with respect to postoperative complication rates.

In the large Dutch Surgical Colorectal Audit study including 1593 patients, patients were divided into three groups in terms of interval from the start of CRT to TME: < 13, 13-14, and 15-16 weeks. The largest pCR (18%) was observed in patients in the 15-16 week group (median time at the end of CRT = 9-10 weeks) [28].

A meta-analysis was conducted that compared two groups of patients: (1) less or equal to the conventional 6-8 week period from CRT to surgery and (2) longer than 6-8 weeks. pCR was the primary end point and was increased from 13.7 to 19.5% in the more than 8 week group [29]. This study included 13 trials inclusive of 3584 patients. Secondary end points (OS, DFS, R0 resection rates, sphincter preservation, and complication rates) were similar in both groups [29]. However, in patients who had a short interval (< 1 week), the rate of perineal wound complication and anastomotic leak was higher [29].

The question of appropriate waiting time periods has also emerged in the context of short course radiation therapy (5 Gy X 5 fractions without concurrent chemotherapy). In the original clinical trials of short-course neoadjuvant therapy, surgery was mandated to be performed within one week of completion of radiation [30]. This regimen has been associated with lower pCR rates relative to long-course neoadjuvant treatment, possibly as a result of the decreased interval between radiation and surgery. In the more recent Stockholm III trial, patients were randomized to one of three arms: short-course radiation followed by surgery within 1 week, short-course radiation followed by surgery at 4-8 weeks, or long-course radiation (2 Gy X 25 fractions, without concurrent chemotherapy) followed by surgery at 4-8 weeks [31]. Interestingly, pCR rates were highest in the short-course radiation group with the extended interval to surgery (12.5%, versus 0.8% in the short interval group and 5% in the long-course radiation group). Patients treated with short-course radiation and delayed surgery had postoperative complication rates that were similar to the two other groups. In an analysis of actual time to surgery, patients treated with short-course radiation followed by surgery at an interval of 11-17 days had the highest rates of postoperative complications.

Many questions remain regarding the appropriate duration of the waiting period in patients undergoing neoadjuvant therapy. Most of the data regarding CRT-TME gap emanate from retrospective studies. Thus, the recommendations of the length of time are largely observational and empirically-driven. However, cCR and pCR has been observed in three randomized controlled trials when the gap is about 8-12 weeks [26;31;32]. Surgery within 3-4 weeks in the long CRT modality should not be performed secondary to radiation reaction. There is currently limited experience in waiting over 12 weeks.

Integration of systemic therapy both during this time period as well as during the induction phase (prior to chemoradiation) remain active areas of clinical interest. In addition, determining which patients are made candidates for sphincter-preserving surgery also remains an imprecise practice. Improvements in imaging technologies and possible use of pre-treatment biomarkers may improve on patient selection for low anterior resection.

5. Current status of the role of non-operative management in rectal cancer for patients with a complete clinical response

Neoadjuvant chemoradiation for the management of patients with stage II and III rectal cancer results in a clinical complete response (cCR), which is defined as the absence of detectable rectal tumor with diagnostic modalities [i.e. endorectal ultrasound (EUS), magnetic resonance imaging (MRI), digital rectal exam (DRE), or proctoscopy] in 10-40% of patients [33]. Can these patients be followed non-operatively?

There have been three sentinel papers that have addressed this issue: one in 2004 published by Habr-Gama's group [34], the second was a reproduction of these results by a Dutch group in 2011 [35], which was followed by a systematic review by Glynne-Jones in 2012 [2]. An editorial summarizes the main aspects of these seminal events [36].

The first manuscript to document a possible approach in observing patients that achieve a cCR was published by Harb-Gama's group in 2004. In this study, 71 patients who had a cCR were compared to 22 patients that had an initial incomplete response, but after surgery, they were found to have no microscopic evidence of tumor in the resected specimen (pCR). Patients who underwent surgery had a 5-year overall survival of 88% compared to the cCR group, which was 100%. Disease free survival was 83% in the surgery group and 92% in the cCR group [34].

Mass et al. documented similar observations in 2011 [34]. This study compared 21 patients who had a cCR and compared them to 20 patients from another observational study that had documented pCR. Only one patient developed a recurrence at a 2-year follow up and they were all alive at this point in time. Comparatively, the 2-year disease free survival for patients in the surgery group was 93% with an overall survival of 91%.

A number of small institutional studies have documented similar observations in small cohort of patients such as in the United States [37] and in the United Kingdom [38] in 2012. A few other papers that demonstrated similar findings was summarized by a systematic review by Glynne-Jones in 2012 [2].

In this systematic review, 30 papers were included that met the primary end point of cCR with secondary end points of local recurrence, overall survival and disease free survival. This analysis demonstrated that 361 patients (56%) were from a single group (Habr-Gama) and the rest (n=289) were from eight different groups. cCR ranged from 11% - 39%. Results of secondary outcomes showed low local recurrence in Habr-Gama studies (~5%), but higher in all other series 33.8% (range 23%-83%). Habr-Gama reported salvage surgery to be possible in most cases, whereas only one quarter of patients could be salvaged surgically in all other groups.

http://dx.doi.org/10.5772/60210

Long-term outcomes (DFS, and OS) in other groups were similar to Habr-Gama's and suggested that patients who achieve cCR have similar outcomes to patients who undergo surgery and are found to have pCR.

The authors of the meta-analysis suggested that there is not enough evidence at this time to support observation in patients who have a cCR [2]. The inability to propose non-operative management for patients with a cCR primarily emanates from an inability to clearly define cCR. However, it is likely that a group of patients with a cCR can be observed without surgery; who those patients are and how we can monitor them closely is a difficult issue in the management of rectal cancer.

6. Appropriate distal margins of resection in the era of neoadjuvant therapy

Following resection of the rectum, current standard procedure is examination of the distal edge to ensure that the cells at this distal margin are free of any tumor characteristics. A positive distal margin is an unequivocal indication for additional treatment as it signifies that the resection has not been adequate.

This length from the tumor to the distal edge is of even greater importance when considering those cancers occurring in the distal or lower portions of the rectum (close to the anal sphincters). In treating patients with lower rectal tumors, a balance of performing an oncologically free operation versus obtaining proper anal sphincter function must be maintained. There is no question that when it comes to patient's preference, an LAR is always preferred to an APR [39-41].

Prior to the era of CRT, substantially large margins of resections were thought to be necessary. A 5 cm margin was widely used, which emanated from studies showing this to result in acceptable outcomes compared to those with greater than 5 cm distal margins [4-10]. In an attempt to perform sphincter preservation operations, this number was rapidly challenged and reduced to the point in which margins less than 5 cm became acceptable [42-47].

With the current tri-modality management of rectal cancer, a 2 centimeter margin has been adopted with excellent oncologic outcomes [48-52]. In 2004, Habr-Gama published results of observing patient who achieved a clinical complete response (cCR) following neoadjuvant CRT [34]. This concept, in a way, challenged the need to obtain a large margin in patients with low rectal tumors who have responded well to pre-operative treatment. Studies have emerged that indicate that even a 1 cm distal margin is oncologically safe [40;48;49;52-58]. This has been considered oncologically acceptable in the literature. The vast majority of work that has examined the question of 1 cm margins has indicated that there is no statistically significant difference in regards to survival or recurrence between groups of patients with margins greater than 1 cm than those with margins less than or equal to 1 cm [40;48;49;52;54-58] Table 1.

More recently, the 1 cm margin has been challenged to be further reduced. Some surgeons have suggested that sub-centimeter margins as small as 2 mm or 5 mm margins are also safe [54].

Paper	% Patients with Neoadjuvant Chemoradiotherapy	Number of local recurrences/total patients by margin (%)		P	% Survival		Years of Follow Up	P
		≤1 cm	>1 cm		≤1 cm	>1 cm		
Andreola et al *(2001)*	61	4/31 (12.9)	3/45 (6.6)	0.4407[a]				
Huh et al *(2008)*	100	1/18 (6)	0/25 (0)	0.058	71.3	81.3	5 years	0.27
Kim et al *(2009)*	71.2	7/167 (4.2)	31/747 (4.1)	0.98				
Kiran et al *(2011)*	40	7/198 (3.5)	19/586 (3.2)	0.821[a]	67.4	66.5	5 years	0.77
Kuvshinoff et al *(2001)*	100	1/16 (6)	0/12 (0)		53	85	4 years	0.06
Moore et al *(2003)*	100	2/17 (12)	7/77 (9)	0.93	82	85	3 years	0.88
Pricolo et al *(2010)*	100	0/10 (0)	0/23 (0)					
Rutkowski et al *(2008)*	100	4/42 (9.5)	17/122 (13.9)	0.597	65.6	68.7	5 years	0.66
Total		22/464 (4.7)	72/1589 (4.5)	0.8995[a]				

A meta-analysis indicated a higher rate of anastomotic recurrence by only 1.6% in the <1cm margin groups, but this small observed difference was not statistically significant. A systematic review of the literature on sub-1 cm distal margins of resection found in only two papers a possible adverse outcome associated with this smaller margin [54]. However, in these two papers, the percentage of patients submitting to neoadjuvant CRT was less than 5% [59;60].

Distal margins of 8 mm or 5 mm have also been proposed [40;54;56;61], but there is currently not enough data to draw definitive conclusions at this time. The results so far seem to point to these margins also being oncologically safe. Published data on possible adverse oncologic outcomes with 8 mm margins has been documented, but this has occurred in the absence of neoadjuvant CRT [62]. In this case, margins below the 8 mm cutoff point were found to correlate with a significantly higher rate of recurrence and lower rate of long-term survival. However, when the same length of distal margin is evaluated within the context of neoadjuvant CRT, 8 mm margins have not been found to have adverse oncologic outcomes compared to patients having more than 8 mm margins. In this study, the authors did find a higher rate of mucosal recurrence in patients with less than 8 mm margins. They concluded that the probable cause of a higher rate of mucosal recurrence was tumor shedding into the anastomosis [40].

Another study evaluated patients who had received neoadjuvant therapy with margins less than or equal to 5 mm in regards to 5 year outcome and local recurrence [61]. There was no difference in local recurrence 5 years after surgical intervention. This finding was echoed by a number of similar studies [48;53;54;56] (Table 2). Additionally, a meta-analysis demonstrated a small non-significant rate of anastomotic recurrence by 1.7% in the 5mm group, but again this also was not statistically significant [54].

Paper	Number of recurrences/total patients by margin (%)		P
	≤0.5 cm	>0.5 cm	
Kuvshinoff et al *(2001)*	1/9 (11)	0/19 (0)	
Kiran et al *(2011)*	2/25 (8)	9/164 (5.5)	0.41
Rutkowski et al *(2010)*	3/29 (10.3)	10/231 (4.3)	0.166
Total	6/63 (9.5)	19/414 (4.6)	0.123

http://dx.doi.org/10.5772/60210

It is important to keep in mind that in all of these retrospective studies, there is a clear aspect of selection bias. Typically, patients that are selected for smaller margins are those that have tumors that are expected to have more favorable outcomes. Low tumors, which have less favorable predicted outcomes are usually treated with an abdominoperineal resection (APR), a procedure that renders the question of margins moot [54]. This makes it difficult to properly match patient populations being compared in these studies. It is also important to emphasize that there is a lack of consistent methodology of measuring the distal margin across all studies. Measurement of the distal margin is done in a variety of circumstances: pinned, unpinned, fixed, immediately after sectioning, etc [54;63;64]. A lack of standardization is disadvantageous to drawing a unified conclusion; however, the broad consensus that exists regardless of this wide range of measurement techniques suggests that the conclusion is nonetheless valid.

Furthermore, while the surgical donuts are oftentimes assessed for tumor cells, they are not included in measurement of the distal margin of resection and therefore the true margin is usually slightly larger than the distal margin of resection. Therefore, a margin reported and measured as 5 mm may in fact be significantly larger, which helps explain why some patients with low margins approaching 0 mm still seem to have acceptable oncologic outcomes.

In conclusion, in the era of neoadjuvant CRT, smaller distal margins are acceptable so long as the overall status of the patient is considered as well as the possible behavior of the tumor. Patients with well differentiated tumors who have achieved an excellent response to neoadjuvant CRT might only need negative margins. However, patients who have poorly differentiated tumors and no response to pre-operative CRT might need greater margins (greater or equal to 1 cm). The distal margin is one of the few that the surgeon can correct and monitor intra-operatively [40;64] and therefore ought to be a constant consideration for all surgeons when performing a rectal resection. This must be done by balancing the desire for sphincter preservation with the need to maintain an oncologically safe and thorough procedure.

Author details

Jeffrey Meyer, Jie J. Yao and Sergio Huerta*

*Address all correspondence to: sergio.huerta@utsouthwestern.edu

University of Texas Southwestern Medical Center, Departments of Radiation Oncology and Surgery, USA

References

[1] Huerta S, Murray B, Olson C, Patel P, Anthony T. Current evidence-based opinions in the management of adenocarcionoma of the rectum. Indian Journal of Surgery 2009; 71(6):356-362.

[2] Glynne-Jones R, Hughes R. Critical appraisal of the 'wait and see' approach in rectal cancer for clinical complete responders after chemoradiation. Br J Surg 2012; 99(7): 897-909.

[3] Ramzan Z, Nassri AB, Huerta S. Genotypic characteristics of resistant tumors to pre-operative ionizing radiation in rectal cancer. World journal of gastrointestinal oncology 2014; 6(7):194.

[4] Huerta S, Gao X, Dineen S, Kapur P, Saha D, Meyer J. Role of p53, Bax, p21, and DNA-PKcs in radiation sensitivity of HCT-116 cells and xenografts. Surgery 2013; 154(2):143-151.

[5] Huerta S, Gao X, Saha D. Mechanisms of resistance to ionizing radiation in rectal cancer. Expert Rev Mol Diagn 2009; 9(5):469-480.

[6] Chen MB, Wu XY, Yu R, Li C, Wang LQ, Shen W et al. P53 status as a predictive biomarker for patients receiving neoadjuvant radiation-based treatment: a meta-analysis in rectal cancer. PLoS One 2012; 7(9):e45388.

[7] Leong KJ, Beggs A, James J, Morton DG, Matthews GM, Bach SP. Biomarker-based treatment selection in early-stage rectal cancer to promote organ preservation. Br J Surg 2014; 101(10):1299-1309.

[8] Garcia-Aguilar J, Chen Z, Smith DD, Li W, Madoff RD, Cataldo P et al. Identification of a biomarker profile associated with resistance to neoadjuvant chemoradiation therapy in rectal cancer. Ann Surg 2011; 254(3):486-492.

[9] Sauer R, Liersch T, Merkel S, Fietkau R, Hohenberger W, Hess C et al. Preoperative versus postoperative chemoradiotherapy for locally advanced rectal cancer: results of the German CAO/ARO/AIO-94 randomized phase III trial after a median follow-up of 11 years. J Clin Oncol 2012; 30(16):1926-1933.

[10] Gerard JP, Azria D, Gourgou-Bourgade S, Martel-Laffay I, Hennequin C, Etienne PL et al. Comparison of two neoadjuvant chemoradiotherapy regimens for locally advanced rectal cancer: results of the phase III trial ACCORD 12/0405-Prodige 2. J Clin Oncol 2010; 28(10):1638-1644.

[11] Gerard JP, Azria D, Gourgou-Bourgade S, Martel-Lafay I, Hennequin C, Etienne PL et al. Clinical outcome of the ACCORD 12/0405 PRODIGE 2 randomized trial in rectal cancer. J Clin Oncol 2012; 30(36):4558-4565.

[12] Aschele C, Cionini L, Lonardi S, Pinto C, Cordio S, Rosati G et al. Primary tumor response to preoperative chemoradiation with or without oxaliplatin in locally advanced rectal cancer: pathologic results of the STAR-01 randomized phase III trial. J Clin Oncol 2011; 29(20):2773-2780.

[13] Schomoll HJ, Haustermans K, Jay T. Preoperative chemoradiotherapy and postoperative chemotherapy with capecitabine and oxaliplatin versus capecitabine alone in

locally advanced rectal cancer: First results of the PETACC-6 randomized phase III trial. J.Clin.Oncol. 31, 3531. 2013. Ref Type: Abstract

[14] Allegra CJ, Yothers G, O'Connell M, Roh MS. Final results from NSABP protocol R-04: Neoadjuvant chemoradiation (RT) comparing continuous infusion (CIV) 5-FU with capecitabine (Cape) with or without oxaliplatin (Ox) in patients with stage II and III rectal cancer. J.Clin.Oncol. 32, 5s. 2014. Ref Type: Abstract

[15] Rodel C, Liersch T, Becker H, Fietkau R, Hohenberger W, Hothorn T et al. Preoperative chemoradiotherapy and postoperative chemotherapy with fluorouracil and oxaliplatin versus fluorouracil alone in locally advanced rectal cancer: initial results of the German CAO/ARO/AIO-04 randomised phase 3 trial. Lancet Oncol 2012; 13(7): 679-687.

[16] Willett CG, Duda DG, di TE, Boucher Y, Ancukiewicz M, Sahani DV et al. Efficacy, safety, and biomarkers of neoadjuvant bevacizumab, radiation therapy, and fluorouracil in rectal cancer: a multidisciplinary phase II study. J Clin Oncol 2009; 27(18): 3020-3026.

[17] Landry JC, Feng Y, Cohen SJ, Staley CA, III, Whittington R, Sigurdson ER et al. Phase 2 study of preoperative radiation with concurrent capecitabine, oxaliplatin, and bevacizumab followed by surgery and postoperative 5-fluorouracil, leucovorin, oxaliplatin (FOLFOX), and bevacizumab in patients with locally advanced rectal cancer: ECOG 3204. Cancer 2013; 119(8):1521-1527.

[18] Heinzerling JH, Huerta S. Bowel perforation from bevacizumab for the treatment of metastatic colon cancer: incidence, etiology, and management. Current surgery 2006; 63(5):334-337.

[19] Huerta S, Li HC. Bevacizumab-associated hypertension: etiology, incidence, and management. Anti-cancer drugs 2009; 20:S22-S24.

[20] Glynne-Jones R, Mawdsley S, Harrison M. Cetuximab and chemoradiation for rectal cancer--is the water getting muddy? Acta Oncol 2010; 49(3):278-286.

[21] Chua YJ, Barbachano Y, Cunningham D, Oates JR, Brown G, Wotherspoon A et al. Neoadjuvant capecitabine and oxaliplatin before chemoradiotherapy and total mesorectal excision in MRI-defined poor-risk rectal cancer: a phase 2 trial. Lancet Oncol 2010; 11(3):241-248.

[22] Fernandez-Martos C, Pericay C, Aparicio J, Salud A, Safont M, Massuti B et al. Phase II, randomized study of concomitant chemoradiotherapy followed by surgery and adjuvant capecitabine plus oxaliplatin (CAPOX) compared with induction CAPOX followed by concomitant chemoradiotherapy and surgery in magnetic resonance imaging-defined, locally advanced rectal cancer: Grupo cancer de recto 3 study. J Clin Oncol 2010; 28(5):859-865.

[23] Schrag D, Weiser MR, Goodman KA, Gonen M, Hollywood E, Cercek A et al. Neoadjuvant chemotherapy without routine use of radiation therapy for patients with locally advanced rectal cancer: a pilot trial. J Clin Oncol 2014; 32(6):513-518.

[24] Glimelius B. Optimal Time Intervals between Pre-Operative Radiotherapy or Chemoradiotherapy and Surgery in Rectal Cancer? Front Oncol 2014; 4:50.

[25] Kaminsky-Forrett MC, Conroy T, Luporsi E, Peiffert D, Lapeyre M, Boissel P et al. Prognostic implications of downstaging following preoperative radiation therapy for operable T3-T4 rectal cancer. Int J Radiat Oncol Biol Phys 1998; 42(5):935-941.

[26] Francois Y, Nemoz CJ, Baulieux J, Vignal J, Grandjean JP, Partensky C et al. Influence of the interval between preoperative radiation therapy and surgery on downstaging and on the rate of sphincter-sparing surgery for rectal cancer: the Lyon R90-01 randomized trial. J Clin Oncol 1999; 17(8):2396.

[27] Garcia-Aguilar J, Smith DD, Avila K, Bergsland EK, Chu P, Krieg RM. Optimal timing of surgery after chemoradiation for advanced rectal cancer: preliminary results of a multicenter, nonrandomized phase II prospective trial. Ann Surg 2011; 254(1): 97-102.

[28] Sloothaak DA, Geijsen DE, van Leersum NJ, Punt CJ, Buskens CJ, Bemelman WA et al. Optimal time interval between neoadjuvant chemoradiotherapy and surgery for rectal cancer. Br J Surg 2013; 100(7):933-939.

[29] Petrelli F, Sgroi G, Sarti E, Barni S. Increasing the Interval Between Neoadjuvant Chemoradiotherapy and Surgery in Rectal Cancer: A Meta-Analysis of Published Studies. Ann Surg 2013.

[30] Improved survival with preoperative radiotherapy in resectable rectal cancer. Swedish Rectal Cancer Trial. N Engl J Med 1997; 336(14):980-987.

[31] Pettersson D, Cedermark B, Holm T, Radu C, Pahlman L, Glimelius B et al. Interim analysis of the Stockholm III trial of preoperative radiotherapy regimens for rectal cancer. Br J Surg 2010; 97(4):580-587.

[32] Pach R, Kulig J, Richter P, Gach T, Szura M, Kowalska T. Randomized clinical trial on preoperative radiotherapy 25 Gy in rectal cancer--treatment results at 5-year follow-up. Langenbecks Arch Surg 2012; 397(5):801-807.

[33] Huerta S, Hrom J, Gao X, Saha D, Anthony T, Reinhart H et al. Tissue microarray constructs to predict a response to chemoradiation in rectal cancer. Dig Liver Dis 2010; 42(10):679-684.

[34] Habr-Gama A, Perez RO, Nadalin W, Sabbaga J, Ribeiro U, Jr., Silva e Sousa AH Jr et al. Operative versus nonoperative treatment for stage 0 distal rectal cancer following chemoradiation therapy: long-term results. Ann Surg 2004; 240(4):711-717.

[35] Maas M, Beets-Tan RG, Lambregts DM, Lammering G, Nelemans PJ, Engelen SM et al. Wait-and-see policy for clinical complete responders after chemoradiation for rectal cancer. J Clin Oncol 2011; 29(35):4633-4640.

[36] Huerta S. Current views on clinical complete response in patients with rectal cancer following neoadjuvant chemoradiation. Colorectal Cancer 2014; 3(2):117-120.

[37] Smith JD, Ruby JA, Goodman KA, Saltz LB, Guillem JG, Weiser MR et al. Nonoperative management of rectal cancer with complete clinical response after neoadjuvant therapy. Ann Surg 2012; 256(6):965-972.

[38] Dalton RS, Velineni R, Osborne ME, Thomas R, Harries S, Gee AS et al. A single-centre experience of chemoradiotherapy for rectal cancer: is there potential for nonoperative management? Colorectal Dis 2012; 14(5):567-571.

[39] Camilleri-Brennan J, Steele RJ. Objective assessment of morbidity and quality of life after surgery for low rectal cancer. Colorectal Dis 2002; 4(1):61-66.

[40] Nash GM, Weiss A, Dasgupta R, Gonen M, Guillem JG, Wong WD. Close distal margin and rectal cancer recurrence after sphincter-preserving rectal resection. Dis Colon Rectum 2010; 53(10):1365-1373.

[41] Zolciak A, Bujko K, Kepka L, Oledzki J, Rutkowski A, Nowacki MP. Abdominoperineal resection or anterior resection for rectal cancer: patient preferences before and after treatment. Colorectal Dis 2006; 8(7):575-580.

[42] Kameda K, Furusawa M, Mori M, Sugimachi K. Proposed distal margin for resection of rectal cancer. Jpn J Cancer Res 1990; 81(1):100-104.

[43] Komori K, Kanemitsu Y, Ishiguro S, Shimizu Y, Sano T, Ito S et al. Adequate length of the surgical distal resection margin in rectal cancer: from the viewpoint of pathological findings. Am J Surg 2012; 204(4):474-480.

[44] Madsen PM, Christiansen J. Distal intramural spread of rectal carcinomas. Dis Colon Rectum 1986; 29(4):279-282.

[45] Shirouzu K, Isomoto H, Kakegawa T. Distal spread of rectal cancer and optimal distal margin of resection for sphincter-preserving surgery. Cancer 1995; 76(3):388-392.

[46] Ueno H, Mochizuki H, Hashiguchi Y, Ishikawa K, Fujimoto H, Shinto E et al. Preoperative parameters expanding the indication of sphincter preserving surgery in patients with advanced low rectal cancer. Ann Surg 2004; 239(1):34-42.

[47] Watanabe T, Kazama S, Nagawa H. A 1cm distal bowel margin is safe for rectal cancer after preoperative radiotherapy. Hepatogastroenterology 2012; 59(116):1068-1074.

[48] Kuvshinoff B, Maghfoor I, Miedema B, Bryer M, Westgate S, Wilkes J et al. Distal margin requirements after preoperative chemoradiotherapy for distal rectal carcinomas: are < or = 1 cm distal margins sufficient? Ann Surg Oncol 2001; 8(2):163-169.

[49] Moore HG, Riedel E, Minsky BD, Saltz L, Paty P, Wong D et al. Adequacy of 1-cm distal margin after restorative rectal cancer resection with sharp mesorectal excision and preoperative combined-modality therapy. Ann Surg Oncol 2003; 10(1):80-85.

[50] Nelson H, Petrelli N, Carlin A, Couture J, Fleshman J, Guillem J et al. Guidelines 2000 for colon and rectal cancer surgery. J Natl Cancer Inst 2001; 93(8):583-596.

[51] Nishioka M, Shimada M, Kurita N, Iwata T, Morimoto S, Yoshikawa K et al. Clinicopathological analysis of distal margin for rectal cancer after preoperative chemoradiation therapy. Hepatogastroenterology 2012; 59(119):2142-2146.

[52] Pricolo VF, Abodeely A, Resnick M. Distal margins in radical resections for rectal cancer after chemoradiation therapy: how short is long enough? Dig Surg 2010; 27(3): 185-189.

[53] Andreola S, Leo E, Belli F, Bonfanti G, Sirizzotti G, Greco P et al. Adenocarcinoma of the lower third of the rectum surgically treated with a <10-MM distal clearance: preliminary results in 35 N0 patients. Ann Surg Oncol 2001; 8(7):611-615.

[54] Bujko K, Rutkowski A, Chang GJ, Michalski W, Chmielik E, Kusnierz J. Is the 1-cm rule of distal bowel resection margin in rectal cancer based on clinical evidence? A systematic review. Ann Surg Oncol 2012; 19(3):801-808.

[55] Kim YW, Kim NK, Min BS, Huh H, Kim JS, Kim JY et al. Factors associated with anastomotic recurrence after total mesorectal excision in rectal cancer patients. J Surg Oncol 2009; 99(1):58-64.

[56] Kiran RP, Lian L, Lavery IC. Does a subcentimeter distal resection margin adversely influence oncologic outcomes in patients with rectal cancer undergoing restorative proctectomy? Dis Colon Rectum 2011; 54(2):157-163.

[57] Mezhir JJ, Shia J, Riedel E, Temple LK, Nash GM, Weiser MR et al. Whole-mount pathologic analysis of rectal cancer following neoadjuvant therapy: implications of margin status on long-term oncologic outcome. Ann Surg 2012; 256(2):274-279.

[58] Tsutsumi S, Tabe Y, Fujii T, Yamaguchi S, Suto T, Yajima R et al. Tumor response and negative distal resection margins of rectal cancer after hyperthermochemoradiation therapy. Anticancer Res 2011; 31(11):3963-3967.

[59] Bokey EL, Ojerskog B, Chapuis PH, Dent OF, Newland RC, Sinclair G. Local recurrence after curative excision of the rectum for cancer without adjuvant therapy: role of total anatomical dissection. Br J Surg 1999; 86(9):1164-1170.

[60] Law WL, Chu KW. Local recurrence following total mesorectal excision with double-stapling anastomosis for rectal cancers: analysis of risk factors. World J Surg 2002; 26(10):1272-1276.

http://dx.doi.org/10.5772/60210

[61] Rutkowski A, Nowacki MP, Chwalinski M, Oledzki J, Bednarczyk M, Liszka-Dalecki P et al. Acceptance of a 5-mm distal bowel resection margin for rectal cancer: is it safe? Colorectal Dis 2012; 14(1):71-78.

[62] Vernava AM, III, Moran M, Rothenberger DA, Wong WD. A prospective evaluation of distal margins in carcinoma of the rectum. Surg Gynecol Obstet 1992; 175(4): 333-336.

[63] Sondenaa K, Kjellevold KH. A prospective study of the length of the distal margin after low anterior resection for rectal cancer. Int J Colorectal Dis 1990; 5(2):103-105.

[64] Tiret E. Assessment of surgical distal margin after rectal resection for cancer. Dis Colon Rectum 2010; 53(10):1353-1354.